The Muscle Energy Manual

VOLUME THREE

Evaluation and Treatment
of the Pelvis and Sacrum

The Muscle Energy Manual

VOLUME THREE

Evaluation and Treatment
of the Pelvis and Sacrum

ᐒ

BY

Fred L. Mitchell, Jr., D.O., F.A.A.O., F.C.A.

Professor Emeritus of Osteopathic Manipulative Medicine
College of Osteopathic Medicine
Michigan State University
East Lansing, Michigan

AND

P. Kai Galen Mitchell, B.A.

ᐒ

MET Press
East Lansing, Michigan
1999

Dedicated to my father's memory.

THE MUSCLE ENERGY MANUAL, VOLUME THREE. Copyright © 1999
by Fred L. Mitchell, Jr. and P. Kai Galen Mitchell First Edition.

Inquiries and requests for permission to reproduce material from this work should
be sent to MET Press, P.O. Box 4577, East Lansing, Michigan 48826-4577.
Fax: (517) 332-4196.

Editors: P. Kai Galen Mitchell, Carol P. Mitchell, & Ann McGlothlin Weller
Design and Layout: P. Kai Galen Mitchell
Photography: Marilyn Fox & P. Kai Galen Mitchell

Printed in the United States of America.
Library of Congress Catalog Card Number: 95–77816
ISBN 0-9647250-1-0 – PB (Volume One)
ISBN 0-9647250-2-9 – PB (Volume Two)
ISBN 0-9647250-3-7 – PB (Volume Three)

MET Press, P.O. Box 4577, East Lansing, Michigan 48826-4577 • Fax: (517) 332-4196.

Preface for The Muscle Energy Manual Series

This series greatly expands upon the concepts presented in the first texts ever published on Muscle Energy (Mitchell, Jr., Moran, Pruzzo; 1973 and 1979). This current work is the culmination of more than thirty-five years of clinical practice, research, and teaching. Muscle Energy Technique (MET) was first introduced by the author into the curriculum of osteopathic colleges in 1964 at the Kansas City College of Osteopathy and Surgery, following a four-year postdoctoral joint practice with Fred L. Mitchell, Sr. (1960–64). Since that time, its concepts and methods have spread to osteopathic colleges in the USA, Canada, and overseas. Today, Muscle Energy is taught at all osteopathic colleges – and many other manual medicine and manual therapy programs worldwide – making the need for an updated, comprehensive Muscle Energy text and manual even more urgent.

Although the 1973 and 1979 Muscle Energy manuals were enthusiastically received at home and abroad, years of teaching have made it apparent that certain deficiencies of the earlier publications have led to incomplete understanding and misapplications of MET. The earlier works did not include sufficient explanation of physiological mechanisms, nor the anatomic detail necessary to provide a rationale for the procedures. Additionally, although some readers no doubt appreciated the brevity of the cookbook approach, the diagnostic and treatment procedure descriptions did not provide enough information for the procedures to be performed reliably and consistently. The new MET series was written to address these omissions.

Possibly because of the name, Muscle Energy has often been perceived as solely a treatment modality for "tight" muscles. Far too often, MET treatment techniques have been taught without sufficient reference to MET's distinctive diagnostic algorithms. MET is more than a method of treatment or therapy; *it is also a biomechanics-based analytic diagnostic system, using precise physical diagnosis evaluation procedures designed to identify and quantify articular range-of-motion restriction.* The unique MET method of evaluation and diagnosis is an essential part of MET, in that it provides the necessary information needed to apply MET correctly, and therefore effectively. Among the algorithms presented in this text is new material on rib-based vertebral joint diagnosis. Expanded also is discussion of the biomechanics of non-neutral ERS and FRS segmental dysfunction.

The series is intended as both a text – especially emphasizing the theory and systematic methods of MET diagnosis – and an evaluation and treatment manual. *The Muscle Energy Manual*, Volume One (1995), covers Muscle Energy concepts and mechanisms, the musculoskeletal screen, and cervical region evaluation and treatment. Volume Two (1998) covers the evaluation and treatment of the thoracic spine, lumbar spine, and rib cage. Volume Three (1999) covers the evaluation and treatment of the pelvis and sacrum.

Fred L. Mitchell, Jr., D.O., FAAO, FCA

Volume Three Preface

There is a widely shared and correct conviction that treatment of somatic dysfunctions of the pelvis and sacrum is complex and has a high priority clinically. In the early days of Muscle Energy Tutorials, in deference to its importance, evaluation and treatment of the pelvis and sacrum was presented first. The transition from pelvis to spine, ribs, and extremities, however, constituted such giant conceptual leaps that the course sequence was changed in the 1980s to begin at the superior end of the axial skeleton. Conceptual development was smoother, advancing in smaller steps with a more logical sequence.

Anticipating that some clinicians will choose to read Volume Three first, we have elected to present, in the Introduction, a brief chronology and history of the development of the Muscle Energy concepts in order to clarify their relevance to pelvic evaluation and treatment.

As with the previous volumes of *The Muscle Energy Manual*, the text begins with the relevant basic anatomy and physiology, proceeds to a general discussion of manipulable disorders, and concludes with the details of clinical evaluation and treatment.

Putting the Muscle Energy approach to evaluation and treatment of the pelvis into specific clinical contexts could be the subject of an entire book. Such a book would discuss clinical applications in many more fields than low back pain management. Until such a book is written, we must trust that all types of clinicians, regardless of specialty, understand the relevance of posture, locomotion, viscerosomatic/somatovisceral reflexes, and microcirculation to their specific fields.

Fred L. Mitchell, Jr., D.O., FAAO, FCA

Acknowledgements

This book would probably have never seen print had it not been for the long and arduous efforts and questionings of my wife Carol and son Kai. Their commitment to this project kept me busy rewriting rewrites and reorganizing reorganized text, until all considered the final work ready for publication. Kai Mitchell created many original graphics for the text, in addition to layout design, editing, and publishing. Many thanks also to Marilyn Fox for her photographic work, to Ann McGlothlin Weller for the precision of her editorial input, and to our loyal model, James Marlow.

My sincere appreciation to Gary Ostrow, DO, FAAO for reading and commenting on the manuscript. As will be obvious to readers, gratitude is also owed to Martin Beilke, DO, Angus G. Cathie, DO, Vladimir Janda, MD, Lawrence Jones, DO, Norman Larson, DO, Karel Lewit, MD, Kenneth Little, DO, Heinz-Dieter Neumann, MD, Charles Owens, DO, A. Hollis Wolf, DO, and J. Gordon Zink, DO, for many important insights and concepts.

I owe my training in cranial osteopathy to the faculties of the Sutherland Teaching Foundation and the Cranial Academy, and especially to Thomas Schooley, DO, FAAO, FCA whose skilled hands and practical mind made cranial motion a reality for me.

Most of all, gratitude is once again expressed to my father, Fred L. Mitchell, Sr., DO, FAAO who, through his teachings, provided me with a lifetime of valuable and knotty problems.

F. L. Mitchell, Jr.

Brief Contents

Preface for the Muscle Energy Manual Series   *v*
Preface for Volume Three and Acknowledgements   *vi*
Brief Contents   *vii*
List of Tables   *viii*
List of Procedures   *ix*
Detailed Table of Contents   *x*
Historical Chronology of Muscle Energy Technique   *xvi*
Introduction   *xvii*
   History of the Development of Muscle Energy Concepts   *xvii*
   Diagnostic Concepts   *xviii*
   Psychophysics of Physical Diagnosis   *xix*
   Treatment Concepts   *xxi*
   A Short History of the Pelvic Axes   *xxiii*
   Some Frequently Asked Questions   *xxiii*

CHAPTER 1 RELEVANT PELVIC ANATOMY   *1*

   •Osteology •Pelvic Landmarks •Pelvic Ligaments •Muscles of the Pelvis •Myofascial Influences

CHAPTER 2 NORMAL SAGITTAL PLANE MOTIONS IN THE PELVISACRAL JOINTS   *21*

   •Weight-bearing and Non-weight-bearing Sagittal Movements of the Sacrum •Transverse Instantaneous Axes of the Pelvis •Sagittal Plane Sacroiliac Motion – Nutation and Counternutation •Paradoxical Sacral Motion •Sacral Flexion vesus Sacral Shear •Iliosacral Motion and Interinnominate Rotation

CHAPTER 3 NORMAL COUPLED MOTIONS IN THE SACROILIAC JOINTS: TORSION AND UNILATERAL SACRAL FLEXION   *33*

   •Sacral Torsion and the Oblique Axes •The Walking Cycle and the Pelvis •Unilateral Sacral Flexion Movement •Lumbosacral Mechanics •Intrapelvic Adaptive Mechanics •The Sacral Base/ILA Paradox

CHAPTER 4 OVERVIEW OF MANIPULABLE DISORDERS OF THE PELVIS   *53*

   •Subluxations of the Pelvis •Sacroiliac Dysfunctions •Iliosacral Dysfunctions •Manipulable Muscle Imbalance •Breathing Movement Impairments •Craniosacral Dysfunction

CHAPTER 5 INTRODUCTION TO EVALUATION AND TREATMENT OF THE PELVIS AND SACRUM   *71*

CHAPTER 6 SCREENING AND LATERALIZATION TESTS FOR THE PELVIS   *75*

   •Relative Leg Length •Iliac Crest Heights Tests •Flexion Tests for Pelvisacral Mobility •Other Pelvisacral Mobility Screening Tests

CHAPTER 7 SUBLUXATIONS AND DISLOCATIONS OF THE PELVIS: EVALUATION AND TREATMENT   *101*

   •Subluxations of the Pubic Symphysis •Upslipped Innominate Lesions •Inflared and Outflared Innominate

CHAPTER 8 EVALUATION AND TREATMENT OF PELVIC ARTICULAR DYSFUNCTION   *121*

   •Diagnosis and Treatment of Sacroiliac and Iliosacral Dysfunctions

APPENDIX: Patient Instructions for Sacroiliac Belt   *159*

BIBLIOGRAPHY and RECOMMENDED READING   *162*

List of Tables

Table 1.A. Pelvic Landmarks for Structural Diagnosis in the Mitchell Model *3*
Table 1.B. Summary of Muscles Related to the Pelvis: Muscles Attached to the Sacrum *15*
Table 1.C. Summary of Muscles Related to the Pelvis: Muscles Attached to the Innominates from Above *16*
Table 1.D. Summary of Muscles Related to the Pelvis: Muscles Attached to the Innominates from Below *18*

Table 4.A. The Six Types of Manipulable Pelvic Disorders, with Possible Variants for Each *54*

Table 5.A. Flow Chart for Evaluation and Treatment Sequence of Manipulable Pelvic Disorders *73*

Table 6.A. Summary of Lateralization and Screening Evaluation Tests for the Pelvis *76*
Table 6.B. Flexion Test Results and Probable Diagnoses *89*

Table 7.A. Age and Sex Distribution of Patients Diagnosed with Upslipped Innominate *108*

Table 8.A. Treatment Sequence for Addressing Pelvic Dysfunction *122*
Table 8.B. Pelvic Diagnosis Table *157*

List of Procedures

I. Diagnostic Procedures   **Page**

A. Iliac Crest Heights Tests   **80**
  1. Standing Iliac Crest Heights Test   80
  2. Seated Iliac Crest Heights Test   81
B. The Standing Flexion Test   **84**
  1. Locating the PSISs/PIPs   85
  2. The Standing Flexion Test Protocol Task Analysis 86
C. The Seated Flexion Test   **88**
  1. The Seated Flexion Test Procedure Protocol   88
D. Other Mobility Screening Tests   **92**
  1. The Fowler Test   92
  2. "Hip Drop" Test   92
E. Recumbent Pelvic Mobility Tests   **94**
  1. Dynamic Leg Length Test Protocol   96
    a. Patient Alignment   96
    b. Leg Shortening Procedure   97
    c. Leg Lengthening Procedure   98
F. Subluxations of the Pubic Symphysis   **102**
  1. The Pubic Crest Heights Test   103
G. Upslipped Innominate Lesions   **107**
  1. Testing for Ischial Tuberosity Heights Procedure Protocol 110
  2. Testing Sacrotuberous (S-T) Ligament Tension Procedure Protocol 111
  3. Prone Leg Length Comparison Procedure Protocol   112
H. Rhomboid Pelvis   **116**
  1. Testing for ASIS Flaring (for Iliac Flare) Procedure Protocol 116
I. Testing for Sacroiliac Dysfunction   **123**
  1. The Prone and Sphinx Tests for ILA Positions Procedure Protocol 124
  2. The Test for Sacral Sulci Depths Procedure Protocol 126
  3. The Lumbar Spring Test   128
J. Evaluation for Rotated Innominate   **142**
  1. Evaluation for Rotated Innominate (AIR ro PIL) Procedure Protocol 142
K. Testing Sacroiliac Respiratory Motion   **150**
  1. Respiratory Motion Test Procedure Protocol   151
L. Evaluation for Coccygeal Rotation   **155**
  1. Examining the Coccyx for Rotation Procedure Protocol 155

II. Treatment Procedures

F. Treatment Procedures for Pubic Subluxations   **104**
  1. Treatment for Superior Pubic Subluxation Procedure Protocol 104
  2. Treatment for Inferior Pubic Subluxation Procedure Protocol 105
  3. Combination Treatment for Superior or Inferior Pubic Subluxation 106
G. Treatment for Superior Innominate Dislocation (Upslipped Innominate) **113**
  1. Upslipped Innominate Treatment Procedure Protocol 113
H. Treatment Procedures for Flare Lesions   **117**
  1. Treatment for Iliac Inflare Lesion Procedure Protocol 117
  2. Treatment for Iliac Outflare Lesion Procedure Protocol 118
I. Treatment Techniques for Unilaterally Flexed Sacrum   **129**
  1. Prone Treatment for Unilaterally Flexed Sacrum   130
  2. Alternate Prone Treatment for a Resistant Unilaterally Flexed Sacrum 132
  3. Self Treatment for Recurrent Unilaterally Flexed Sacrum 132
I. Treatment Techniques for Forward Torsioned Sacrum   **134**
  1. Mitchell Sr. Procedure Protocol for Treatment of Forward Torsioned Sacrum 134
  2. Mitchell Jr. Treatment for Forward Torsioned Sacrum – Operator Seated Method 136
  3. Self Treatment for Forward Torsioned Sacrum   138
I. Treatment Techniques for Backward Torsioned Sacrum   **139**
  1. Treatment for Backward Torsioned Sacrum Procedure Protocol 140
J. Treatment Techniques for Anterior Rotated Innominate   **143**
  1. Lateral Recumbent Technique for Anterior Innominate (Right) (AIR) 144
  2. Prone Treatment for AIR   146
  3. Self Treatment for Anterior Innominate (Right) (AIR) 147
J. Treatment Techniques for Posteriorly Rotated Innominate **148**
  1. Prone Treatment for Posterior Innominate (Left) (PIL) Protocol 148
  2. Lateral Recumbent Technique for Posterior Innominate (Left) (PIL) 149
K. Treating Restricted Sacroiliac Respiratory Motion   **152**
  1. Treatment for Restricted Sacroiliac Respiratory Motion Protocol 152
L. Treatment for Coccygeal Dysfunction   **156**
  1. Ischiorectal Fossa Technique for Coccygeal Dysfunction 156
  2. Kegel's Exercise   156

Detailed Table of Contents

Introduction

CHAPTER 1 RELEVANT PELVIC ANATOMY *1*

Osteology *1*

Pelvic Landmarks *3*

  Bony Landmarks for Determining Anatomic Leg Length or Assessing Pelvic Dysgenesis *4*
  Iliac Crests – Superior Surfaces

  Bony Landmarks Indicating Innominate Position or Movement *4*
  Locating the Posterior Superior Iliac Spines (PSIS) and Posterior Iliac Prominences (PIP) 4
  Locating the Anterior Superior Iliac Spines (ASIS) 6
  Umbilicus 6
  Ischial Tuberosities – Inferior Surfaces 8
  Sacrotuberous Ligaments 8
  Medial Malleoli –Inferior Surfaces 9
  Heel Pads – Inferior Surfaces 9
  Pubic Crests – Superior Surfaces 9

  Landmarks for Assessing Sacral Position *10*
  Finding the ILAs 10
  Anatomic Considerations when Palpating for Sacral Sulcus Depth 11

Pelvic Ligaments *12*

Muscles of the Pelvis *14*
  Muscles attached to the Sacrum *15*
  Muscles attached to the Innominates *16*

Myofascial Influences *20*
  Piriformis: The Sacroiliac Muscle *20*
  Influence of the Fibula on the Pelvis *20*

CHAPTER 2 NORMAL SAGITTAL PLANE MOTIONS IN THE PELVISACRAL JOINTS *21*

Transverse Axes and Sacroiliac Motion *23*
  Sacral Middle Transverse Axis *23*
  Sacral Motion with Trunk Flexion and Extension *24*
  Instantaneous Axes and the Sacroiliac Ligaments *24*
  The Superior Transverse Axis *25*
  How the Axis Shifts from Middle to Superior *26*
  The Great Controversy: To Nutate or Counternutate *27*
  Non-Weight Bearing Sagittal Movement *27*
  Translatory Sacral Motion *28*

Transverse Axes and Iliosacral Motion *29*
  Pubic Transverse Axis *29*
  Iliosacral Inferior Transverse Axis *29*
  Summary of Pelvic Axes *30*
  Medio-lateral Displacement of PSISs with Nutation/Counternutation *31*
  Voluntary *versus* Involuntary Sacral Motion *31*
  Causes of Sacroiliac Motion *31*

Craniosacral Motion   *31*
Amplitude of Craniosacral Motions   *32*

CHAPTER 3   NORMAL COUPLED MOTIONS IN THE SACROILIAC JOINTS: TORSION AND UNILATERAL SACRAL FLEXION   *33*

Sacral Torsion and the Oblique Axes   *34*
The Four Sacral Torsion Movements   *36*
Spinal Forces and Sacral Torsion   *37*

The Walking Cycle and the Pelvis   *41*
Original Walking Cycle as Described by Fred Mitchell, Sr.   *41*
Kinesiology of the Walking Cycle   *42*
Phases of the Gait Cycle   *42*
Role of Striated Muscles in Movements of Passive Pelvic Joints   *46*

Unilateral Sacral Flexion Movement   *46*

Lumbosacral Mechanics   *47*

Intrapelvic Adaptive Mechanics   *49*

The Sacral Base/ILA Paradox Revisited   *50*

CHAPTER 4   OVERVIEW OF MANIPULABLE DISORDERS OF THE PELVIS   *53*

Subluxations of the Pelvis   *55*
Pubic Symphyseal Dislocation or Subluxation   *55*
Upslipped Innominate   *56*
Rhomboid Pelvis   *58*

Sacroiliac Dysfunctions   *59*
Unilaterally Flexed Sacrum   *60*
Mechanism of Injury in Sacral Flexion   61
Torsioned Sacrum   *62*
Forward and Backward Sacral Torsions   62
Effects of Sacral Torsion Dysfunction   63
Comparison of a Unilaterally Flexed Sacrum on the Left and a Torsioned Sacrum to the Left   64

Iliosacral Dysfunctions   *65*
Anterior or posterior rotated innominate   65

Manipulable Muscle Imbalance   *66*
Functional Relationship between Weakness-Prone and Tightness Prone Muscles   66

Breathing Movement Impairments   *68*
Sacroiliac Respiratory Restriction   *68*

Craniosacral Dysfunction and Relationships   *68*
Functional Relationship of the Pelvis to the Cranium   *68*
Sacral Oscillation   *69*

CHAPTER 5 INTRODUCTION TO EVALUATION AND TREATMENT OF THE PELVIS AND SACRUM *71*

CHAPTER 6 SCREENING AND LATERALIZATION TESTS FOR THE PELVIS *75*

Relative Leg Length *76*
Measuring Anatomic Leg Length *77*
Trunk Adaptations to Sacral Base Asymmetry *78*

Iliac Crest Heights Tests *80*

Standing Iliac Crest Heights Test *80*
Procedure Task Analysis *80*

Seated Iliac Crest Heights Test *81*
Interpreting Crest Heights Tests *81*

Flexion Tests for Pelvisacral Mobility *81*

The Standing Flexion Test *84*
Prior to Performing the Standing Flexion Test *84*
Task Analysis for Finding the PSISs/PIPs *85*

The Standing Flexion/Extension Test Protocol Task Analysis *86*
Interpretation of Results *87*

The Seated Flexion Test *88*
The Seated Flexion Test Procedure Protocol *88*
Interpretation of Results *89*
Biomechanical Events of the Flexion Tests *90*
Effect of Pubic Subluxation on Pelvic Flexion Tests *91*

Other Mobility Screening Tests *92*

Stork Test: The Fowler Test *92*

Hip Drop Test *92*
The "Hip Drop" Test Protocol *93*
Interpretation of Results *93*

Recumbent Pelvic Mobility Tests *94*

Functional Leg Length *94*
Dynamic Leg Length Tests *94*
The Dynamic Leg Length Test of Pelvic Motion Symmetry *95*
Dynamic Leg Length Test Protocol *96*
A. Patient Alignment *96*
B. Leg Shortening Procedure *97*
C. Leg Lengthening Procedure *98*
– Interpretation of the Dynamic Leg Length Test *99*

CHAPTER 7 SUBLUXATIONS AND DISLOCATIONS OF THE PELVIS: EVALUATION AND TREATMENT *101*

Subluxations of the Pubic Symphysis *102*

Testing for Pubic Crest Heights Asymmetry *102*
The Pubic Crest Heights Test *102*
The Pubic Crest Heights Test Procedure Protocol *103*

– Interpretation of Results *103*

Treatment Procedures for Pubic Subluxation *104*
Treatment of Superior Pubic Subluxation *104*
Treatment of Superior Pubic Subluxation Procedure Protocol *104*
Treatment of Inferior Pubic Subluxation *104*
Treatment of Inferior Pubic Subluxation Procedure Protocol *105*
Combination Treatment for Superior or Inferior Pubic Subluxation *106*

Upslipped Innominate Lesions *107*
Incidence of Upslipped Innominate *107*
Diagnostic Criteria for Upslipped Innominate *108*
Using Mobility Tests for Lateralization and comfirmation of Upslipped Innominate *109*

Testing for Superior Subluxation or Dislocation of the Innominate *110*
Testing for Ischial Tuberosity Heights Procedure Protocol *110*
Testing Sacrotuberosity Ligament Tension Procedure Protocol *111*
– Interpretation of Results *111*

Prone Leg Length Measurement *112*
Prone Leg Length Comparison Procedure Protocol *112*
– Interpretation of Results *112*

Treatment of Superior Innominate Dislocation (Upslipped Innominate) *113*
Procedure Protocol *113*
– Significance of Results *114*
Sacroiliac Belt *114*

Rhomboid Pelvis *116*
Testing for Inflare-Outflare of the Innominate – a Subluxation *116*
Testing for ASIS Flaring (for Iliac Flare) Procedure Protocol *116*
– The Results of ASiS Flare Testing (for Iliac Flare) *116*

Treatment Procedures for Flare Lesions *117*
Treatment of the Iliac Inflare Lesion Procedure Protocol *117*
Treatment of the Iliac Outflare Lesion Procedure Protocol *118*

CHAPTER 8 EVALUATION AND TREATMENT OF PELVIC ARTICULAR DYSFUNCTION *121*
Sacroiliac Dysfunction *121*
Torsioned Sacral Dysfunction *121*
Flexed Sacral Dysfunction *122*
Respiratory Sacral Dysfunction *123*

Sacroiliac Dysfunction *123*
Evaluation for Sacroiliac Dysfunction *123*
Testing for Sacroiliac Dysfunction *124*
The Prone and Sphinx Tests for ILA Positions Procedure Protocol *124*
The Test for Sacral Sulci Depth Procedure Protocol *126*
– Interpretation of Results for the ILA Position and Sacral Sulci Depths Test *127*
The Lumbar Spring Test *128*
The Lumbar Spring Test Procedure Protocol *128*
The Lumbar Component of Sacroiliac Dysfunction and the Sphinx Test *128*

Treatment for Unilaterally Flexed Sacrum *129*
Prone Treatment for Unilaterally Flexed Sacrum *129*
Prone Treatment for Unilaterally Flexed Sacrum Procedure Protocol *130*
Alternate Prone Treatment of a Resistant Unilaterally Flexed Sacrum *132*
Self Treatment for Recurrent Unilaterally Flexed Sacrum *132*

Treatment for Sacral TorsionDysfunctions *133*
Diagnostic Criteria for Torsioned Sacrum *133*

Treatment Techniques for Forward Torsioned Sacrum *134*
Mitchell Sr. Procedure Protocol for Treatment of the Forward Torsioned Sacrum
    (Left-onLeft) Protocol Task Analysis *134*
Mitchell Jr. Treatment of the Forward Torsioned Sacrum – Operator Seated Method *136*
Self Treatment of Forward Torsioned Sacrum *138*
Task Analysis Protocol *138*

Treatment Techniques for Backward Torsioned Sacrum *139*
Treatment of the Backward Torsioned Sacrum Procedure Protocol *140*

Rotated Innominate Dysfunction *142*

Evaluating for Rotated Innominate *142*
Evaluation for Anterior or Posterior Rotated Innominate Procedure Protocol *142*
– *Interpretation of Results* *142*

Treatment Techniques for Anterior Rotated Innominate *143*
Lateral Recumbent Technique for AIR *143*
Lateral Recumbent Technique for AIR Procedure Protocol *144*
Prone Treatment for Anterior Innominate (AIR) Procedure Protocol *146*
Self-Treatment for Anterior Innominate Right – Standing Technique Procedure Protocol *147*

Treatment of Posteriorly Rotated Innominate *148*
Treatment for Posterior Innominate Left (PIL) *148*
Prone Treatment for Posterior Innominate Procedure Protocol *148*
Lateral Recumbent Treatment for Posterior Innominate Procedure Protocol *149*

Sacroiliac Respiratory Dysfunction *150*

Testing Sacroiliac Respiratory Motion *151*
Procedure Protocol *151*

Treating Restricted Sacroiliac Respiratory Motion *152*
Treatment of Restricted Sacroiliac Respiratory Motion Procedure Protocol *152*

Coccygeal Dysfunctions *154*

Evaluation for Coccygeal Rotation *155*
Examining the Coccyx for Rotation Procedure Protocol *155*

Treatment for Coccygeal Dysfunction *156*
Procedure Protocol for Ischiorectal Fossa Technique *156*

Kegel's Exercise *156*

Pelvic Diagnosis Table *157*

APPENDIX   Patient Instructions for Sacroiliac Belt *159*
            Of Clinical Interest *161*

BIBLIOGRAPHY and RECOMMENDED READING *162*

Historical Chronology of Muscle Energy Technique

1909   Birth of Frederic Lockwood Mitchell, Sr. (FLM, Sr.), the originator of MET, on December 3, 1909.

1929   Frederic Lockwood Mitchell, Jr. (FLM, Jr.) is born on January 10, 1929.

1934   FLM, Jr. suffers third-degree burns over 50 percent of his body (considered uniformly fatal at that time). After witnessing the family physician, Charles Owens, D.O., reverse renal failure using Chapman's Reflexes – thereby saving "Freddie's" life – FLM, Sr. makes the decision to become an osteopath.

1935-37   FLM, Sr. studies with Dr. Owens before entering the Chicago College of Osteopathy in 1937.

1941   FLM, Sr. graduates from the Chicago College of Osteopathy.

1941   FLM, Sr. sets up private practice at 517 James Building, Chattanooga, Tennessee.

1948   FLM, Sr. publishes the article *The Balanced Pelvis in Relation to Chapman's Reflexes* in the Yearbook of the Academy of Applied Osteopathy.

1958   FLM, Sr. publishes the article *Structural Pelvic Function* in the Yearbook of the Academy of Applied Osteopathy (reprinted in 1965).

1959   FLM, Jr. graduates from the Chicago College of Osteopathy.

1960-64   FLM, Jr. joins FLM, Sr. in private practice, studying osteopathic principles and techniques intensively with FLM, Sr. for several years.

1964   FLM, Jr. joins the faculty at the Kansas City College of Osteopathy and Surgery (KCCOS – now University of Health Sciences College of Osteopathic Medicine); introduces Muscle Energy Technique into the curriculum, making KCCOS the first osteopathic college to include MET in the curriculum.

1970   FLM, Sr., teaches the first of six Muscle Energy Tutorials at Fort Dodge, Iowa. The tutorial was hosted by Sarah Sutton, D.O., who was later very active in the development of the posthumous Muscle Energy tutorials.

1973   Publication of *An Evaluation and Treatment Manual of Osteopathic Manipulative Procedures* by FL Mitchell, Jr., PS Moran, and NA Pruzzo – the first text to include Muscle Energy evaluation and treatment. Text based on class notes taken by PS Moran from lectures given by FLM, Jr. at KCCOS.

1973   FLM, Jr. joins the faculty at Michigan State University College of Osteopathic Medicine.

1974   FLM, Sr. dies on March 2, 1974.

1974   The Muscle Energy Tutorial Committee is formed to develop a Continuing Medical Education course on MET. Principally taught by FL Mitchell, Jr., the first posthumous MET course was offered in December by the College of Osteopathic Medicine at Michigan State University.

1979   FLM, Jr., PS Moran, and NA Pruzzo publish the first strictly Muscle Energy textbook, *An Evaluation and Treatment Manual of Osteopathic Muscle Energy Procedures* (out of print 1991).

1980   Paul Kimberly, D.O. includes "muscle force (energy)" techniques in "Outline of Osteopathic Manipulative Procedures," the Kirksville College of Osteopathic Medicine's OMT syllabus.

1995   Volume 1 of *The Muscle Energy Manual* (FL Mitchell, Jr. & PK Mitchell) is published by MET Press.

1998   Volume 2 of *The Muscle Energy Manual* (FL Mitchell, Jr. & PK Mitchell) is published by MET Press.

1999   Volume 3 of *The Muscle Energy Manual* (FL Mitchell, Jr. & PK Mitchell) is published by MET Press.

Introduction

The History of the Development of Muscle Energy Concepts

The development and refinement of what is now known as Muscle Energy Technique has been a process in evolution over the past fifty years. Muscle Energy Technique (MET), which originated with Fred L. Mitchell, Sr., continues to develop and evolve, first in the hands and minds of those who were privileged to study and learn the method directly from Fred Sr. (the 'second generation'), and now, as the third and fourth generation of students of the method apply it in their practices.

In the late 1940s while I was still in high school, Fred Mitchell and Paul Kimberly discovered that they had much in common and became close friends. As a result of their association Mitchell, Sr., was challenged to write one of his few published papers, "The Balanced Pelvis in Relationship to Chapman's Reflexes" (1948), a monograph attempting to explain what Charles Owens, author of "An Endocrine Interpretation of Chapman's Reflexes" (1937), had meant by "balanced pelvis" in relation to Chapman's Reflexes. My father's paper generated so much controversy that he was driven to research and develop a unified kinematic model of the pelvis. The paper explaining this paradigm was published in 1958 under the title "Structural Pelvic Function," and was slightly revised and reprinted in 1965. This model of the pelvis remains a central concept in manipulative medicine. Its consistency and predictability have stood for over 40 years.

Inspired in the late 1940s and early 1950s by T. J. Ruddy, DO, and Carl Kettler, DO, Mitchell, Sr., began developing what he later called "muscular energy" techniques, first to treat movement impairments of the pelvisacral joints, and later to treat other joints in the body, utilizing the same simple principles: first position the joint *at* its movement restriction, and then put a force, generated by the patient's own voluntary muscle contraction exerted against "a precisely executed counterforce (Kettler)," through the joint to alter its form and function. During the post-contraction relaxation, the joint could be repositioned, and the contract-relax sequence repeated, if necessary.

I have always suspected that my father developed what I chose to call (ungrammatically) Muscle Energy Technique after he realized that I, like most of my classmates, had learned few OMT skills in my four years of osteopathic education, and that he needed something simple and safe to teach to me.

The application of muscular energy technique principles to spine, ribs, and extremity joints began developing shortly before I joined him in practice in 1960, and continued through the years of our joint practice (1960-64), and on until his death in 1974. Many times my time with a patient was interrupted by more pressing clinical education issues – a new method he had devised, or a condition I had never seen before.

As I subsequently discovered, learning is a two-way street between teacher and student. Much fleshing-out of the MET concepts, which began as a simple paradigm, occurred during the ongoing dialogue between my father and myself, especially after I began my academic career at the Kansas City College of Osteopathic Medicine and Surgery in 1964 and discovered how difficult it was to teach a half-formed idea. The refinement of MET concepts has been, in fact, an ongoing process continuing to the present, including the years of dialogue with my son and co-author, and new information that came to light during the writing of this series.

The years from 1958 to 1969 saw the Mitchell – Kimberly team teaching courses at state conventions (one such course was "The Pelvis and Its Environs," sponsored by the Academy of Applied Osteopathy), and Mitchell, Sr., conducting private tutorials in his practice in Chattanooga. By 1970 the demands for teaching Muscle Energy had imposed some structured organization on the content of the tutorials, and in March of 1970 a class of six attended a five day Muscle Energy tutorial hosted by Dr. Sarah Sutton in Fort Dodge, Iowa. The class included Drs. Sutton, John Goodridge, Philip Greenman, Rolland Miller, Devota Nowland, and Edward Stiles. Before his death in 1974, Mitchell, Sr. taught five more of these hosted tutorials in various locations around the country. One tutorial was hosted by the College of Osteopathic Medicine at Michigan State University as inservice training for the Departments of Biomechanics and Family Medicine.

In 1974, a task force chaired by Sarah Sutton, DO, was organized to perpetuate the teaching of Muscle Energy technique. I was a member of this task force, along with some educational resource people from the Office of Medical Education Research and Development at MSU-COM. Most of the task force com-

---

*Included in this manual are brief excerpts, which have been adapted and reprinted with the permission of the publishers, from: Mitchell FL Jr.: Elements of muscle energy technique, in Basmajian JV, Nyberg R (eds.) Rational Manual Therapies. Baltimore, Md. Williams & Wilkins, 1993, 285-321.

mittee members were osteopathic physicians who had attended Mitchell, Sr's tutorials and believed that the concept was vital and important enough to justify spending time away from their busy practices. After days of intensive effort, this committee organized the first posthumous Muscle Energy Tutorial, which was sponsored jointly by The College of Osteopathic Medicine at Michigan State University and the American Academy of Osteopathy. With myself as the principal teacher, the course was presented in December of 1974 to a class of 12. By 1985 more than sixty 40 hour Muscle Energy Tutorial CME courses had been presented by Mitchell, Jr., Paul Kimberly, DO, John Goodridge, DO, Ed Stiles, DO, and others.

The labors of the task force continued for several years under the able chairmanship of David Johnson, DO, as the AAO Muscle Energy Tutorial Committee, with the expenses of the meetings funded by the American Academy of Osteopathy and the National Osteopathic Foundation. Other hard-working members of that ongoing committee included S.D. Blood, DO, Martha I. Drew, J.P. Goodridge,DO, R.E. Gooch, DO, R.C. MacDonald, DO, N.A. Pruzzo, DO, Sarah Sutton, DO, and myself. Analyzing the educational challenge before them, the task force restructured the curriculum content into one forty hour Basic and two forty hour Advanced tutorials, Muscle Energy IIA (above the diaphragm) and Muscle Energy IIB (below the diaphragm).

Diagnostic Concepts

As one might suspect, the diagnostic concepts of Muscle Energy were based on the manipulative techniques Mitchell, Sr., learned in the 1930s from Charles Owens and in medical school at the Chicago College of Osteopathy. Charles Owens had earned his mentorship by saving my life when I was five years old and had been severely burned. In 1934 such burns were uniformly fatal, usually terminating life shortly after renal failure occurred. Owens treated my kidneys and my uremic projectile vomiting with Chapman's Reflexes, restoring renal function and saving my life, which was supposed to have ended the following morning.

The osteopathic lesion had been defined and redefined by osteopathic authors such as Downing (1923) and Fryette (1935) who came after Still. Basic to the concept of the osteopathic lesion was geometric malposition of a bone, referred to by some authors as a 'subluxation'. Correct position of the bone was thought of in terms of static geometric symmetry and postural harmony. This static concept lingers on in the minds of patients and even some manipulative practitioners, who still think that manipulation is a process of putting bones back in place. Worse still, manipulators were once known as "lightning bone setters." In spite of the static nomenclature, movement restriction was considered by some authors to be a primary feature of the osteopathic lesion, and the anatomic, physiologic and pathologic mechanisms of the restrictions were considered important.

A more functional concept of the osteopathic lesion gradually evolved and rather rapidly matured as the Muscle Energy concepts developed. Malposition was thought of as what happened to a bone when a portion of its range of motion was taken away. If a part of a bone's ability to flex (forward bend) on another bone is lost, then attempts to actively or passively flex the bone completely will result in the bone coming to rest in a position which is more extended than it should be. Hence, the bone could be said to be 'extended.' Such positional descriptions of the osteopathic lesion were, in a sense, carry-overs from the older static concepts. They seemed a natural way to describe a visible malposition of a bone, and were used widely, even by those more analytic practitioners who understood the dynamic nature of the osteopathic lesion.

The concepts of spinal kinematics as worked out by Halladay (1957) and Fryette (1950) were rather widely understood (and, apparently, also widely misunderstood) and were a part of the curriculum taught to my father by Martin Beilke, D.O. and Frasier Strachan, D.O. at the Chicago college. I recall that he used the "ERS" and "FRS" notations in his office progress notes from the very start of his practice. This notation continued after he had begun to use more Muscle Energy techniques than thrust (high velocity–low amplitude) techniques. This understanding of the behavior of lesioned vertebral joints was basic to the diagnostic analysis necessary for applications of Muscle Energy technique, or mobilization by thrust, for that matter.

One of the important ideas Mitchell got from Ruddy was the concept of restrictors as unnaturally shortened muscles. The deeper ones ("short restrictors") abnormally limiting movement of one joint, larger muscles ("long restrictors") affecting more than one joint. It didn't matter that other mechanisms: edema, fibrosis, or joint malcongruence might also restrict joint movement, since the Muscle

Energy techniques seemed to be effective even when these elements were demonstrably present.

The short muscle paradigm, in other words, while it was an over-simplification, was clinically and heuristically useful. Muscle Energy technique is effective treatment for somatic dysfunctions of the pelvic joints, even though they are passive joints. The forces which are indirectly applied to the sacroiliac ligaments by specific muscle contractions in specific body positions work to restore function to these joints.

The Psychophysics of Physical Diagnosis

Teaching Muscle Energy technique has brought into focus the importance of understanding our own sensory/perceptual nervous systems in order to conduct valid physical examinations of the musculoskeletal system with reasonably dependable inter-rater reliability. In terms of the morale of beginning students attempting to acquire the psychomotor skills of physical diagnosis, there is great heuristic advantage to the notion that the human nervous system is analogous to a sophisticated, high technology scientific instrument. Before one begins to use a scientific instrument, it is usually a very good idea to read the instruction manual first, and then calibrate the instrument. Like any fine precision instrument, the human nervous system must be calibrated and used according to a set of instructions in order to obtain reliable data with it. The rules for Observation, Palpation, Percussion, and Auscultation are determined by the anatomy and physiology of the perceptual systems involved.

Observation is a basic and necessary part of Muscle Energy diagnosis. I believe, however, that the art and science of manipulation has become conceptually and linguistically over linked to palpatory diagnosis. There was a time when one went to OMT class to learn "manips". So much emphasis was put on the *treatment techniques*, that we thought we were extraordinarily enlightened when we appended "*and palpatory diagnosis*" to the catalog description of the course content. Having learned the new catechism of "Manipulation *and Palpatory Diagnosis*," we congratulated ourselves on having entered the scientific age, and felt rather complacent until we were confronted with our failure to integrate manipulation into the rest of the curriculum.

Perhaps this largely unexamined historical perspective explains why observation, auscultation and percussion have nearly been excluded from the teaching of structural diagnosis. Clearly, this linguistic association of "manipulation" and "palpation" has had profound effects on osteopathic college curricula. Some instructors have even taught their students to close their eyes when examining a patient for somatic dysfunction, in order to focus concentration on palpatory data. In itself, this is a valid approach to teaching the art of palpation. The trouble is, the instructors sometimes forget to tell the students to also *look at the patient*.

Some modalities of manipulation, for example, the indirect cranial and functional techniques, depend almost entirely on *palpatory* data for physical diagnosis. {The tapping, taught by Bowles (1981) and Johnston (1972), proponents of Functional Technique, could be regarded as an application of percussion. Exclusive of the "cracked pot note" of skull fracture (DeGowin, 1981), I have no knowledge of applications of auscultation or percussion in cranial diagnosis.} In my opinion, the indirect cranial and functional techniques are valid and clinically useful paradigms, and yet one must speculate on the impact they have had on the teaching of the more widely used modalities of manipulation, namely, thrust and Muscle Energy. Most practitioners of these indirect styles of manipulation emphatically maintain that their palpatory data are qualitatively the same as visually observable data, but, in general, are quantitatively more sensitive, since the phenomena accessible to palpation are so hard to see. As you will soon see, I take exception to this generalization.

Let me give an example of this generalization. The diagnostic data of Functional technique considers only three describable phenomena: (1)"ease" and (2)"bind", which are characteristic of "lesion" behavior, and are not detectable in (3)"non-lesion" – normal compliant – behavior. The conceptual leap occurs when "bind", which is a manifestation of "lesion" behavior detectable by introducing passive movement from any starting position and palpating the local tissue response to the movement, is assumed to be evidence that the range of motion of the specific part being examined is abnormally restricted in the *same* direction of movement which evokes the "bind" reaction. If right rotation produces a sense of "bind", then it is assumed that right rotation is restricted. In terms of theoretical parsimony, and in the interests of theoretical unification, it would be nice if this were so. It does tend to muddy the conceptual waters, however, when confronting the problems of the interpretation and the physiology of pain in relation to joint mobility.

In order to demonstrate the error of this assumption, all one need do is examine the same structure both for "ease and bind" and for altered range of motion. This was, in fact, done as an informal experiment by William Johnston (the Functional examiner), Lon Hoover (the gracious volunteer subject), and myself (the range-of-motion examiner). We met once a week for several weeks. After many hours of comparing Johnston's "ease-bind" palpatory findings with my palpatory-visual range of motion findings, I concluded that about two out of three times, when Johnston reported "bind" in one direction I would find range of motion restriction *in the other direction*. Direction agreements tended to be about flexion and extension movements. These findings were never published. Since I had the very poor inter-rater reliability of a tyro in Functional technique, and Johnston could not do MET examination procedures reproducibly, a communication impasse was reached. Given that I have a high regard for Johnston's skill, I accept the intrarater reliability of his findings. So, for me, the problem of interrater disagreement does not go away.

I prefer to believe that there is a qualitative as well as a quantitative difference between the "ease-bind" data and the range-of-motion data. For one thing, range-of-motion data is partly visual. For another, end-field quality and quantity is included in range-of-motion measurement, but is rarely examined in Functional technique. I would be willing to postulate that "ease-bind" data would correlate closely with any measurement of segmental facilitation, e.g., galvanic skin response or infrared thermography; and, therefore, is more closely related to segmental pain syndromes. Range-of-motion data, on the other hand, is less directly related to these phenomena and more closely related to trauma history and the ensuing chronic adaptations to those injuries.

Because of the importance of visual observation to Muscle Energy diagnosis, teaching Muscle Energy leads to an increased appreciation of the special characteristics of visual perception, especially as it applies to physical diagnosis. Taking eye dominance into account often resolves the problems of inter-rater UN-reliability. For example, when the eyes are used to make quantitative geometric judgments, the dominant eye should be positioned so that it is the closer eye to the subject. The theory is that the visual information from this perspective is more manageable by the analytic left cerebral hemisphere. Picture, if you will, two right eyed examiners looking at the same subject lying supine on an examining table, but from different sides of the table. They are both trying to decide if the positions of the anterior superior spines of the ilia are symmetrical in some geometric frame of reference. They disagree. Instead of one of them feeling threatened by the other, and deciding to agree with him, they switch sides and make the observation again. To their surprise, they now find that they disagree with themselves!

What being right eyed means is that the right eye looks straight at the object being regarded while the left eye converges on the same object. The slight difference in angulation of the eyes is interpreted as depth perception. It also means that optic nerve impulses generated by the right visual field go to the *dominant* (left) cerebral cortex. Eye dominance may be "mixed", i.e., not on the same side as the dominant hand. Eye dominance may be alternating, one eye dominant for near vision, the other eye for far vision. The test for eye dominance for the intermediate distances involved in physical diagnosis is done as follows: With both eyes open and both elbows straight place the index fingers and thumbs together to form a diamond shaped aperture. Look through the aperture at a small object across the room, and then close one eye. If the object disappeared, the closed eye is the dominant one. If it did not disappear, the open eye is dominant.

Because we exist in a gravitational field our eyes are extremely good at detecting small variations (1 or 2 degrees) from perfect horizontal or perfect vertical. This ability and other abilities derived from it, such as angle mensuration, have many applications in physical diagnosis. For example, vertebral rotation is much easier to see from a superior tangent view of the back than it is to perceive with depth perception or palpation.

Our peripheral vision is especially sensitive to small movement variations. For example, when two simultaneous movements are being quantitatively compared, as in evaluating respiratory movements of the rib cage, it is best NOT to watch the movements with the eyes' central vision, but to use the peripheral vision, instead.

The importance of relaxation for palpation has taken on new meaning through experiences in teaching others Muscle Energy diagnosis. The textbooks admonish us to relax our palpating hand, and even suggest pushing the palpating hand in with the other hand to avoid exerting the palpating hand. The basic principles of physical diagnosis which medical students have the hardest time with are the ones which are most essential in the learning process in Muscle Energy technique. When we teach palpation in the Physical Diagnosis skills courses, we emphasize how important it is to relax the palpating hand. In Muscle Energy technique, as in cranial technique, you had better have more than your hand relaxed, if you expect to even find the transverse processes or other bony landmarks. In fact, the degree of relaxation required for accurate diagnostic palpation of the musculoskeletal system often produces a warming of the hands and a cooling of the face, similar to the effect produced by biofeedback training.

Because teaching Muscle Energy skills often involves a one to one student teacher ratio, the relationship between postural BALANCE AND RELAXATION is easy to observe. We began teaching students to do their palpating from a balanced posture, which enabled them to relax better.

Bony landmarks are best found by using the stereognostic palpatory sense of the palms of the hands instead of the fine epicritic palpatory senses of the finger pads, which are especially designed to discriminate variations in tissue texture and firmness.

Treatment Concepts

The treatment concepts of Muscle Energy technique originated with Carl Kettler and T.J. Ruddy. At a convention attended by my father Kettler was demonstrating his famous "airplane" technique. As he demonstrated and talked about what he was doing, he used the expression, "The patient pushes against a distinctly executed and controlled counterforce provided by the operator." These words were still ringing in his head when my father returned to his office. At another convention, T.J. Ruddy was demonstrating his Rapid Resistive Duction technique applied to decongesting the orbit. He instructed the patient to turn his eyeball against the resistance which he provided with a finger against the eyelid. Resistive Duction suggested a whole spectrum of techniques employing the muscular efforts of patients, against a "distinctly executed counterforce".

The *basic* physiologic mechanisms of Muscle Energy techniques fell into place in a short time. The post-isometric relaxation phenomenon, in which the myotatic response of the muscle is apparently inhibited, was conceived mostly by serendipity. Mitchell initially thought of the isometric contraction as a way to get the muscle to mechanically stretch itself. After all, Mitchell had majored in Mechanical Engineering in college, not Neurophysiology. However, he immediately saw the application of Sherrington's second law (specifying the mutual reciprocal inhibition of antagonist muscles) in the instant suppression of muscle spasm by strong antagonist contraction.

One way to make a muscle longer is to inhibit its alpha motor nerve supply by forcefully contracting its antagonist. Reciprocal inhibition of antagonist muscles was first announced as a neurologic principle by Sherrington. Clearly, this method would be especially effective in lengthening spastic or hypertonic muscles. To maximize the inhibition, the antagonist muscle should be concentrically contracted isotonically against a very resisting (only slowly yielding) counterforce.

The correction of somatic dysfunction by isometric contractions is the primary basic technique in Muscle Energy. The patient is asked to exert a force against an unyielding counterforce for a few seconds and then relax it. During the post-isometric relaxation phase the muscle can be passively stretched longer without eliciting any myotatic reflex response. We came to understand that there was more than a neurologic event involved in this new lengthened state of the muscle. Since striated muscle contractions are venous/lymphatic pumps, some fluid must have been squeezed from the muscle when it contracted.

The force of the contraction might also have altered the structure of the muscle's endomysium, perimysium, and epimysium. While densely organized collagen tissue strongly resists deformation, the loose areolar fascia separating the planes of deep fascia deforms more easily, and thus the muscle may become longer by changing the shape of its fascia.

Both isometric and isotonic procedures were used by my father, sometimes combined, to more effectively mobilize a restricted joint. And, of course, he never forgot how to pop a joint. Because of its precision and inherent gentleness, Muscle Energy Technique has proven to be a safe, efficient, and effective alternative to joint mobilization by thrust. Under some circumstances, the techniques characterized as "high velocity low amplitude" (thrust) techniques are sometimes more efficient and, in the absence of contraindications, equally safe when applied skillfully and with precision. In my own practice thrust technique became considerably more precise once I had mastered Muscle Energy Technique. I now use thrust less than one percent of the time.

Other concepts and mechanisms grew out of the necessities of teaching people with inquiring minds. It soon became apparent that treatment effectiveness with Muscle Energy technique was dependent on getting the *correct* muscles to contract. Clearly, if flexion movement is restricted, then the extensor muscle must be too short. And to get the patient to contract the extensor muscle you tell the patient to extend. But is it really that simple? Which extensor muscle are we talking about? Spinalis? Longissimus? Multifidus? Rotatores? The functional classification of muscles into TONIC and PHASIC and the roles they play in spinal movement seems quite relevant. Phasic muscles are strong and have greater leverage on the vertebrae. Phasic muscles are disproportionally influenced by events affecting the tonic muscles.

In a single vertebral joint dysfunction the mono-articular tonic muscle is abnormally short. To contract it isometrically requires only light voluntary effort. By varying the force of the patient's contractions different layers of muscles may be activated.

The concept of localization underwent some refinement as the method developed. At first, precise localization, in the sense we now understand it, was not regarded as especially important. If a joint could not flex, then one flexed it to treat it. The more one flexed it the more the extensor muscles got stretched.

The term 'barrier' came into use, at first indicating generally the direction that movement was *not* permitted. As Mitchell. Sr., attempted to teach the Muscle Energy method to me and to others, it soon became clear that getting the desired results with Muscle Energy technique required a much more precise concept of the Barrier and of Localization. In coming to terms with my initial failures to get as good results as he was able to, he came to understand that precise localization required being in precisely the right position in relation to the Barrier, before introducing any corrective force. Of course, after years of clinical practice, when he treated patients, he did that intuitively; but intuition is very hard to teach to someone else.

In our discussions of localization he tried to explain to me what it meant to be at the 'feather edge' of the barrier, and I set about trying to learn what it felt like when I had encountered the 'feather edge'. The complicating feature of this learning process, I discovered, was the qualitative and quantitative variability of barriers. In the process of defining what 'barrier' meant precisely, recognition of these variations became heuristically important. The nature of the restrictive mechanism clearly determined the quality of the barrier 'end-field' (or some prefer to spell it 'end-feel'). Barrier properties could be discriminated by palpation: viscosity, elasticity, rigidity, hysteresis effects, and non-Newtonian variabilities characteristic of colloidal substrates. At times one could say with some conviction that the restriction felt like it was due to edema, or fibrosis, or muscle spasm, or muscle hypertonus, or intra-articular locking (although the latter seemed indistinguishable from the 'end-feel' of fibrosis).

The localization question then became, "Where must one be in relation to each of these barriers, or combinations of them, in order for the treatment to be sufficiently localized?" The 'feather edges' of each type of barrier were unique!

Additionally, it became clear that some lesioned joints were more restricted than other lesioned joints. Sometimes the barrier was encountered before one had traversed half of the normal range of motion. Such an extreme loss of joint mobility in a somatic dysfunction came to be called a 'major restriction', in contradistinction to the 'minor restriction' in which less than half of the normal range of motion has been lost. After years of applying Muscle Energy concepts to treat my patients, I discovered that I had been making a crucial localization error very often. I had simply not taken into account the magnitude of the restrictions when setting up the dysfunctions for correction! Consequently, the minor restrictions were always easy to treat, and the major restrictions often resisted correction. Once I began positioning the lesioned joint at the 'feather edge' of its restrictive barrier, correction of the major restrictions became as easy as it was for the minor ones.

In much of my earlier writing I have parroted the phrase, "...engage the barrier in all three planes," just as my father had taught many of his students. I continued to do so even after I changed the way I localized treatment procedures. Karel Lewit, MD (personal communication, 1999) made me aware of the discrepancy between what I was saying and what I was doing. To simultaneously engage all three planes of barrier would be difficult, if not impossible. Axial rotation is not a localizable movement. What I actually have been doing for the treatment of spinal segmental dysfunction is approaching the sidebending barrier from joint neutral, and during post-isometric (flexion or extension) relaxation, testing for a release of segmental sidebending. If the sidebending release is sufficient, I find that there is no longer a restriction of rotation or sagittal plane motion; those pathologic barriers are no longer present.

Fortunately, manipulation is a very forgiving art, permitting us a certain measure of success even when we do not do it perfectly correctly. Still, there is more personal satisfaction in being able to predict how things will come out. One great strength of Muscle Energy technique is its predictive power. Even complex patterns of somatic dysfunction have a logic which may be analyzed, permitting predictions of the outcomes of treatments. This is the fun part of manipulation for me.

I conclude by acknowledging the debt of gratitude we all owe to the dedicated people – students and colleagues – who contributed to the dissemination of this knowledge and skill, and to its refinement and development.

A Short History of the Pelvic Axes

Fred Mitchell, Sr.'s motivation to construct a theoretical model of pelvic joint biomechanics grew out of his need to explain apparent paradoxical clinical findings in physical examination of the pelvis. The relationship between findings of sacral base positions and findings of sacral inferior lateral angles (ILAs) positions was inconsistent. Sometimes the findings were ipsilateral, and sometimes contralateral. His resolution of these paradoxes led him to postulate two different dysfunctions of the sacrum which he named sacral torsion lesions and unilateral sacral flexion lesions. This entailed assigning an oblique axis to the rotation of the sacrum which he termed sacral torsion. He conceived two instantaneous oblique axes, which he arbitrarily named "left" and "right" according to the side of the superior end of the axis.

The oblique axis had been postulated by Harold Magoun, D.O. in 1939 (Magoun, HI. A method of sacroiliac correction. In*Academy of Applied Osteopathy Yearbook,* 1954, pp. 113-116). Magoun credits C.B.Atzen of Omaha and D. L. Clark of Denver for developing the treatment techniques described in this article, which was delivered before the Orthopedic Section at the Forty-Third Annual Convention of the American Osteopathic Association, Dallas, Texas, June 29, 1939. However, neither Atzen nor Clark refer to an oblique axis in the osteopathic literature. Magoun appears to have been the first to reason that a sacrum found in a rotated position must have turned on an oblique axis.

The mistake that these pioneers made was in assuming that the rotated sacrum was held that way entirely by intra-articular restriction, instead of an arrested spinal ambulatory undulation. Their manipulative procedures were clearly designed to untwist the sacrum.

In sacral torsion, sacroiliac articular mobility is restricted primarily at the inferior pole of the oblique axis. The sacrum is free to derotate as soon as the spine straightens. This principle is the basis for the Sphinx test, in which the forward torsion dysfunction straightens with lumbar backward bending, and the backward torsion becomes more rotated.

Other axes had already been described by early anatomists. Bonnaire (cited in Kapandji, 1974) placed an axis for sagittal plane sacral motion (between the ilia) within the articular facet between the cranial and caudal segments. Bonnaire's axis probably corresponds to Mitchell's middle transverse axis. Mitchell credited Magoun with describing what Mitchell termed the superior transverse axis, although Farabeuf, referenced by Kapandji, undoubtedly preceded Magoun. It is likely that controversy about these two transverse axes has an even longer history, possibly dating back to Albinus (1677-1770) or John Hunter (1718-1783), or possibly von Luschka (1814). Farabeuf located the axis (superior transverse) at the axial interosseous ligament (the short posterior sacroiliac ligament).

Mitchell, Sr., considered the middle and superior transverse axes, plus the two oblique (diagonal) axes, sufficient to describe *sacroiliac* motion – movements of the sacrum between the ilia caused by forces from the spine above. The oblique axes enabled him to describe sacral torsion (rotated) positions. He made no attempt to describe an axis for unilateral sacral flexion (sidebent) position other than to suggest that the superior transverse axis was involved in the downward and backward swing of the sacrum – sacral nutation – and the lesion occurred when one side of the sacrum could not swing the other way, up and forward.

To account for the often-observed clinical evidence of asymmetric displacement of one innominate relative to the other as indicated by anterior superior iliac spine positions, Mitchell, Sr. proposed a transverse axis through the symphysis pubis, and an iliosacral axis through the inferior pole of the sacral auricular surface. This pubic axis was later demonstrated by Lavignolle, et al (1983) and Frigerio, et al (1974). Frigerios's large amplitude interinnominate motion findings were consistent with clinical observations (several centimeters of iliac crest movement), but were questioned by many in the scientific community whose measurements of intrapelvic motion tended to be smaller.

Some Frequently Asked Questions

What is the relationship between the Mitchell model of the pelvis and Muscle Energy?

Although both originated with Mitchell, Sr., and Muscle Energy bases its diagnostic criteria for pelvic dysfunction on the Mitchell model of the pelvis, the model is not Muscle Energy, *per se.* Mitchell Sr.'s pelvisacral model predates the formulation of Muscle Energy, and can be considered independently. The model presents a way to *analyze* the pelvis and is applicable to both thrust treatment and MET treatment. However, MET offers an alternative, highly specific, non-traumatic way to treat somatic dysfunctions of the pelvis, and it addresses those dysfunctions in a more direct physiologic manner. The Mitchell model of the pelvis is based on general mechanical principles which can be viewed independently of any given treatment modality; this includes the principles of MET treatment. In fact, prior to the development of MET – but after he had laid the foundation for his model of the pelvis – Mitchell, Sr., like many of his contemporaries, treated the pelvis with Thrust technique.

Mitchell, Sr.'s greatest creative effort went into developing the pelvic model. When he began using muscular cooperation of patients to treat their lesions, what he did was based on how he understood Kettler and Ruddy, plus a large measure of mechanical intuition. From this a few basic principles of MET were conceived.

What causes sacroiliac/iliosacral motion?

Muscles do not *directly* move the sacrum between the ilia. Instead, sacral movement is the result of gravitational, inertial, and elastic forces resulting from spinal movements, which are indeed the result of muscular activity. The role of elasticity is discussed by Dorman (1992). Similarly, muscles do not directly move the innominate bones in relation to each other, or in relation to the sacrum. Again, such movements result from gravitational, inertial, and elastic forces from the legs.

The bones of the pelvis are moved by the elasticity of the connective tissue comprising the pelvic ligaments and fascial continuity of the trunk, pelvis and lower limb.

Likely the association of the pelvis model with Muscle Energy Technique has misled many students who were not aware that the sacroiliac is a passive joint, i.e., not *directly* moved by muscle contraction. If they lacked a rational explanation for what could be observed in the pelvis, some individuals "invented" muscles capable of moving ilium on sacrum, sacrum on ilium, or ilium on ilium. Understandably, some students began trying to figure out what muscle they needed to make longer in order to restore movement to the sacroiliac joint. Unsuspecting, they were led into this error by first being exposed to Muscle Energy for the treatment of spinal or extremity joints, where muscles do move joints. If a spinal or extremity joint has restricted motion, then to eliminate the restriction, the shortened muscle must be lengthened. The students should have been told that this principle does not apply to the pelvis. *In the pelvis the bones are pushed around in relation to each other by bone on bone compression or ligament and fascial tensions and elasticity.*

How can MET affect passive joints?
One may well wonder how dysfunction of the sacroiliac joint can be treated with Muscle Energy Technique. Unlike the isometric techniques used to treat vertebral or extremity joints, the Muscle Energy techniques for treating pelvic joint dysfunctions do not use muscle contractions to lengthen short muscles. Instead, the muscle contractions exert forces on the ligaments, capsule, and intra-articular structures which result in increasing the range-of-motion of the joint.

How did the oblique axes get their names?
The rationale for naming the oblique axes originally was based on Mitchell, Sr.'s hypothesis that the upper end of the axis was the stable end. He hypothesized that the upper end of the oblique axis was stabilized on the side of the stance leg by the weight of the spine on the sacrum, and therefore, the stance leg and the named axis were ipsilateral. His description of the walking cycle was, therefore, "out of step" with the current description. This nomenclature persists even though the model has since been modified by Mitchell, Jr.

What is the goal of MET treatment, as it relates to the Mitchell model of the pelvis?
1. Restoring and maintaining normal anatomic relationships for the functional axes of the pelvis.
2. Restoring physiologic mobility to the joints of the pelvis by reducing friction or hysteresis in the sacroiliac joint.
3. Increasing the efficiency of the physiologic functions of the pelvis: locomotion, breathing, circulation, and visceral support – both mechanical and neuro-endocrine.

What is unique about MET's approach to evaluation of the pelvis?

Because MET's evaluation is based on the Mitchell Model of pelvic mechanics, it has the following advantages:

■ Permits more specific and effective treatment by discriminating more discrete lesion possiblities, as well as distinguishing between sacroiliac and iliosacral *functions* of the joint;
■ Uses more axes to describe physiologic movement;
■ Distinquishes between subluxation and dysfunction;
■ States reasons why subluxations must be treated before dysfunctions.

What other modalities address Pelvic dysfunction?

Thrust, Cranial, Myofascial, Functional Technique, Strain-Counterstrain, Respiratory-Circulatory Technique, and Exercise Therapy, among others.

How do they differ from MET in evaluation and treatment of Pelvic dysfunction?

With the exception of Thrust technique, none of the techniques mentioned above consider the axes or planes of pelvic mechanics relevant in their evaluation or treatment of the pelvis.

Thrust technique, as it is generally understood, is based on a model simpler than that of MET. In the early days, the goal of Thrust technique was thought to be "putting the bones back in place." The idea of restricted intraarticular mobility grew out of this static malposition concept, and is the rationale for Thrust technique. MET views somatic dysfunctions of the pelvis as involving complex interactions of pelvic components with spine, cranium, and legs, and includes these influences in the MET treatment procedures.

Cranial evaluation assesses the Primary Respiratory Mechanism as a component in the manifestation of pelvic dysfunction. This would include cerebrospinal fluid dynamics, dural tensions, and osseous articular mechanisms.

Myofascial Technique is the most similar to cranial inasmuch as it follows tension states in the myofascia, and considers the sacrum as part of a fascial continuity. The axes or planes of movement, however, are not considered.

Jones Strain-Counterstrain defines the sacroiliac lesion in terms of tender points at or near the sacrum which can be made non-tender through the use of correct positioning. Strain-Counterstrain terminology tacitly assumes biomechanic factors are at work in pelvic dysfunction, but makes no reference to axes or planes of motion, and no landmarks are used to confirm the efficacy of the treament.

Functional Technique diagnosis of the pelvis is based on the assessment of three guiding criteria: Ease, Bind, and Normal. These criteria guide and determine the treament of the pelvis, without consideration for the axes and planes of motion or range-of-motion.

The Respiratory-Circulatory Model defines dysfunction in the pelvis (as it does with other parts of the body) as breathing motion impairment. If there is impaired breathing motion of the pelvis, the clinician will then relate the impairment in the pelvis to impairments that exist in other parts of the body as well. But, as with many of the other modalities, consideration of the axes and planes of motion in the pelvis are not relevant to evaluation and treatment.

Exercise Therapy is concerned with the pelvic stabilizing functions of trunk and limb muscles and their coordination. Retraining cerebellar and spinal cord reflexes to reprogram spinal effector mechanisms is often an important adjuct to manual therapy for the pelvis, both to correct pelvic dysfunction and maintain normal function.

What are the similarities and differences between the European Post-Isometric Relaxation (PIR – Lewit, 1999) and Muscle Energy Technique (MET – Mitchell, Jr., 1995, 1998, 1999)?

The Muscle Energy concept probably was introduced to Karel Lewit, MD, by the late Fritz Gaymans, MD, who had learned of it from American colleagues. Heinz-Dieter Neumann, MD brought Lewit and Gaymans together because he knew both had been working on self-mobilization techniques. Based on whatever information or germinal ideas Gaymans, and possibly others, communicated about Muscle Energy, Lewit was able to creatively and systematically develop the concept into structured courses on post-isometric relaxation techniques.

In 1977 Lewit and Mitchell, Jr. met for the first time at Michigan State University, and had an opportunity to share ideas and observe each other's methods. Lewit's lectures on PIR to the faculty of the College of Osteopathic Medicine were illustrated with slides he used in teaching his European courses. Mitchell, Jr. was astonished at the similarity, and observed that he could have taught his own MET courses using Lewit's slides. The following year Mitchell, Jr. began teaching MET courses to European osteopaths in France, Belgium, and England.

Considering the chain of secondary communications involved in introducing the Muscle Energy concepts to Lewit, it is reasonable to expect that there would be differences between PIR and MET. It is indeed remarkable that there are so many similarities.

Mitchell, Jr. sent Lewit the 1979 revision (*An Evaluation and Treatment Manual of Osteopathic Muscle Energy Procedures*) of his original 1973 *An Evaluation and Treatment Manual of Osteopathic Manipulative Procedures* as soon as it was published.

In Volume 1 of the Muscle Energy Manual series, differences between PIR and MET were briefly commented on. However, in the years since Lewit and Mitchell, Jr. met in 1977, they have learned from each other. The force of muscle contraction is no longer a major difference, if it ever was. In each system the force varies according to the specific application, although the majority of applications will be light force isometric for both MET and PIR.

Mitchell, Jr. and Lewit also agree (personal communication, 1999) that approaching the barrier(s) in all three planes simultaneously, usually before isometric contraction, is neither realistic nor necessary. Motion restriction is addressed *one* plane at a time, usually resulting in consequent restored mobility in the other two planes as well. As Lewit states, "In practice I found that mobilizing successfully in one plane, I usually succeed in freeing the entire joint."

There has also been rapprochement in the barrier terminology; Mitchell Jr.'s approach is now in close agreement with Lewit's approach. The expression, "engaging the barrier" has been supplanted by the less aggressive "localization to the barrier," and the English authors' "taking up the slack." The concept of treatment localization appears to be very similar in other respects as well. Lewit: "In taking up the slack, we try to bring the joint into its extreme position ... of normal function ... to the first slight increase of resistance." Localization is described only slightly differently by Mitchell, Jr. for MET: (Volume 1) "... passively introducing motion in the direction of mobilization, stopping just before the adjacent bone moves." In re-localization, Mitchell and Lewit both agree that the important thing is to wait and not move to the new barrier until the patient is sufficiently relaxed.

MET and PIR differ mainly in how they view the indications. PIR sees its *primary* application in muscle tightness, spasm, and myofascial trigger points, with joint mobilization the consequence of muscle relaxation. MET sees its *primary* application in mobilization of both active and passive joints, and regards muscle spasm and tightness, when they occur, as neurological consequences of postural and locomotor *adaptation* to articular dysfunction usually located elsewhere in the body. MET is occasionally used to lengthen tight or short muscles, strengthen weak muscles, remove peripheral tissue edema, reduce articular subluxations, or stretch deep fascia, but vertebral articular mobilization is the principal application for MET.

Another important difference is in the criteria used for *diagnosing* articular restriction. PIR includes movement restriction, spasm, soft tissue abnormalities, asymmetry, and pain or tenderness in the *diagnosis* of somatic dysfunction. MET bases diagnosis entirely on motion restriction as determined by assessing changes in the *static* positions of bony landmarks before and after movement. In MET diagnostic analysis, soft tissue states may be impediments to diagnosis, which is based on assessing change in bony landmark position. It is not assumed that articular motion restriction can be accounted for by *palpable* muscle or tissue tightness.

Fred L. Mitchell, Jr., DO, FAAO, FCA

"The pelvic girdle is the cross-roads of the body, the architectural center of the body, the meeting place of the locomotive apparatus, the resting place of the torso, the temple of the reproductive organs, the abode of the new life's development, the site of the two principal departments of elimination, and, last but not least, a place upon which to sit .... When the osteopathic physician appreciates the relationship of the bony structures of the pelvic girdle to good body mechanics, circulation to the pelvic organs and lower extremities, reflex disturbances to remote parts of the organism through endocrine or neurogenic perverted physiology, and can master the diagnosis and manipulative correction, he has the basic tool from which all therapy can begin." (Mitchell, Sr., 1958)

"...pelvic imbalance will prevent normal function of the body in both directions: toward the feet and toward the head..." (Mitchell, Sr., 1948)

"Whenever we study body mechanics we are forced to recognize that the sacroiliac articulation is the real mechanical base of body structure. Often the feet are referred to as the foundation of the body but from a real mechanical study we must admit that all foot activity is dependent on the mechanics of the hip and pelvis. Therefore, there is no doubt that the sacroiliac forms a logical starting point for all osteopathic study." (Northup, 1943-4)

"Fryette had this to say of the sacrum: 'Little wonder that the ancient Phallic Worshippers named the base of the spine the Sacred Bone. It is the seat of the transverse center of gravity, the keystone of the pelvis, the foundation of the spine. It is closely associated with our greatest abilities and disabilities, with our greatest romances and tragedies, our greatest pleasures and pains.' " (Mitchell, Sr.,1958)

CHAPTER 1

Relevant Pelvic Anatomy

This chapter will review those aspects of pelvic anatomy relevant to the evaluation and treatment of dysfunctions of the pelvis using Muscle Energy technique (MET). Familiarity with the osteology of the pelvis is essential because MET diagnosis is based on the evaluation of *static* bony landmark relationships – before and after movement. Knowledge of the muscles and ligaments is also important in order to understand the mechanics of intrapelvic movement, which will be discussed in Chapters 2 and 3.

Osteology

The pelvis is composed of three bones: two innominate bones (*os coxae*) and the sacrum. The innominates are paired and symmetrical structures, each one formed from three embryological parts: the ilium (which interfaces the sacrum), pubis, and ischium. The sacrum is a solid inverted pyramid-shaped bone whose base faces superior and anterior. It develops from the fusion of (usually) five sacral vertebrae.

On the most superior portion of the sacrum is the sacral base, which articulates with the body of the most inferior lumbar vertebra (presumably L_5) through an intervening fibrocartilage disc. On its left and right sides, the L-shaped auricular (*latin* for "ear-shaped") articular surfaces (approximately located between S_1 and S_3) of the sacrum articulate with the articular (auricular) surfaces of the ilia. The left and right innominates also directly articulate with each other, anteriorly and medially, at the pubic symphysis. The acetabulum of the pelvis provides the articular surface for the head of the femur, and is located laterally on that portion of the pelvis where the ilium, pubis, and ischium join.

Located on the superior edge of the first (superior) sacral segment on each side of the sacral canal are the two zygapophyseal facets facing posteromedially. The inferior zygapophyseal facets of the fifth lumbar fit against them, forming two synovial joints. The superior interlumbar facets are shaped to fit a vertical cylinder, the posterior part facing medially and the anterior part facing posteriorly. Unlike the interlumbar zygapophyseal joints, the lumbosacral facets are nearly flat planes oriented 45 degrees to the coronal and sagittal planes.

There is individual variation in lumbosacral facet orientation. Those facets which are closer to the coronal plane permit more sidebending and rotation of L_5 on the sacrum. The more sagittal facets permit less sidebending and rotation, and allow mainly flexion and extension. At times the facet orientation is not symmetrical. This condition is called "zygapophyseal trophism," and is suspected in the presence of asymmetric gait patterns, or can be detected radiographically.

In this chapter:

■ *Osteology*

■ *Pelvic landmarks*

■ *Pelvic ligaments*

■ *Muscles of the pelvis*

■ *Myofascial influences*

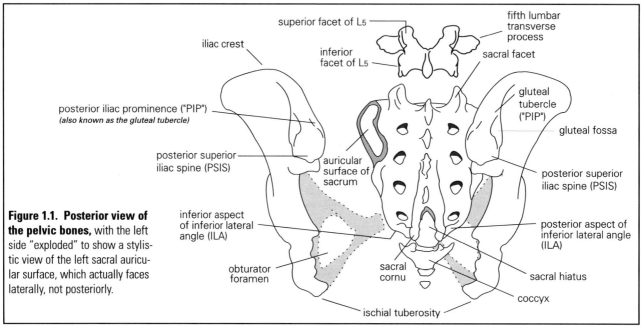

Figure 1.1. Posterior view of the pelvic bones, with the left side "exploded" to show a stylistic view of the left sacral auricular surface, which actually faces laterally, not posteriorly.

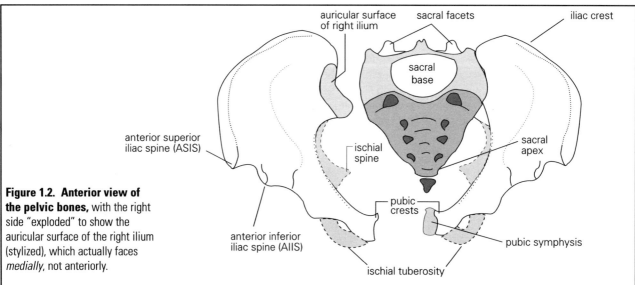

Figure 1.2. Anterior view of the pelvic bones, with the right side "exploded" to show the auricular surface of the right ilium (stylized), which actually faces *medially*, not anteriorly.

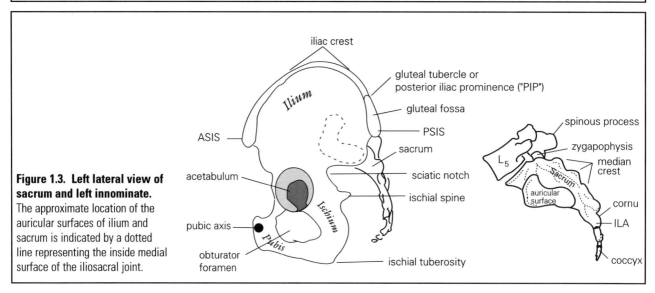

Figure 1.3. Left lateral view of sacrum and left innominate. The approximate location of the auricular surfaces of ilium and sacrum is indicated by a dotted line representing the inside medial surface of the iliosacral joint.

Pelvic Landmarks

Virgil Halladay, D.O. (1957) had this to say about landmarks:

"Before making any attempt at diagnosis, we must first discover the palpable structures of the pelvis that change their position with movement."

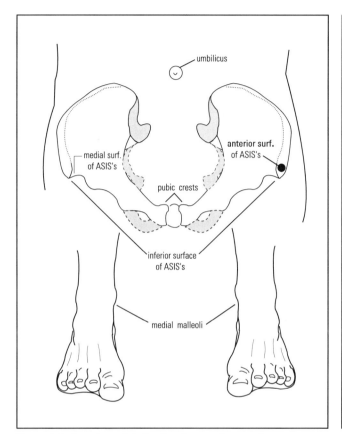

Figure 1.4. Anterior pelvic landmarks – patient supine.

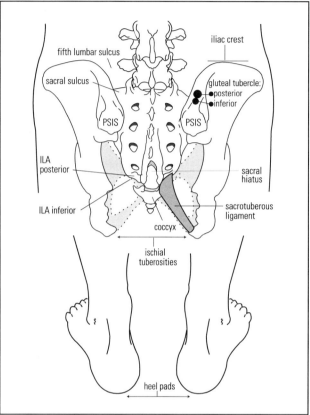

Figure 1.5. Posterior pelvic landmarks – patient prone.

Table 1.A.

Pelvic Landmarks for Structural Diagnosis in the Mitchell Model

Landmark	Purpose
1. Iliac Crests – superior surfaces	To evaluate anatomic leg length
2. Medial Malleoli – inferior surfaces	To evaluate functional leg length
3. Heel Pads – inferior surfaces	To evaluate functional leg length
4. Pubic Crests – superior surfaces	To evaluate for pubic subluxation
5. Ischial Tuberosities – inferior surfaces	To evaluate for innominate subluxation
6. Sacro-tuberous Ligaments – inferior surfaces	To evaluate for innominate subluxation
7. Inferior Lateral Angles (ILA) – posterior surfaces	To evaluate for a torsioned sacral lesion
8. Inferior Lateral Angles (ILA) – inferior surfaces	To evaluate for a unilaterally flexed sacrum lesion
9. Gluteal Tubercle (PIP) – inferior surface	Used in performing standing and seated flexion tests
10. Gluteal Tubercle (PIP) – posterior surface	Used in evaluating sulcus depth measurement
11. Posterior-Inferior Iliac Spine (PSIS) – inferior surface	Used in performing flexion tests or to evaluate for innominate rotation
12. Sacral Sulcus	To evaluate for sacroiliac dysfunction
13. L5 Transverse Processes – posterior surfaces	To evaluate for lumbosacral and sacroiliac dysfunction
14. Anterior-Inferior Iliac Spine (ASIS) – inferior surface	To evaluate for innominate rotation
15. Anterior-Inferior Iliac Spine (ASIS) – anterior surface	To evaluate for innominate rotation
16. Anterior-Inferior Iliac Spine (ASIS) – posterior surface	To evaluate for flare subluxation
17. Umbilicus	Used as a mid-line marker for flare evaluation

Pelvic Landmarks (*continued*)

Bony Landmarks for Determining Anatomic Leg Length or Assessing Pelvic Dysgenesis

Iliac Crests – Superior Surfaces. These most *superior* surfaces of the ilia are usually easily found in the standing subject. They are located below the indentations at the waistline which are just above the level of the highest points on the iliac crests.

The iliac crest is the top margin of the hip bone (innominate). Commencing at the anterior superior iliac spine, it arcs up and back to terminate at the posterior superior iliac spine. In young people ages 15 to 20 the iliac crest is separated from the body of the ilium by a hyaline cartilage diaphysis (not palpable). In adults, the iliac crest epiphysis (i.e. the growth center of the bone) is fused to the body of the ilium. The apex of the iliac crest is at or near the midaxillary line of the body.

By placing the palmar surfaces of the index and middle finger of each hand on the apex of each iliac crest, the examiner can use this hand position as the visual target with which to assess potential leg length asymmetry. Using ones own hands as the visual target greatly enhances the accuracy of the examiner's measurement of leg length asymmetry. Positioning the hands so that they accurately represent the heights of the iliac crests is best done by pushing the soft tissues below and lateral to the iliac crests in a superior direction to avoid trapping the soft tissue between the examiner's hands and the iliac crests. In order to pull fat up from the lateral aspect of the hip, the skin must be slack. To create skin slack pull some skin down from the waist before placing your palms firmly on the lateral hip surface. To assess the levelness of the hands, it is important that the examiner's eyes be positioned in the same horizontal plane as the visual target.

Bony Landmarks Indicating Innominate Position or Movement

The bony landmarks used to assess innominate position or monitor movement are as follows:

■ Posterior superior iliac spines (PSISs) or posterior iliac prominences (PIPs), also known as the gluteal tubercles;
■ Ischial tuberosities and the sacrotuberous ligaments;
■ Anterior superior iliac spines (ASISs);
■ Pubic crests.

Locating the Posterior Superior Iliac Spines (PSISs) and Posterior Iliac Prominence (PIP)

On most pelves, two prominences may be palpated on the posterior aspect of each iliac crest; the more *inferior* of which is the posterior superior iliac spine (PSIS), and the more *superior* is the posterior iliac prominence (PIP). The distance between the PIP and the PSIS is variable, but is often as much as 2 cm. The PIP occurs at the level of S_1 and is the point from which the sacral sulcus is measured. The PSIS is usually at the level of S_2.

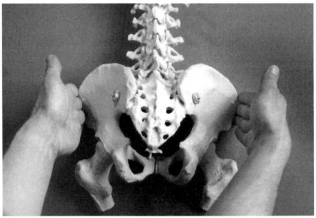

Figure 1.6 Lateral contacts for the iliac crests – landmark palpation.
It is best to avoid compressing thick soft tissues when palpating and observing the positions of the iliac crests. First place the hands below the iliac crests and push the skin and soft tissue up until the index fingers top the crests.

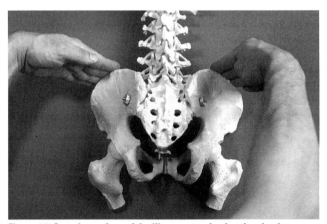

Figure 1.7 Superior surface of the iliac crests – landmark palpation.
The flat palms are turned horizontal with the index fingers resting on top of the iliac crests at their apices. Examiners eyes should be horizontal with the hands.

The dimple of Michaelis can be used as an aid in locating the PSIS and PIP (Figure 1.8). The bony prominence on the posterior aspect of the iliac crest that can be felt deep to the dimple of Michaelis is the PIP. The PIP is formed on the iliac crest by the origin of the *gluteus maximus*, and hence is located at the superior margin of the *gluteus maximus* fossa on the iliac crest. The PIP is the point where the lumbodorsal fascia meets the gluteal fascia, and the subcutaneous deep fascia is firmly anchored to the skin, creating a dimple. The actual posterior superior iliac spine (PSIS) is often a centimeter or more inferior to the dimple of Michaelis. Because the PSIS is located at the extreme posterior end of the iliac crest, the overlying *gluteus maximus* musculature sometimes makes the PSIS difficult to find and to stay on while performing motion tests. If this is the case, the PIP is the preferable landmark.

When the dimple is not visible, the PIP and/or PSIS can be found by stereognostic palpation. Place three fingers pressed flat against the skin over the place where the dimple should be, and move the skin around in a small circle (this is called a "friction"). The bony contour of the tubercles can be easily felt, even through thick adipose tissue. The opposite hand may be used to stabilize the pelvis against the pressure of the palpating hand. If more than one knot is felt, the extra knots are usually fibrolipomas, benign subcutaneous tumors composed of encapsulated fat, which are somewhat softer than bone and more movable, but are sometimes rather firmly attached to the periosteum of the bone and cannot be easily pushed aside.

When palpating for the PIP with the circular movement of the flat finger pads against the back of the pelvis at the dimple, more than one knot may be felt. Two of them should feel like hard bone, the PIP at the dimple and the PSIS just below the dimple, anywhere from a few millimeters to 2 centimeters. Many practitioners call the landmark at the dimple "the PSIS." It is a trivial error; the two are sometimes so close together they may feel like one bump. It makes sense to choose the landmark with the greatest prominence – PIP or PSIS – which, therefore, will be easier to follow when doing the flexion test.

The PIP or the PSIS may be used for several diagnostic purposes. In addition to using them to *confirm* rotated positions of the ilia (best diagnosed with the ASISs), they are the points against which to hold one's thumbs while observing articular motion of the sacroiliac joints. Such articular motion tests include the standing and seated flexion tests, the Stork tests, and testing of sacroiliac respiratory motion. When the PIPs are used for the standing or seated flexion tests, the thumbs are kept firmly against their inferior slopes and observed as they move with the ilia, just as if they were the PSISs.

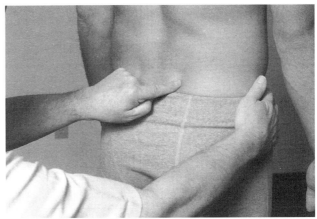

Figure 1.8. Examiner pointing to the dimple of Michaelis on the right. The dimple at the right hand corner of the the rhomboid of Michaelis is often a visible landmark.

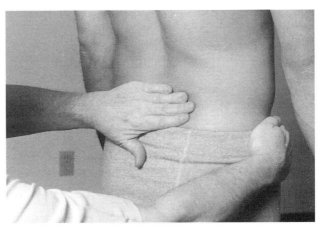

Figure 1.9. Examiner locating the PSIS/PIP using stereognosis. In palpating the PIP and the PSIS using circular friction stereognosis, firm pressure can be applied while the other hand is used to stabilize the pelvis.

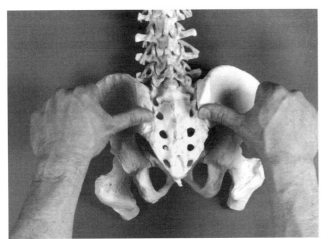

Figure 1.10 Inferior surface of the Posterior Superior Iliac Spine (PSIS) – landmark palpation. These landmarks are in the same horizontal plane as S_2.

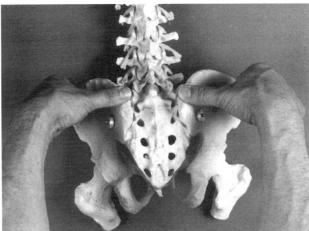

Figure 1.11 Posterior surface of the gluteal tubercle (PIP) – landmark palpation. These landmarks are in the same horizontal plane as S_1..

Locating the Anterior Superior Iliac Spine (ASIS)

The ASISs are usually examined with the patient lying supine. Evaluation of innominate rotations is accomplished most accurately by establishing bilateral contact with the pads of one's thumbs on the inferior slope of the anterior superior iliac spines. **As indicators of anterior/posterior innominate rotation, the ASISs are preferred over the PSISs, because their amplitude of displacement is greater.** These most anterior parts of the ilia are found easily and quickly by stereognostic palpation with the palms of the hands. The slight bumps in the superior-lateral area of the iliac region of the abdomen are readily discerned. Palmar stereognosis is the fastest and most reliable way to locate the ASISs. Standing at the side of the examining table one simply places the palms of the hands on each side of the front of the pelvis. The relatively sharp points of the ASISs will be immediately felt with the palms. The thumbs are then placed on the landmarks on the appropriate surface. Visual comparison of these points is best made with the dominant eye nearest the patient.

For comparative measurement purposes three different surfaces are contact points for the thumbs: inferior, anterior, and medial. The inferior slopes of the ASIS landmarks are the best indicators of anterior or posterior innominate rotation. Comparative inferior displacement of the ASIS, in the absence of pubic subluxation or sacral torsion, means the ilium is rotated anteriorly (crest anterior). The inferior side has its iliac crest rotated anteriorly, or the superior side is rotated posteriorly. The anterior surfaces of the ASISs can be used to confirm the findings on the inferior slopes. When looking at the thumbs on the inferior slopes, the eyes must be positioned vertically above the supine patient. When looking at the thumbs on the anterior surfaces, the eyes should be sighting horizontally.

The medial surfaces of the ASISs are used to evaluate inflare and outflare subluxations of the innominates. Thumbs are placed against the medial edges of the ASIS and visual comparison of their distances from a midline structure, such as the *umbilicus*, is made with the eyes sighting vertically.

Umbilicus

This is an important anterior surface landmark of the abdomen, as it is almost always located in the midsagittal plane at the level of the third lumbar vertebra. Therefore, it can be utilized as a quick and accurate reference point to the midline of the body when evaluating ilial flare, provided surgical scars have not pulled it off-center.

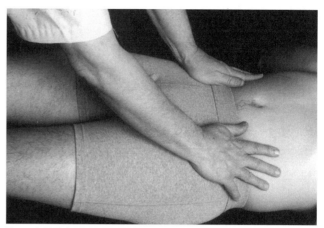

Figure 1.12 Palmar stereognostic location of the anterior surface of the Anterior Superior Iliac Spines – landmark palpation.

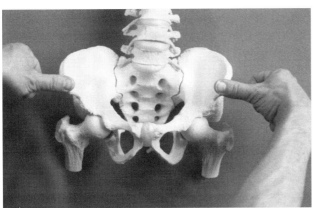

Figure 1.13. Anterior surface of the Anterior Superior Iliac Spines – landmark palpation. Examiner's gaze should be horizontal.

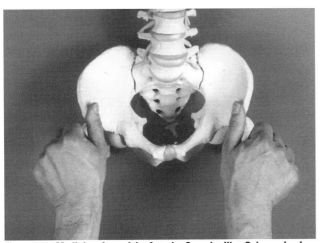

Figure 1.14. Medial surface of the Anterior Superior Iliac Spines – landmark palpation. Examiner's gaze should be vertical, as the distances of the left and right medial surfaces of the ASISs are compared relative to the umbilicus – which is used as the midline reference point.

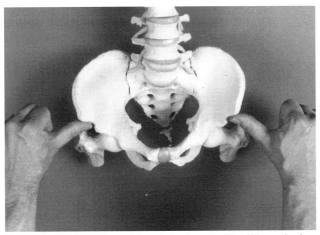

Figure 1.15. Inferior surface of the anterior Superior Iliac Spines – landmark palpation. Examiner's gaze should be vertical.

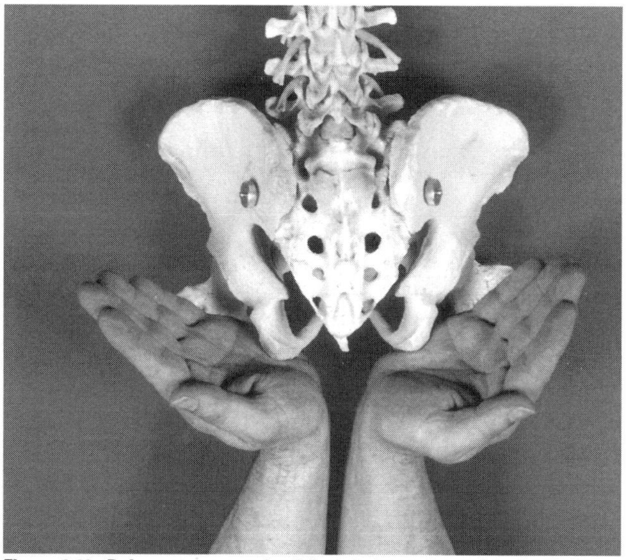

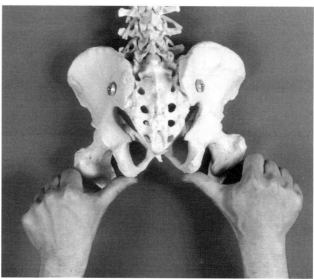

Figure 1.16. Palmar stereognosis of the inferior surface of the ischial tuberosities – landmark palpation. Palmar stereognosis should be used to precisely identify the ischial tuberosities.

Figure 1.17. Palpating the inferior surface of the ischial tuberosities. Examiner's thumbs are placed on the inferior points of the ischial tuberosities to make their positions visible.

Ischial Tuberosities, Inferior Surfaces

These most inferior portions of the ischium are palpated at the level of the horizontal gluteal fold. This part of the hip bone supports the weight of the body in the sitting position. The inferior edges of the tuberosities are compared bilaterally to evaluate for superior subluxation of the ilia (also known as "upslipped innominate"). Stereognosis is essential for accurate location of this landmark. The palms and heels of the hands, facing cephalad, are placed on the inferior gluteal folds and moved in small circles while pressing first anterior and then superior. The lowest points on the ischial tuberosities can be felt stereognostically before placing the thumbs on them for visual comparison of their relative inferior-superior positions. To reduce the resistance of skin to the palpating thumb, draw skin down from the buttocks to the posterior thigh before pressing the thumbs into the gluteal fold.

Sacrotuberous Ligaments

The sacrotuberous ligaments run in a straight line from the ischial tuberosities to the sacral apex and should also be used to evaluate iliac subluxations (upslipped innominate). One method of evaluation is to place one's thumbs midway between the sacral apex and the ischial tuberosities, pressing the thumbs superolaterally to test the tension of the sacro-tuberous ligaments. A preferred method is to slide the thumbs off of their inferior contacts on the tuberosities medial and superior, keeping lateral pressure against the bone. If the sacrotuberous ligament is slack on one side, the thumb will be permitted to slide farther on that side before its progress is checked by the ligament. Slack in the skin of the posterior thigh is especially important for this maneuver.

Other landmarks have been used to assess the pelvis for upslipped innominate subluxation, i.e., recumbent iliac

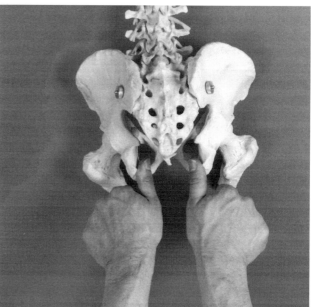

Figure 1.18. Sacrotuberous ligament – landmark palpation. Tensions of the sacrotuberous ligaments can be compared by sliding the thumbs up them toward the sacrum. Tension of the ligament normally prevents the thumb from staying in contact with the ischial bone.

crests, PSIS and ASIS. While these are logical choices, they are less practical than the ischial tuberosities and sacrotuberous ligaments. The visual perspective of the iliac crests in the recumbent position is a disadvantage for quantitative comparison. The PSIS can be be an imprecise landmark for a number of reasons. It may be near a fibrolipoma. It may have a thick covering of gluteal muscle. Or the gluteal tuberosity may be mistaken for it. The ASIS is a fairly precise landmark, but its use in diagnosing upslipped innominate depends on the position of the ipsilateral PSIS which cannot be simultaneously observed.

Medial Malleoli, Inferior Surfaces

The medial malleoli are used to measure functional leg length in the supine position. They are at the distal end of the tibia where it overlaps the talus on the medial side of the ankle. Their inferior surfaces present easily palpable shelves against which the edges of the thumbs can be firmly positioned for visual comparison of leg length. Using the medial malleoli for measurement purposes in this fashion requires that the patient lie supine and straight on the examining table with the legs visually aligned with the long axis of the body parallel with the edges of the table.

Heel Pads, Inferior Surfaces

Measuring functional leg length in the prone position is most easily accomplished by comparing the inferior surfaces of the heel pads. Ideally, the feet should be off the end of the table, so that the ankles can be symmetrically dorsiflexed. Differences in the malleoli or heel pads may indicate such variants as anatomic or apparent short leg, innominate rotations and subluxations, pubic subluxations, sacral torsion, and unilateral sacral flexion. Leg length measured supine or prone is best referred to as "apparent leg length," to acknowledge the multiple factors, in addition to anatomic leg lengths, which influence this measurement.

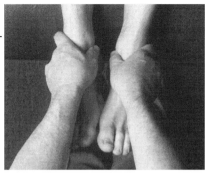

Figure 1.19. Inferior surfaces of the medial malleoli – landmark palpation position. Examiner's gaze should be vertical. This photograph demonstrates a short right leg.

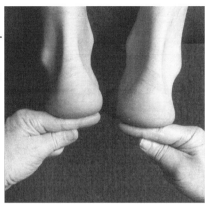

Figure 1.20. Inferior surfaces of the heel pads – landmark palpation position. Examiner's gaze should be vertical. This photograph demonstrates a short left leg.

Pubic Crests, Superior Surfaces

These small, raised, osseous projections are located on the medial-superior surface of the pubic bones . In the ectomorph, the pubic crests can be visualized as the superior edge of the mons pubis. Pubic crests should not be confused with the pubic tubercles which are located more laterally and project laterally along the line of the inguinal ligament which attaches to them. Palpation of the pubic crests entails placing index finger tips at the anterior center of the mons pubis, gently sliding the fingers superiorly to push the adipose tissue out of the way so that bilateral con-

tact can be established on the crests, and sliding the fingers back and forth laterally to ensure comparison of identical points of each crest. To make the palpatory search for the pubic crests as brief as possible, the palm should be placed flat on the midline of the lower abdomen and the upper margin of the pelvis identified stereognostically with the heel of the hand before placing the fingers on the patient. Evaluation consists of comparing the crests for superior or inferior subluxation in the frontal plane.

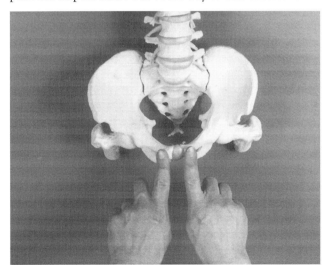

Figure 1.21. Anterior surface of the pubic crests – landmark palpation position. Finger tips will push the *mons veneris* away from the pubic crests.

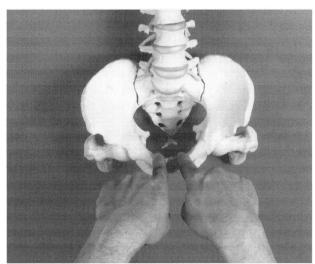

Figure 1.22. Superior surface of the pubic crests – landmark palpation position. Examiner's gaze should be vertical.

Landmarks for Assessing Sacral Position

Finding the ILAs

The inferior lateral angles (ILAs) are the alae, or transverse processes analog, of the fifth sacral segment (vertebra). They lie in the same transverse plane as the sacral hiatus, which is the inferior opening of the sacral canal, and are just lateral to the sacral cornua, which are the bifid spinous process analogs at the inferior end of the median crest of the sacrum. Their left and right posterior surfaces can be palpated just lateral to the sacral cornua and observed for rotated positions of the sacrum. The ILA inferior surface can be palpated (avoiding the coccyx) and observed for sidebent positions of the sacrum. Posterior displacement of one of the ILAs represents rotation of the sacrum toward that side. Inferior displacement of one of the ILAs represents sidebending of the sacrum toward that side.

There are two palpation ways to find the ILAs. One method is to palpate with a finger pad the median crest of the sacrum from the top of the natal cleft to the bifurcation of the median crest which creates the sacral cornua. Finger pad stereognosis is then used to identify the *sacral cornua*, which are the bifid spinous processes on each side of the midline *sacral hiatus*, which is the inferior opening of the *sacral canal*, normally opening at S_5. If the hiatus is wide enough to accommodate one finger pad, the sacral cornua can be felt on each side of the finger. Since the coccyx also has cornua, care must be taken to detect the most superior opening of the sacral canal along the *median crest* of the sacrum. Occasionally the hiatus commences as high as S_3, or more rarely it is open the entire length of the sacrum. The two cornua are often different sizes, and this may mislead the examiner to believe a sacral positional fault exists, unless the bone is palpated lateral to the cornu.

The ILAs are immediately lateral to the sacral cornua. The examiner's thumb pads are placed symmetrically in the same transverse plane 1.0–1.5 cm. lateral to the midline of the hiatus, i.e., far enough lateral to avoid the cornua, whose size and shape may not be symmetrical, but not so far lateral as to fall off the sides of the sacrum. The thin soft tissues which cover the ILAs are then compressed with anterior pressure of the thumbs – <0.5 kilogram – to experience the relatively unyielding hardness of the bone. Lowering the head to make the line of sight nearly horizontal, the thumbs are observed for posterior displacement on one side. Gluteal muscle tensions can influence this observation.

The alternative way to find the ILAs is to use stereognostic palpation with the palm of the hand on the posterior surface of the sacrum to identify the most posterior part of the sacrum, which is the S_5 segment. Palmar stereognosis may be necessary if the hiatus is too narrow to accommodate a finger pad. S_5 projects posteriorly more than any other part of the sacrum or the coccyx, and therefore can be easily identified on the prone patient using this method.

The assessment of the ILAs is part of a routine screening test for sacroiliac dysfunction. If the ILAs are symmetrical, there is probably no sacroiliac dysfunction. The rare excep-

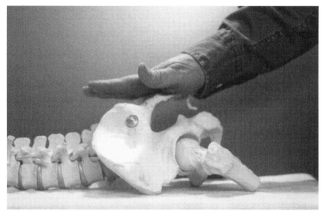

Figure 1.23. Palmar stereognosis to locate the most posterior aspect of the sacrum – landmark palpation position.

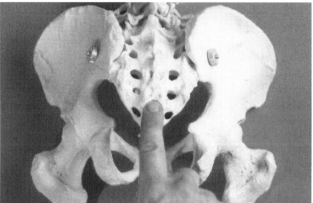

Figure 1.24. Examiner's index finger palpating the sacral hiatus.

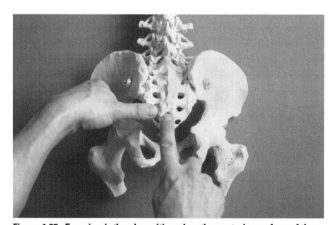

Figure 1.25. Examiner's thumb positioned on the posterior surface of the ILA, just lateral to the index finger palpating the sacral hiatus.

tion is when bilateral symmetrical dysfunctions of the sacroiliac joints exist. The respiratory functions of the sacroiliac joints may also be impaired without showing any ILA asymmetry. In every case, when the ILA is *more posterior* on one side, that side will also be *more inferior*. The reason is that the caudal portion of the sacroiliac joint surface is a wide track which runs posteriorly and inferiorly. This fact can be used to validate palpatory and visual findings. If inferior does not agree with posterior, one of them is not a valid finding.

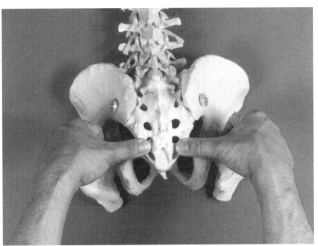

Figure 1.26. Posterior surface of the Inferior Lateral Angles – landmark palpation. With thumb pads flat on the posterior surface of the ILAs, the examiner's gaze should be horizontal.

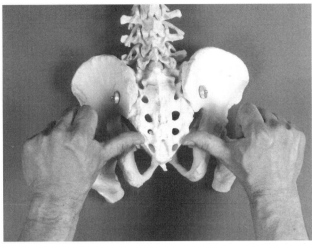

Figure 1.27. Inferior surface of the Inferior Lateral Angles – landmark palpation. With thumb pads pushing superior on the inferior surface of the ILAs, the examiner's gaze should be vertical.

Anatomic Considerations when Palpating for Sacral Sulcus Depth

The sacral sulcus measurement is the distance from the posterior surface of the gluteal tubercle to the posterior ala of S_1. It is measured by palpation, not visually. Thumb pads are placed on the gluteal tubercles of the iliac crests and the thumb tips are curled mediad and anteriorly toward the base of the sacrum while the thumb pads remain in contact with the iliac crests to determine which thumb sinks in deeper *from the iliac crest*. Attempts to palpate the sacral base directly should be discouraged. However, the presence of fibrolipomata near the iliac crest may sometimes make it necessary. In palpating the sacral base, one should remember that the position of the palpating thumbs or fingers is to be compared to the two points on the iliac crests at the gluteal tubercle and not to the coronal plane of the body.

Obviously the palpating thumb never reaches the posterior ala of the sacrum, because of the thickness of the soft tissues. Most of the time this thickness is dependably uniform left to right, and, therefore, does not compromise the accuracy of the test. The tips of the pressing thumbs are stopped at the same depth. However, soft tissue anomalies are common in this area. The most common of these are fibrolipomata (fibromas, for short), small balls of adipose tissue encapsulated in fibrous tissue. Fibrolipomata usually attach themselves firmly to deep fascia or periosteum and can get in the way of palpating the sacral sulcus. Sometimes they are as hard as bone, but they usually can be pushed and moved aside a little.

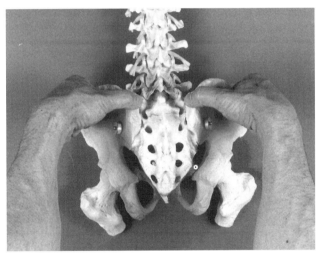

Figure 1.28. Sacral sulcus – landmark palpation. Examiner should avoid making a visual assessment, but rather should rely on the felt sense of sulcus depth.

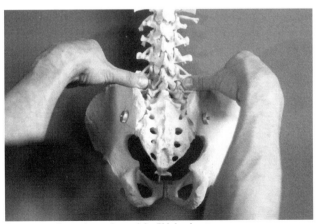

Figure 1.29. Posterior surface of the fifth lumbar transverse processes – landmark palpation. Examiner's gaze should be slightly horizontal.

Figure 1.30. The anterior pelvic ligaments link the ilia to the sacrum and the fourth and fifth lumbars to the ilia and sacrum. Most of the ventral sacroiliac ligaments are just thickenings of the capsule of the joint. But as they near the inferior part of the joint they are stronger, probably to stabilize the iliosacral pivot. The iliolumbar ligaments couple spinal motion to motion of the iliac crests. Thus, when L_5 rotates to the left (arrow), the right innominate is rotated anteriorly and/or the left innominate rotates posteriorly (paired arrows). The horizontal lines B–B' and A–A' drawn across the inferior slopes of the anterior superior iliac spines (ASISs) show their asymmetric positions. The sacrotuberous and sacrospinous ligaments restrict nutation of the sacrum. The superior pubic ligament helps hold the pubic bones together anteriorly. They cannot offer much resistance to vertical shearing of the pubic symphysis.

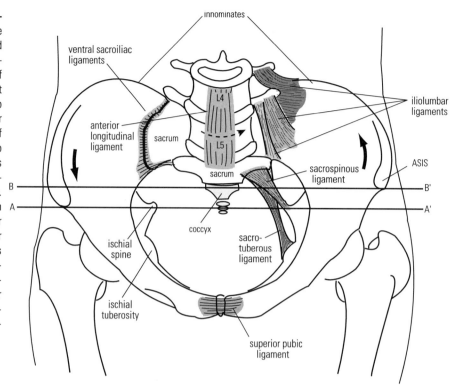

Pelvic Ligaments

The ligaments of the pelvis are described in various ways in different anatomy texts. This has resulted in some confusion and ambiguity concerning their structure. In the following descriptions the ligaments are considered from a functional perspective.

The function of ligaments is to limit bone movement to a physiologic range of motion, not to prevent motion altogether. When ligaments are said to restrict or resist movement, "limit" is the proper interpretation. It would be just as realistic to say that ligaments *permit* movement. The following lists the ligaments which are important for our purposes, and the motion(s) that they permit and/or resist:

1. The sacrotuberous ligaments arise from the tuberosities of the ischia and the hamstring tendons and pass superior, posterior, and medial to attach to the coccyx and the apex of the sacrum – the S_5 alae. From the sacrum they appear to continue cephalad, accompanied by the long dorsal sacroiliac ligaments, to attach to the posterior superior iliac spine (PSIS). The portion inferior to the sacrum resists sacral nutation, mostly on the middle transverse axis. The part attached to the PSIS resists counternutation.

Recommended anatomy texts are Kapandji *Physiology of the Joints*, (1974), Anson *Morris' Human Anatomy*, (1966), and Warwick and Williams *Gray's Anatomy 35th British Edition* (1973). An excellent discussion of pelvic arthrology may be found in Lee's *The Pelvic Girdle, 2nd Edition* (1999). In this text, axes and pelvisacral motion are discussed in Chapters 2 and 3.

2. The sacrospinous ligaments arise from the ischial spines to attach, along with the sacrotuberous ligaments, posteromedially to the sides of the sacrum and coccyx below the sacroiliac facets. They resist sacral nutation, mostly on the superior transverse axis.

3. The ventral sacroiliac ligaments are mostly thickenings of the synovial capsules of the sacroiliac joints. However, they become stronger near the posterior inferior iliac spine (PSIS) where they attach S_3 to the lateral margin of the pre-auricular surface, reinforcing the iliosacral pivot points, or inferior transverse axis.

4. The iliolumbar ligaments arise from broad areas on the transverse processes of the fourth and fifth lumbar vertebrae. They consist of five parts which link the vertebrae to the iliac crests. One of their functions is generally conceded to be stabilization of the lumbosacral articulation [Bogduk, 1991; Kapandji, 1974; Willard, 1997]. Their ability to convert axial rotation of the spine into *x-axis* rotations of the innominates is speculative. There must be a fair amount of slack in that system, since most of the time innominate rotations and lower lumbar rotations are relatively independent.

5. The anterior longitudinal ligament of the spine extends past the lumbosacral joint onto the sacral promontory where it attaches to the first sacral segment. Its fibers blend into the sacral periosteum, but it becomes distinguishable again as the **ventral sacrococcygeal ligament.** It limits extreme backward bending of the trunk (Anson, 1966).

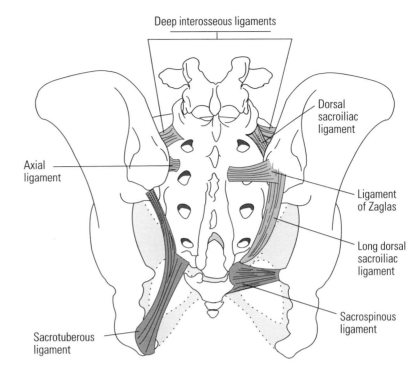

Figure 1.31. The posterior sacroiliac ligaments. The deeper ligaments include the deep interosseous ligaments, the axial ligament, and the sacrotuberous and sacrospinous ligaments. Most of the interosseous ligaments are hidden from view by the iliac crests. Three divisions of the dorsal sacroiliac ligaments (labeled and shown on the right) are the dorsal and long dorsal sacroiliac ligaments, and the Ligament of Zaglas. The superior transverse axis for sacral nutation and counter-nutation is stabilized by the axial ligament and/or the ligament of Zaglas.

6. **The superior pubic ligament** extending across the top of the symphysis pubis, and the **arcuate pubic ligament** passing below the symphysis, hold the two halves of the pelvis together in front. They are not designed to limit vertical shearing motions of the pubic symphysis.

7. **The inguinal ligament** is not really a ligament; it is a fold of muscular raphe providing attachment for the oblique abdominal muscles. It does not support any specific joints.

8. **The interosseous sacroiliac ligaments** attach to the dorsal alae of the sacrum lateral to the neural foramina (the sacral tuberosities) uniting them to large medial anterior surfaces on the ilia. They resist anterior and inferior translation of the sacral base while permitting a small amount of nutation on either the middle or superior transverse axis.

9. **The short axial ligament** consists of the most horizontal fibers of the deep posterior interosseous ligament, which attach to the ala of the second sacral segment deep to the superficial dorsal sacroiliac ligaments. Its position is close, or corresponds, to the superior transverse axis for sacral nutation and counternutation.

10. **The superficial dorsal sacroiliac ligaments** have three main parts – the **superior dorsal,** the **ligament of Zaglas,** and the **long dorsal** – all of which converge on the posterior superior iliac spine (PSIS). The superior portion ascends from the PSIS anteromedially to attach to the first sacral segment, and resists nutation on the middle transverse axis. The **ligament of Zaglas** reinforces the axial ligament which lies just deep to it. The **long dorsal ligament**

extends down to the sacral apex at the S_5 inferior lateral angle and resists counternutation on the middle transverse axis.

11. **The posterior longitudinal ligament** covers the posterior surfaces of the vertebral bodies. At the cranial end of the spine it becomes continuous with the *membrana tectoria* which blends with the **craniospinal dura** on the superior surface of the basiocciput.

Caudally, it reestablishes a relationship to the **spinal dura** by attaching to the inside of the sacral canal just above the dural attachments. At the coccyx it is renamed the **lateral and dorsal sacrococcygeal ligaments**.

In craniosacral theory (Sutherland, 1939), the **craniospinal dura** is said to link the inherent motions of the occiput to the sacrum, which is passively moved by the cranial rhythmic impulse. This mechanical connection is proposed because of the inelasticity of the dural membrane, which is certainly less elastic than the posterior longitudinal ligament. However, empirically it does appear that there is considerable slack in this mechanism permitting a lot of independence of sacrum from occiput.

12. Vleeming et al (1995) point out that the **thoracolumbar fascia** plays a critical role in the transference of load from the trunk to the lower extremity. It is the origin of several important postural muscles, and has fascial continuity to the upper limb through the *latissimus dorsi* and to the lower limb through the sacrotuberous ligament, the hamstrings, and the *fascia lata*.

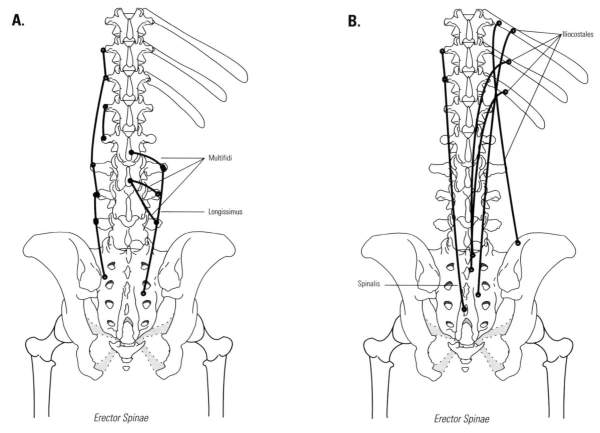

Figure 1.32. A, B, C, D, and E. Muscles attaching to the sacrum and coccyx. A. and B. The *erector spinae* muscles are arranged in three vertical columns: *spinalis, longissimus, and iliocostalis*. All are attached to the sacrum, but iliocostalis also attaches to the iliac crest. Deep to the erector muscles are the *multifidi* muscles. **C.** *Piriformis* arises from the anterior-lateral surfaces of the sacrum, passes through the greater sciatic notch to insert on the femur trochanter. **D. and E.** The pelvic diaphragm (*levator ani* and *coccygeus*) forms the floor of the pelvis.

Muscles of the Pelvis

The sacroiliac joints are classified as *passive joints* because, under normal circumstances, the joints of the pelvis are not directly moved by muscle contractions. Except for some *gluteus maximus* fascia, the only other muscle which crosses the sacroiliac joint is the *piriformis*, and its function is clearly to stabilize the sacrum on the ilium, not to move it. The sacrum moves between the ilia solely because the lumbar spine load on the sacral base changes direction.

The trunk and leg muscles do, however, have profound indirect effects on pelvic joint functions. The actions of muscles changes the configuration of the lumbar spine in ways which alter the load on the sacral base. In this sense, the lumbar musculature must be considered an important part of pelvic mechanics.

Clearly the trunk and leg muscles determine the positional relationship of the pelvis as a whole to gravity and to other body masses. Such pelvic region postural positioning profoundly affects the loading of the sacral base, and how that load is transferred through the pelvis to the legs.

Sacroiliac dysfunction may occur when such postural dynamics become static through failure of muscles to relax appropriately. The details of this principle will become clear in a later discussion of sacral torsion dysfunction.

The MET classical tradition holds that there are only six muscles in the body: flexors, extenders, right sidebenders, left sidebenders, right rotators, and left rotators. Although this oversimplification of myology is heuristically somewhat useful, there are times when other classifications of muscles are necessary for a clear understanding of function. Janda's (1996) tightness-prone and weakness-prone classification of muscles is quite relevant to understanding functions of the pelvis. Muscles can also be classified as joint stabilizers, postural support muscles, and phasic action muscles. Histologic classification of muscle fiber types pertains to these other systems of classification, which at this time cannot be combined into one unified theory of myology/kinesiology.

The following summary tables present the muscles associated with pelvic function with their actions.

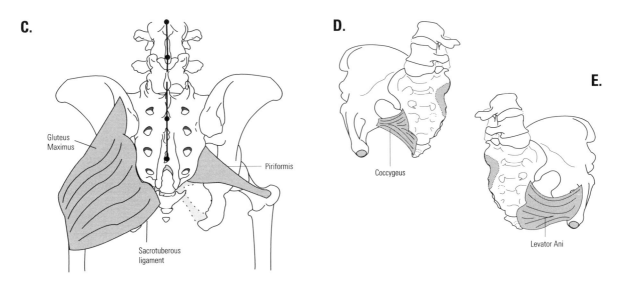

Table 1.B. Summary of muscles related to the pelvis.

Muscles Attached to the Sacrum

Muscle	Origin and Insertion	Innervation	Action
Attached to the sacrum (from above):			
erector spinae: iliocostalis lumborum, longissimus, spinalis, multifidi	The erector spinae divide into longitudinal columns which include branches of the iliocostalis lumborum, longissimus thoracis, and the spinalis thoracis. Arising from the sacrum and iliac crests, it has various attachments to the spinous and transverse processes of the lumbar and lower thoracic segments, as well as the rib angles of the lower six ribs.	Posterior primary rami of spinal nerves	Extends, laterally flexes, and rotates the vertebral column. As the lumbars go into hyperflexion, the erector spinae pulls the sacrum cephalad.
Attached to the sacrum (from below):			
piriformis	The piriformis attaches to the sacrum along the pars lateralis, lateral to the anterior sacral foramina. From there it passes through the sciatic foramen and attaches to the upper border of the greater trochanter with the common tendon of obturator internus and gamelli.	1st and 2nd sacral nerves	Rotates the thigh laterally; close-packs and stabilizes the sacroiliac joint at the inferior pole of the oblique axis, which is necessary for sacral torsion movements.
levator ani and coccygeus	The levator ani originates at the back of the pubis, pelvic fascia, and the spine of the ischium – inserts along the pars lateralis and lower portions of the sacrum and coccyx, the perineum, and external sphincter ani. The coccygeus originates at the spine of the ischium and sacrospinous ligament, and attaches to the sides and lower portion of the sacrum and upper portion of the coccyx.	3rd and 4th sacral nerves	Assists in raising and stabilizing the pelvic floor and the actions of the anal sphincter; stabilizing the sacrum and coccyx; milks the venous plexus in the ischiorectal fossa; assists in coughing.
gluteus maximus	Parts of the gluteus maximus originate on the dorsal surface of the sacrum and coccyx, and the posterior gluteal line. Some fibers of the gluteus maximus have been observed to cross the sacroiliac joint. Most of gluteus maximus muscle arises from the sacrotuberous ligament and a small diamond shaped fossa about one or two inches long on the posterior iliac crest immediately above the PSIS. At the superior corner of this fossa, the overlying skin is more tightly tethered to the deep fascia, creating a dimple. Gluteus maximus inserts into the iliotibial band and along the gluteal line of the femur.	inferior gluteal nerve	Extends and externally rotates the femur.

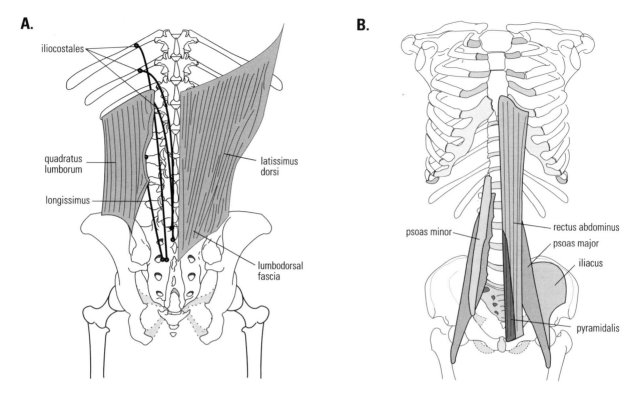

Figure 1.33 Posterior (A) and anterior (B) views of trunk muscles attaching to the pelvis.

Table 1.C. Summary of muscles related to the pelvis.

Muscles Attached to the Innominates from Above

Muscle	Origin and Insertion	Innervation	Action
longissimus and iliocostales	Both are branches of the erector spinae, and attach to the median crest of the sacrum, the medial dorsal aspects of the ilium, and the lateral sacral crest. The longissimus thoracis attaches to the transverse processes of the lumbar vertebrae, the lumbodorsal fascia, and the transverse processes of all of the thoracic vertebrae and the lower 10 ribs between the rib angle and tubercle; the iliocostalis attaches to the inferior borders of the lower 7 ribs via tendons.	Thoracic and lumbar spinal nerves	Bends the spine backwards and laterally; provides lateral stabilization of the lumbar spine.
ilio-psoas– (major and minor)	The ilio-psoas is comprised of the psoas and the iliacus muscle (a fan shaped muscle covering the superior and medial aspects of the iliac fossa, parts of the sacral ala). The psoas major muscle attaches to the lateral aspects and vertebral discs of the lumbar vertebrae, and has tendinous attachment to the lesser trochanter of the femur. The psoas minor muscle attaches to the vertebral bodies of T_{12} and L_1, running anterior to the psoas major, eventually attaching to a ridge on the iliac portion of the pelvic brim.	Anterior primary rami of the upper 3 lumbar segments	Assists rectus abdominis in flexing the lumbar segments, and assists the iliacus in flexing the hip joint; flexes and externally rotates the femur on the pelvis; flexes and lateral bends individual lumbar segments. The psoas major and minor flex the pelvis on the spine.
quadratus lumborum	Quadratus lumborum runs from the iliac crest and iliolumbar ligament to the transverse processes of the upper 4 lumbar vertebrae and the lower border of the 12th rib.	12th thoracic and 1st, 2nd, and 3rd lumbar	Involved in flexing and/or sidebending the trunk; approximates the iliac crest and 12th rib during the gait cycle. May be considered an extension of the diaphragm.
latissimus dorsi	Lower six thoracic spinous processes, lumbosacral fascia, iliac crest to bicipital groove of humerus. (Figure does not show all thoracic attachments.)	cervical nerve roots 7 and 8 via the thoracodorsal nerve	Adducts, internally rotates, and extends the humerus. Stabilizes the ilia and the lumbosacral aponeurosis. Co-contracts with quadratus lumborum.

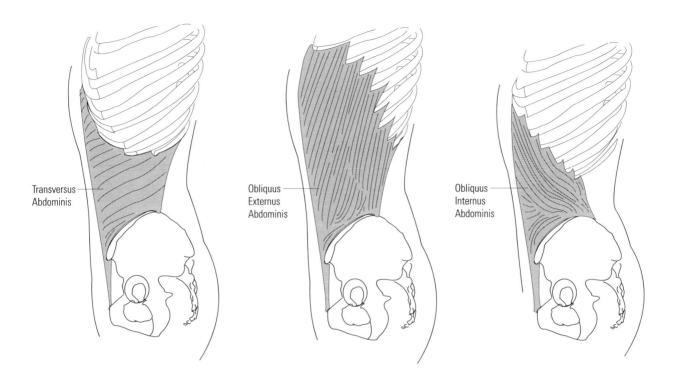

Figure 1.34 The transversus and obliquus abdominal muscles. Blending posteriorly with the lumbodorsal fascia and anteriorly with the rectus abdominis and linea alba, they are the walls of the abdominal cavity, as well as extensions of the pelvic fascias.

Table 1.C. Summary of muscles related to the pelvis – *(continued)*

Muscles Attached to the Innominates from Above

Muscle	*Origin and Insertion*	*Innervation*	*Action*
obliquus abdominis externus	Interdigitates on the lower 8 ribs to attach to anterior portions of the iliac crest, and inserts into aponeurosis of anterior abdominal wall.	Anterior primary rami of lower 6 thoracics and upper 2 lumbar	Rotates the thoracic spine in relation to the pelvis; active in forced exhalation; may inappropriately substitute for rectus weakness.
obliquus abdominis internus	From the anterior two-thirds of the iliac crest, lateral portions of the inguinal ligament, and the lumbar fascia, to the outer surface of the cartilages of the last 3 ribs, fanning into an aponeurosis which extends from 10th costal cartilage to the pubic bone, forming linea alba in the ventral mid-line.	Anterior primary rami of lower 6 thoracics and upper 2 lumbar	Rotates the thoracic spine in relation to the pelvis; active in forced exhalation; may inappropriately substitute for rectus weakness.
transversus abdominis	From the anterior two-thirds of the iliac crest, lateral portions of the inguinal ligament, and the lumbar fascia, to the inner surface of the cartilages of the lowest 6 ribs, fanning into an aponeurosis with obliqi and the linea alba.	Anterior primary rami of lower 6 thoracics	Rotates the thoracic spine in relation to the pelvis; active in forced exhalation; may inappropriately substitute for rectus weakness.
rectus abdominis	From the pubic symphysis (medial tendon) and the crest of the pubis (lateral tendon), it runs to the xiphoid process and costal cartilages of the 5th, 6th, and 7th ribs.	Anterior primary rami of lower 6 thoracics	Flexes the thoracic/lumbar spine and the pelvis; active in forced exhalation; may inappropriately substitute for rectus weakness (prone to inhibition and weakness due to tight lumbo- sacral multifidi).
pyramidalis	From the anterior aspect of the pubis and the pubic ligament, it runs along the linea alba between the pubis and the umbilicus.	12th thoracic	Supports abdominal viscera; active in forced exhalation; may inappropriately substitute for rectus weakness.

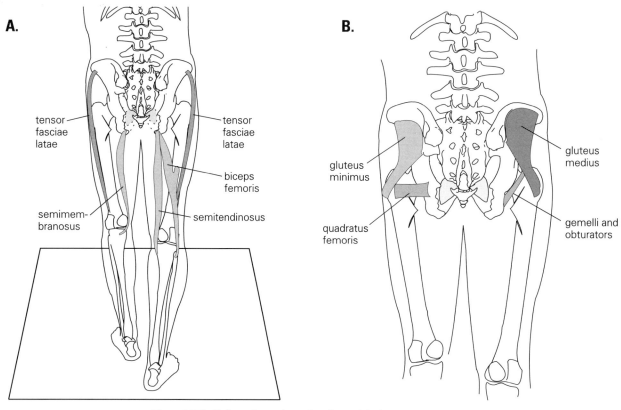

A.

tensor
fasciae
latae

tensor
fasciae
latae

biceps
femoris

semimem-
branosus

semitendinosus

B.

gluteus
minimus

gluteus
medius

quadratus
femoris

gemelli and
obturators

Figure 1.35.A.–E. Posterior and anterior views of the leg-pelvis muscles.

Table 1.D. Summary of muscles related to the pelvis.

Muscles Attached to the Innominates from Below

Muscle	*Origin and Insertion*	*Innervation*	*Action*
iliacus	(see ilio-psoas)	(see ilio-psoas)	(see ilio-psoas)
obturator internus *obturator externus*	The obturator internus and externus both attach near the margin of the obturator foramen and parts of the obturator membrane, to the greater trochanter.	obturator nerve	Stabilizes the femur in the acetabulum; both are weak external rotators.
gemellus superior and inferior	The gemellus inferior originates on the tuberosity of the ischium; the gemellus superior originates on the ischial spine and the margin of the sciatic notch. Both insert on the tendon of the obturator internus.	obturator nerve	Stabilizes the femur in the acetabulum; both are weak external rotators.
quadratus femoris	Originates on the lateral border of the ischial tuberosity and attaches to the intertrochanteric ridge.	obturator nerve	Stabilizes the femur in the acetabulum; externally rotates femur; adducts the leg.
rectus femoris	The rectus femoris is the only branch of the quadriceps femoris which attaches to the pelvis. The more superior portion attaches to the anterior inferior iliac spine and a groove on the upper brim of the acetabulum, and runs anterior to the femur to attach to the upper border of the patella.	a branch of the femoral nerve	Assists in flexing the thigh and extending the leg. When tight, it tilts the pelvis forward on the femur, creating lordotic postural stress.

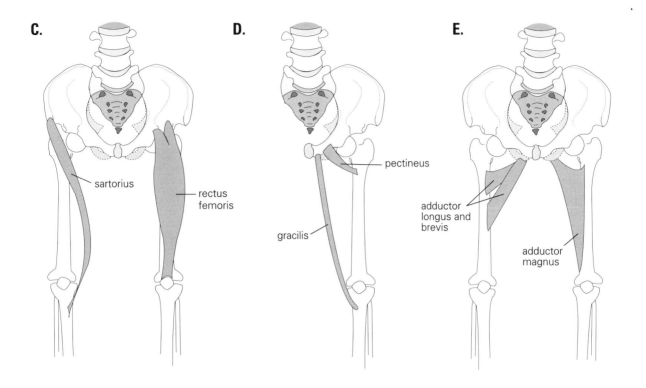

C.

sartorius

rectus femoris

D.

pectineus

gracilis

E.

adductor longus and brevis

adductor magnus

Table 1.D. Summary of muscles related to the pelvis – *(continued)*

Muscles Attached to the Innominates from Below

Muscle	Origin and Insertion	Innervation	Action
gluteus maximus	The gluteus maximus originates along the gluteal line on the lateral surface of the iliac crest and the pars lateralis and ILA of the sacrum as well as along the sacrotuberous ligament. It attaches to the gluteal tuberosity of the femur, and to the ili-otibial band.	inferior gluteal nerve	A powerful external rotator of the femur, the gluteus maximus also is involved in extension of the thigh, and assists in adduction. Depending on its action, it also can participate in extension of the trunk.
gluteus medius and minimus	The gluteus medius and minimus originate on the outer surface of the ilium from the iliac crest and gluteal line down to margin of the greater sciatic notch; both attach to the lateral and anterior surfaces of the greater trochanter.	superior gluteal nerve	Abducts the thigh and rotates the thigh medially (particularly when the thigh is extended).
tensor fasciae latae	Originates just posterior to the ASIS along the antero-lateral border of the ilium, and inserts along the upper 1/3 of the lateral aspect of the femur.	superior gluteal nerve	Abducts the femur and transmits tension from the fibular head to the iliac crest; assists in flexing and medially rotating the thigh.
adductor group: gracilis pectineus adductor brevis, longus, and magnus	The gracilis originates at the lower half of the pubis symphysis, and attaches to the medial surface of the tibia close to the knee. The other adductors listed originate along parts of the pubis and ramus of the ischium, and attach along the medial surface of the femur with tendon/fascia extension to the medial tibia just below the knee.	obturator, femoral, and sciatic nerves	All are involved in adduction of the thigh, as well as flexion. With the exception of the gracilis (which is involved in internal rotation of the thigh), all participate in external rotation of the leg.
sartorius	Sartorius originates at the ASIS, and attaches to the medial surface of the tibia close to the knee.	femoral nerve	External rotator of the thigh, and participates in flexion of the leg on the thigh and the thigh on the pelvis.
hamstrings: biceps femoris semitendinosus semimembranosus	All originate on the ischial tuberosity, and attach medially to the tibia, with the biceps inserting laterally on the head of the fibula.	sciatic nerve	Extends the hip joint and flexes the knee joint. This group of muscles is very prone to tightness.

Myofascial Influences

Specific myofascial continuities exist that affect pelvic function. Although this chapter has primarily focused on static anatomy, some correlations will be drawn in the following discussion between myofascial anatomy and functional influences on the pelvis.

Piriformis: The Sacroiliac Muscle

The sacroiliac or iliosacral joints (same joint, different function) are passive joints, i.e., movements of these joints is not directly caused by muscle actions. The only muscle which, in its entirety, crosses the sacroiliac joint is the *piriformis*, which runs from a broad attachment on the anterior-lateral surface of the middle three sacral segments, the sacroiliac joint capsule, the PSIS, and the sacrotuberous ligament to a tendinous attachment on the superior-medial aspect of the femoral trochanter, where it is often united with tendons of the *gemelli, obturator internus,* or *gluteus medius.* The *piriformis* is variously described as a femur external rotator with the hip extended, and a femur abductor with the hip flexed to 90° and beyond. Its action on the sacrum is obviously to pull the sacrum obliquely toward the inferior pole of the sacroiliac joint, where it is theorized there is an intersection of the innominate rotation axis, or pivot, and one of the oblique axes of sacral torsion movement. *It therefore seems reasonable to ascribe a sacroiliac stabilizing function to the piriformis,* which is anatomically capable of setting a pivot on the inferior pole of the sacroiliac joint, allowing for simultaneous innominate rotation and sacral torsion movements. Based on this theory, one would anticipate the histologic composition of the population of muscle fiber types in the *piriformis* would show a preponderance of slow-oxidizing fibers and possibly a dense population of proprioceptors.

Influence of the Fibula on the Pelvis

Joint play motion impairment of the proximal fibula (restriction or hypermobility) can alter tensions in the *fascia lata* through its iliotibial band attachment to the fibula. This can initiate or sustain *iliosacral* dysfunction – impaired movement of one innominate in relation to the sacrum and to the other innominate. The *biceps femoris* part of the hamstring muscle also attaches to the fibula. Thus myofascial tensions in the hamstrings may be altered by proximal fibular joint dysfunction. In addition, there is probably hamstring myotatic reflex reaction to the changed input from joint mechanoreceptors in the proximal fibular joint, increasing its natural tendency to contracture. The resulting tensions, transmitted from the hamstring tendon attachment to the ischial tuberosity through the sacro-

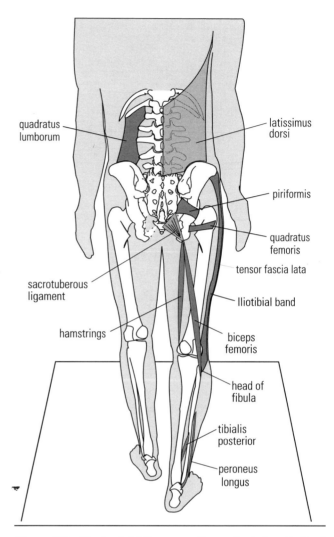

Figure 1.36. Myofascial Influences. The mechanical continuity of muscle fascia and ligaments is illustrated, showing the connection from the fibula to the lumbodorsal fascia *(latissimus dorsi)*. The fibula is linked to the deep lumbodorsal fascia through the *biceps femoris*, sacrotuberous ligament, sacrum, and fifth lumbar. It is linked to the superficial lumbodorsal fascia through the iliotibial band, fascia lata, gluteal fascia, and iliac crest.

tuberous ligament can affect sacroiliac (sacral movement in relation to the ilia – normally sacral adaptations to movements of the spinal column) motion, predisposing to dysfunction. Vleeming (1995) has demonstrated mechanical continuity from the fascia lata through the sacrotuberous ligament and sacrum to the lumbodorsal fascia.

CHAPTER 2

Normal Sagittal Plane Motions in the Pelvisacral Joints

In order to understand dysfunctions and subluxations of the pelvic joints, it is necessary to first understand normal sagittal plane translatory and rotatory motions of the sacrum in relation to the ilia. Translatory movement is linear displacement in any plane of one bone in relation to another, and rotation is turning about an axis.

Movements of pelvic joints are caused either by changes in vertebral column position or by leg movements. Movements caused by changes in vertebral column position are characterized in the Mitchell model as "*sacro*iliac motion*," conceived as movement of the sacrum in relation to stationary ilia. In this model "*ilio*sacral motion," caused by leg movements, is conceived as movement of either ilium on a stationary sacrum. The "sacroiliac versus iliosacral" distinction is clinically relevant inasmuch as diagnostic and treatment methods for somatic dysfunctions of each type are different.

Mechanisms which cause the spine to move the sacrum are:

- Trunk bending movements;
- Changes in body position relative to gravity;
- Respiration;
- Movements of cranial bones.

Transmission of motion from vertebrae to sacrum occurs through:

- Shifting gravitational or inertial loads on the sacral base;
- Changing myofascial tensions in erector spinae muscles and vertebrosacral ligaments, which include the anterior and posterior longitudinal ligaments, parts of the iliolumbar ligaments, ligamenta flava, and the spinal dura.

Controlling influences determining directions and amplitudes of movements include:

- Sacroiliac, sacrotuberous, sacrospinous, and iliolumbar ligaments;
- The anatomic position of the sacrum relative to spinal posture and loading;
- Sacroiliac joint surface morphology;
- Inter-innominate compliance mobility to adapt to changes in sacral position.

As stated above, other movements of pelvic joints result from leg movements. Because locomotion movements of the legs are usually reciprocal, except for hopping, inter-innominate motion requires mobility at the *symphysis pubis* as well as on the two lateral surfaces of the sacrum.

In this chapter:

- *Weight-bearing and non-weight-bearing sagittal movements of the sacrum*

- *Transverse instantaneous axes of the pelvis*

- *Paradoxical sacral motion*

- *Sacroiliac motion – nutation and counternutation*

- *Iliosacral motion and interinnominate rotation*

- *Sacral flexion versus sacral shear*

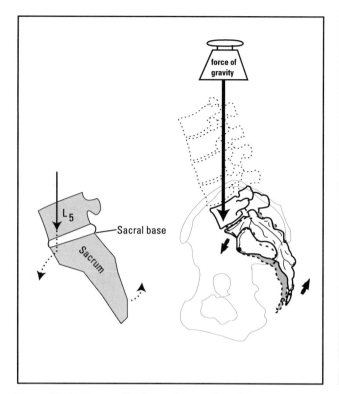
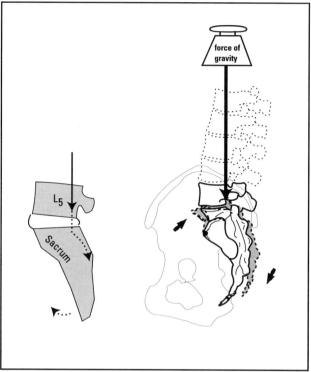

Figure 2.1. Mid-range flexion and extension of the trunk causes the sacrum to tip forward **(nutation)** and backward **(counternutation)** on its middle transverse axis, as the load on the sacral base shifts forward or backward.

Physiologic (symmetrical) rotatory movement of the sacrum between the ilia in the sagittal plane, caused by forward and backward bending of the trunk, is the focus of this chapter. Such movements of the sacrum are best labeled **nutation** and **counternutation**, since meanings of the terms flexion and extension have been muddied by their contradictory use in various systems. **Nutation** (from the Latin *"nutare"* – to nod) means anterior-inferior tilting of the **sacral base** (the superior part of the sacrum). **Counternutation** is the opposite – backward-superior movement of the sacral base.

With forward bending of the trunk, the gravitational load carried by the fifth lumbar onto the sacral base shifts anteriorly, increasing the leverage moment (force times lever length), thereby causing the sacrum to nutate relative to the ilium. Backward bending of the trunk shifts the gravitational load posteriorly, which causes the sacrum to counternutate. For both flexion and extension of the trunk, the ilia are prevented from following the moving sacrum by myofascial attachments from the legs, i.e., the *fascia lata* and the tendons of the muscles, such as hamstrings (Fig. 2.2). These myofascial tensions stabilize the ilia which keeps them relatively stationary until the sacroiliac joint has moved as far as the sacroiliac ligaments will permit. Sacral movement beyond this point will be accompanied by the ilia.

As the sacrum moves relative to the ilia in response to trunk flexion and extension, the sagittal motions of the

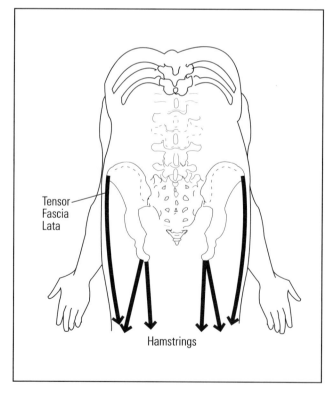

Figure 2.2. Muscles and fascia of the thigh have a stabilizing effect on the ilium, restraining it from moving with the sacrum in the act of forward bending, until the sacrum reaches its nutation limit and pulls the ilium with it.

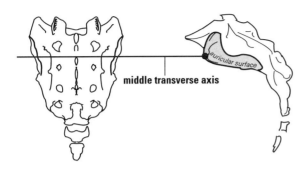

Figure 2.3. The middle transverse axis for nutation and counternutation of the sacrum lies in the transverse plane at the level of S$_2$ through the auricular surfaces anteriorly. This instantaneous axis functions in both sacroiliac respiratory movement and in trunk flexion and extension. Craniosacral motion may also use this instantaneous axis, at times.

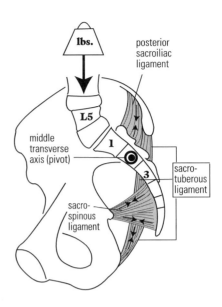

Figure 2.4. The middle transverse axis around which the forces of gravity are opposed by the sacrotuberous ligaments which prevent anterior nutation of the sacrum from the gravitational force of the spine. (Adapted from Grant, JCB. A Method of Anatomy. 6th Ed, 1958. Williams & Wilkins. Baltimore. Used by permission of Lippincott–Williams & Wilkins).

sacrum can be described as rotation about a transverse axis. The term "rotation" has previously been defined anatomically as turning in a transverse plane about a vertical *y-axis* (in reference to the anatomic position) as the anterior surface moves to the left ("+") or to the right ("–"). **In the pelvis and cranium "rotation" means turning around *any* axis.** Therefore, the location of the axes must be identified for all rotatory pelvic (or cranial) joint movements.

Just as in intervertebral biomechanics, **all pelvic joint movement axes are *instantaneous*,** i.e., axes which change their location (or orientation) by translating or rotating around another axis during different phases of the movement.

Temporary stability of a pelvic axis is a function of anatomic configuration of the bones and joints, ligamentous restraints, and gravitational and/or other inertial loads.

It should be emphasized that muscles do not *directly* move the sacrum between the ilia. Rather, sacral movement is the result of gravitational, inertial, and elastic forces secondary to spinal movements (which are the result of muscular activity). Similarly, muscles do not *directly* move the innominate bones in relation to the sacrum. Again, such movements result from gravitational, inertial, and elastic forces from the legs. In this sense, **the pelvisacral joints are classified as passive joints.**

Transverse Axes and Sacroiliac Motion

The Mitchell model describes two transverse sacral axes: the **middle transverse axis** and the **superior transverse axis.** Other models consider only one axis, if any. Although opinions vary among different researchers, the proposed axis for nutation and counternutation which seems to have the greatest historical consensus in biomechanics and anatomy is the *middle transverse axis* (Fig. 2.3).

Sacral Middle Transverse Axis

The middle transverse axis passes through the sacroiliac joint surface at the anterior portion of the second sacral segment near the junction of the short arm and the long arm of the sacroiliac auricular surface. This junction usually corresponds to a slight change in the bevel of the sacroiliac joint, creating a natural anatomic pivot at the second sacral segment. It appears that the middle transverse axis serves several **movement functions: (1)** It is the principle nutation axis for the sacrum during trunk forward and backward bending in mid-range. The range of this movement with trunk forward and backward bending has not been satisfactorily measured; it could possibly be greater than Kottke's (1962) figures, especially if one takes the terminal range reverse nutations into account. **(2)** It is the axis for sacral movements which accompany voluntary respiratory movements of the spine (Mitchell, Jr. and Pruzzo, 1971). **(3)** It is probably one of the axes for the craniosacral primary respiratory mechanism.

In addition to these three movement functions, a *static function* has been assigned to the middle transverse axis. Grant (1952) places an axis in this location as the center of postural support (Figs. 2.4 and 2.7), showing that without the restraining influence of the sacrospinous, sacrotuberous, and posterior sacroiliac ligaments the sacrum would nutate on this axis due to the weight of the spine on the sacral base.

Sacral Motion with Trunk Flexion and Extension

When the lumbar spinal column flexes and extends, the gravitational load on the sacral base shifts forward and backward, and some nutational sagittal plane movement of the sacrum can be expected. The transverse axes for these nutatory sacral motions must be characterized as instantaneous axes, i.e., axes which change their location during different phases of the movement.

For the *mid-range motions* of **sacral flexion and extension**, as well as for the *respiratory motions* of the sacrum, the sacrum rotates about a middle transverse axis which is located at the second sacral segment. However, when lumbar flexion or extension come to the *extremes* of sagittal plane range of motion, the sacral transverse axis may shift to a new location, designated the *superior transverse axis*. The timing of this axis shift is quite variable. In some individuals it may occur early in the trunk bend. It usually occurs very near the completion of the bend. In some cases it may not occur at all.

Rotation about the *middle transverse axis* involves arcuate sliding of the sacrum at the sacroiliac joint about a fixed pivot point which is located within the joint at the junction of the long arm and short arm of the auricular surface. The sacrum in this case does *not* track the arc of the auricular surface of the ilium (Fig. 2.5). Rotations of the sacrum about the *superior transverse axis*, however, do involve the sacrum sliding along the arc of the L-shaped auricular surface of the ilium (Figures 2.11.A and B, and Figures 2.9.A and B).

Halfway between the extremes of flexion and extension the sacral auricular surfaces are approximately bilaterally congruent with the auricular surfaces of the ilia, assuming no dysfunction or dislocation exists. As the sacrum moves toward flexion (nutation), the sacral base (the superior portion of the sacrum) moves anterior and inferior while the **apex of the sacrum** (the inferior portion of the sacrum) moves posterior and superior; the opposite is true of sacral extension (counternutation). Because the axis is closer to the base of the sacrum (and farther from the apex), there is greater displacement of the apex than of the sacral base with the movements of flexion and extension.

Instantaneous Axes and the Sacroiliac Ligaments

The resistance provided by the ligaments, along with the geometry of the joint surfaces, determines how the sacrum will move in response to spinal forces. Temporary stabilization of the middle transverse, or the superior transverse, axis is a function of three elements:

1. The contours of the osteoarticular facet surfaces, especially the change in bevel at the second sacral segment;
2. The vector of load force applied to the sacrum;
3. The specific restraints of ligaments.

The function of the ligaments (Fig. 2.4) is to provide (temporary) stability at the sacroiliac joint and to limit

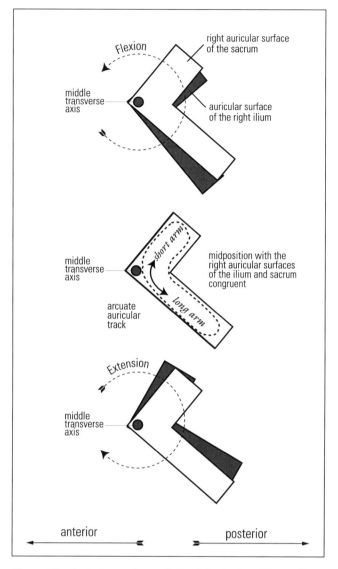

Figure 2.5. Auricular surface relationships in the midrange flexion/extension of the sacrum. Note that the upper and lower parts of the sacral auricular surface simply slide in shearing arcs and do not follow the arcuate track of the short arms and long arms of the iliac auricular surfaces.

motion of the sacrum to a safe range. Movement beyond a certain range would result in avulsion of the ligamentous tissues if the axis did not shift. In addition, by virtue of their position and spatial orientation, ligaments serve a functional role in relation to the arthrokinematics of the sacroiliac joint, as well as to the gravitational and inertial forces (the mechanics of load displacement).

This triadic relationship between the vector forces, the stabilization provided by ligaments, and the geometry of the joint surfaces increases the likelihood that the sacrum will consistently pivot around a given point (axis) for a given movement. In other words, every time these three elements line up in the same way the rotational axis will always be in the same place. Thus, guided by the restraints of the superior sacroiliac, sacrospinous, and sacrotuberous

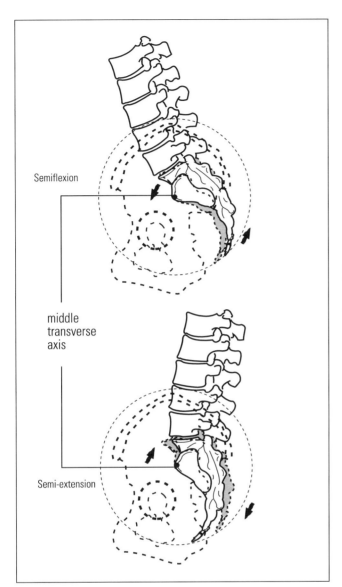

Figure 2.6. Mid-range flexion-extension of the trunk. With small flexion-extension movements of the trunk the sacrum nutates and counternutates on the middle transverse axis. The grey outline of the sacrum represents its position with the spine erect.

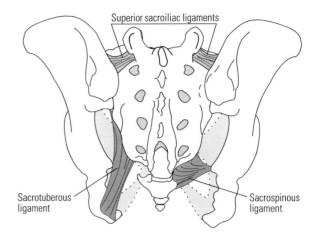

Figure 2.7. The superior sacroiliac ligaments and the sacrospinous and sacrotuberous ligaments. These ligaments limit the amount of possible nutation of the sacrum due to the gravitational load on the sacral base, while permitting a small amount of *x-axis* rotation in the sagittal plane (on the middle transverse axis).

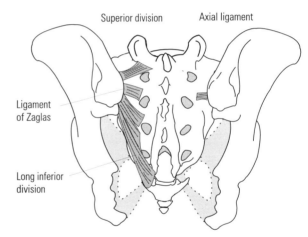

Figure 2.8. The posterior sacroiliac ligaments resist sagittal movement on the superior transverse axis, while preventing inferior and anterior sacral translation. At the level of S_2 are two components of the posterior sacroiliac ligaments, a short axial ligament which is anterior and deep to the ligament of Zaglas. The superior transverse axis is located near these short ligaments. The more superior division of the posterior sacroiliac ligaments, attached to S_1, resist nutation on the superior transverse axis. The long inferior fibers of the posterior sacroiliac ligaments, extending down to the sacral apex and coccyx from the PSIS, resist counternutation on the superior transverse axis.

ligaments, and guided by the planes of available osteoarticular motion on the auricular facets, when the forward bending trunk shifts the L_5 load on the sacral base forward, the sacrum nutates on the middle transverse axis (Fig. 2.6). As this occurs, the iliac crests fall medially, decreasing tension on the superior sacroiliac ligaments (Fig. 2.15). The dynamic relationship between these elements contributes to the formation of a natural instantaneous axis (i.e., the middle transverse axis) about which rotation of the sacrum is likely to occur for these motions.

The Superior Transverse Axis
Motion of the sacrum about the superior transverse axis can be visualized as a swinging action with the center of the arc

of the swing located in the posterior sacroiliac ligaments. Both middle and superior transverse axes are located at the S_2 level, but the tilted anatomic position of the sacrum puts the superior axis above the middle axis.

The **ligament of Zaglas** is the second digitation of the intermediate layer of the posterior sacroiliac ligaments, suspending the sacrum from the iliac crests. The **short axial ligament** is deep to it. Either of these ligaments can serve

Figure 2.9.A Transverse axis shift.
With extreme flexion the erector spinae muscles exert traction on the back of the sacrum, drawing it up along the short arm, which guides the sacral base posteriorly, reversing the nutation. This sometimes causes the distance between the PSISs to spread. In the standing position the pelvis shifts back increasing the posterior vector of the gravitational load force on the sacral base. **Figure 2.9.B. (Far right)** Extreme backward bending of the trunk can shift the load on the sacral base and drive it forward and down along the short arm of the auricular surface. Again the transverse axis shifts from middle to superior. Such nutation is very different from mid-range flexion nutation, and can produce unilateral wedging of the joint (sacral flexion lesion).

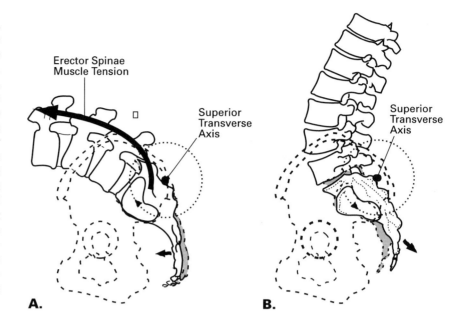

A. B.

Erector Spinae Muscle Tension

Superior Transverse Axis

Superior Transverse Axis

as the stabilizer of the superior transverse axis (Fig. 2.8).

The location of the superior transverse axis is posterior and superior to the middle and inferior transverse axes. It is the axis for paradoxical (e.g., spine bends forward, sacrum bends backward or *vice versa*) movements of the sacrum. This axis becomes functional *only* in the extremes of backward and forward bending of the trunk, at the moment when the sacrum begins to rotate in a direction opposite to the movements of the vertebrae.

How the Axis Shifts from Middle to Superior
As trunk flexion/extension moves from the mid-range into hyperflexion or hyperextension, the load on the sacral base is increased significantly through the increase in spinal leverage. With mid-range flexion the load force is directed inferiorly on the anterior sacral base – causing the sacrum to nutate. Conversely, with mid-range extension the load force is directed inferiorly on the posterior sacral base – causing the sacrum to counternutate. Paradoxically, as the trunk continues into the hyper-ranges of flexion and extension, instead of continuing to nutate in response to increased flexion, and counternutate in response to increased extension, the sacrum does just the opposite. Hyperflexion causes the sacrum to counternutate, and hyperextension causes the sacrum to nutate. (Figure 2.9, A.& B.)

Several factors must be taken into account to explain the counterintuitive response of the sacrum. One factor is that, by the time the sacrum reaches the limit of its range with respect to the sacrotuberous, sacrospinous, and superior sacroiliac ligaments, the load force transferred through L_5 has not only increased, but is applied to the sacrum more off-center. As the direction and force of load on the sacral base changes, other ligaments are invoked to stabilize or

resist the change in forces. As was mentioned, the ligaments that stabilize the sacrum in mid-range flexion/extension are the sacrotuberous, sacrospinous, and superior sacroiliac ligaments. However, at some point these ligaments – having reached the limit of their available slack – will allow no further movement of the sacrum consistent with the middle transverse axis. In order for the sacrum to accommodate the increase in force and continue moving, it must rotate about a different transverse axis – the superior transverse axis.

In the case of hyperflexion, the primarily inferiorly directed load force associated with mid-range flexion begins to push the anterior sacral base posterior. This is because – in the hyperflexed position – the body of L_5 is more anteriorly positioned in relation to the sacral base. In addition, the counternutation associated with hyperflexion is facilitated by increased tension in erector spinae muscles, which pulls the posterior sacral base superiorly. In order for the sacral base to move superiorly and posteriorly, the sacrum slides up along the path of the auricular L-shaped surface.

In the case of hyperextension, the load applied through L_5 shifts more posteriorly, exerting an anteriorly directed force vector onto the posterior portion of the sacral base; this in opposition to the posterior movement that the sacral base has already done. In the hyperextended position, the sacral base slides anteriorly and inferiorly along the auricular surface, as the sacrum becomes the lowest segment in an increasing lordotic curve. For this to occur, the location of the transverse axis had to change to allow for compliant movement of the sacrum permitted by ligaments other than the tight sacrospinous and anterior sacroiliac ligaments. Of course, the reversal of sacral movement relative to the ilia creates slack in the sacrotuberous ligament as other ligamentous components of the sacroiliac joint tighten.

Why does not the reversal of sacral counternutation caused by hyperextension of the spine simply nutate on the middle transverse axis instead of the shifting to the superior transverse axis? The best answer is probably that the inferiorly directed vector of the gravitational load is tremendously increased, calling for more inferior sacral movement than the ligamentous attachments associated with the middle transverse axis will allow.

The Great Controversy: To Nutate or Counternutate

Having described how sagittal forward bending of the spine can produce both nutation and counternutation, it would be well here to explain the mechanisms whereby the sacrum sometimes moves with the fifth lumbar and sometimes moves counter to the fifth lumbar. In forward bending of the trunk, the *erector spinae* muscles are active in an isotonic eccentric contraction throughout the movement. This is undoubtedly the mechanism in what we have called midrange flexion/extension – when the sacrum, coupled to the spine by the active *erector spinae* muscles, follows the direction of movement of the spine. When flexion becomes extreme, these same muscles cause the sacral axis to shift and the sacrum to counternutate – at least sometimes.

However, when discussing sacroiliac osteokinematic diagnosis, the principle of lumbosacral contrary motions is presented. This principle states that whatever the fifth lumbar does, the sacrum does the opposite, in contradiction to the mechanism of trunk flexion described above. The contrary motion principle applies to the balanced sidebending relationship between the fifth lumbar and the sacrum, not to the act of flexing the trunk, which unbalances the sagittal load on the sacral base and elicits myotatic contraction of the *erector spinae*. The sacral nutation with trunk hyperextension represents a reversal of direction, and a shift of axis, especially when weight support is predominantly on the posterior sacroiliac ligaments.

Non-Weight Bearing Sagittal Movement

Studies of non-weight bearing sagittal movements are too few to confidently assign transverse axes to activities like situps or hands-and-knees cat stretches. However, one variant of non-weight bearing sagittal movement which has been studied is **respiratory sacroiliac motion**. (Fig. 2.10)

The functional relationship of the pelvis to voluntary and involuntary respiration is clinically important. Respiratory motion impairment at the sacroiliac joint increases the work of breathing significantly; if the sacrum – independent of the ilium – is not free to follow the breathing movements of the spine, each breath must move the entire bone-muscle mass of the hemipelvis. Breathing motions of the pelvic and urogenital diaphragms are possibly due to passive stretch and recoil of these muscular tissues. The author is not aware of any EMG evidence to indicate whether or not there is active neuromuscular contraction

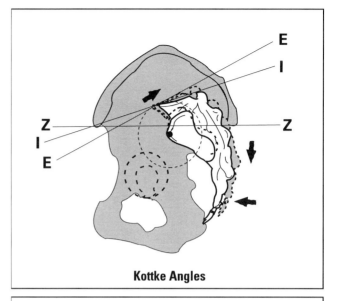

Kottke Angles

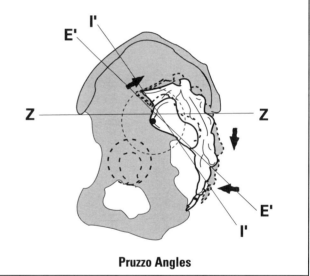

Pruzzo Angles

Figure 2.10. Sacroiliac respiratory motion measured roentgenographically. In an experiment by Kottke (1962), the lines I-I (sacral position with trunk hyperextension) and E-E (sacral position with trunk hyperflexion) were drawn across the sacral base, and intersected the line Z-Z drawn from ASIS to PSIS, forming 2 pelvi-sacral angles. Subtracting one pelvisacral angle from the other equals the net change in pelvisacral angle from the hyperflexed to the hyperextended position. It also equals the angle formed at the intersection of lines I-I and E-E (Kottke's angle).

Pruzzo (1971) used Kottke's measurement method to quantify sacroiliac respiratory motion. To evaluate the reliability of the measurement method he also drew lines (I'-I' for inhaled and E'-E' for exhaled) on the anterior margin of the first sacral segment, creating Pruzzo's angle at their intersection with Z–Z. On the same subject, Pruzzo's angle equalled Kottke's angle ±0.1 angular degrees, indicating a high degree of reliability for the method.

Lead (Pb) markers attached to the skin at the gluteal tubercle dimple and over the sacral median crest followed the movements of the bony landmarks precisely, radiogrammetrically validating photogrammetric research on sacroiliac respiratory mobility.

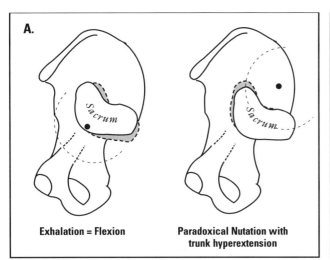

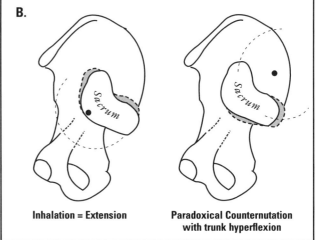

Figure 2.11. A and B. Comparison of sacroiliac respiratory motion with nutation and counternutation of the sacrum caused by extreme trunk backward and forward bending. The respiratory axis through the second sacral segment near the anterior edge of the auricular surface is probably the axis of sacral nutation and counternutation as it occurs in the mid-range of trunk flexion and extension.

and relaxation of the pelvic diaphragms with breathing. A myotatic response to stretch during inhalation would be inefficient and add to the work of breathing; one might assume their proprioceptor population is rather small. Mindful observers can document that the pelvic diaphragm muscles contract with sudden forceful exhalation, as in coughing, along with the abdominal and internal intercostal muscles.

Respiratory sacroiliac motion may seem to be paradoxical. Given that the sacrum is moved by the lumbar spine, which straightens its lordotic curve with inhalation, why does the sacrum counternutate instead of nutating as it does in weight-bearing spinal flexion, which also straightens the lumbar lordotic curve?

Obviously, the force vectors do not load the sacral base in the same way. In weight-bearing flexion the gravitational load on the sacral base increases with spinal flexion, causing sacral nutation.

Inhaling increases the internal pressure of the abdominopelvic region. The lumbar and sacral base compliance to this pressure is to move posteriorly as the straightening lumbars apply a caudal pressure against the sacral base.

The superior transverse axis is regarded by some to be the axis for **craniosacral primary respiratory motion**. However, Magoun (1976) locates the primary respiratory axis of the sacrum "...at the level of the second sacral segment, probably somewhere near the angle of the two auricular arms." Radiogrammetric studies by Mitchell, Jr. and Pruzzo (1970) on voluntary respiratory motion in the sacroiliac joints confirm the respiratory axis in this location, which appears to correspond to the middle transverse axis.

Translatory Sacral Motion

With no rotational axis stabilized, linear displacement of the sacrum can, and does, occur (Figure 2.12), usually in the direction of the acceleration of gravity, as in slip-and-fall

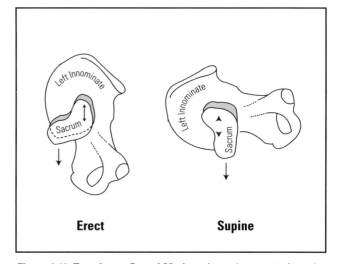

Figure 2.12. Translatory Sacral Motion. A certain amount of translatory displacement of the sacrum does occur with changes in body position from recumbent to erect. Normal limits of such displacement have not been clearly established, but shearing greater than 5 mm. probably represents hypermobility. Normal ligamentous slack permits a small amount of both vertical and horizontal translation.

injuries.

The purpose for physiologic translatory mobility of the sacrum can be understood in terms of the complex simultaneous events that occur in the pelvis during walking. While one innominate rotates on a stable sacral pivot point (the supporting leg), the other innominate, lacking a stable pivot point, must, nevertheless, derotate, and must find another way to move posteriorly. The path of movement it takes is determined by the ballistics of the swinging leg, and the planes of the auricular surfaces. The instantaneous axes involved must constantly change as the position of the sacrum changes and the ligamentous tensions vary. The slack in the system which allows these complex adaptive

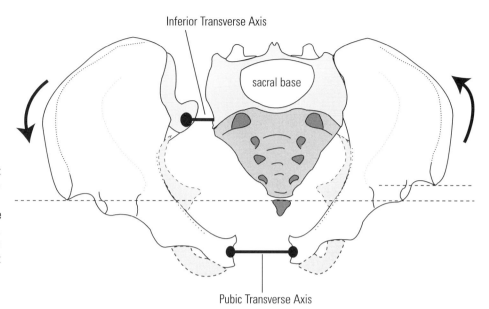

Inferior Transverse Axis

sacral base

Pubic Transverse Axis

Fig. 2.13. Interinnominate rotation – anterior rotation of the right innominate in relation to the posterior rotation of the left innominate. In order for innominate bones to follow leg motion in walking, they must turn in opposite directions in relation to each other. While rotating around a transverse inter-pubic axis an ilium must pivot on the sacrum. Side-tipping of the whole pelvis on a pubic A-P axis keeps the sacral base more level.

movements is demonstrated by linear displacement of the sacrum in relation to the innominates as body position changes from recumbent to standing (Colachis, 1963).

Translatory and rotatory movements are not mutually exclusive; they may occur together or sequentially.

Transverse Axes and Iliosacral Motion

The two innominate bones (os coxae) normally rotate in relation to each other on a transverse axis which passes through the symphysis pubis. The terms "anterior" and "posterior" are used to describe these rotations and refer to the direction of iliac crest movement. Anterior or posterior innominate rotation obviously necessitates movement in one or both sacroiliac joints. **While pivoting on the transverse pubic axis, each innominate must also move on the sacrum. Such sacroiliac motion is best labeled "iliosacral"** to distinguish it from pelvic joint movements generated by the spine load on the sacral base.

Pubic Transverse Axis

The **pubic transverse axis** constitutes the *locomotion axis of the pubis*, i.e., the axis between the two innominates upon which they rotate in opposite directions as they accompany the movement of the legs. In the walking cycle, independent rotation of the ilia in directions opposite to each other requires movement at the pubic symphysis as well as at the iliosacral joint. In normal walking cycle motion, the pubic bones rotate on a shared transverse axis. The normal amplitude of this rotatory motion can displace the anterior superior iliac spines in opposite directions, anteroinferiorly and superoposteriorly producing an asymmetry of 2 centimeters or more. As the innominates rotate on this axis the entire pelvis tips from side to side so that the anteriorly rotating innominate is lowered in space.

Note: The pubic bones do not normally shear vertically on each other during walking. To do so would produce a ligamentous strain in the sacroiliac joints which would interfere with the physiologic movements of sacrum and ilium.

Stability of the pubic transverse axis is provided by abdominal and upper thigh muscles. Maintenance of the stability of this axis is important in order that the physiologic axes of the sacroiliac joints line up, i.e., are not sheared. Vertical shears at the pubic symphysis are prevented by normal balanced muscle tonus maintained in several muscles including the *rectus abdominis* and *adductors femores* muscles. When the tonus of one or more of these muscles gets out of balance, they have the potential to pull a pubic bone out of place. Orthopedic literature from the early 1930s indicates that surgical fusion of the pubic symphysis to treat pubic instability demonstrated by one-leg-stand posterior/anterior X-rays was once a popular procedure. However, the disastrous consequences of the fusion were soon evident, and the procedure was abandoned.

Iliosacral Inferior Transverse Axis

When the sacroiliac joint is loaded, as in one leg standing, or during walking, a stable pivot point exists for the weight-bearing ilium to rotate physiologically on the sacrum. The axis for such innominate rotation has been labeled the "inferior transverse axis." The **inferior tranverse axis is** actually **two separate and independent left or right pivot points, operating only on one side at a time.** It would be more accurate to say that there are two independent inferior transverse axes, each one instantaneous, and neither of them corresponding to a perfect anatomic *x-axis*.

When the sacrum is loaded symmetrically, as it is when

2.14. A. and B. The transverse axes in relation to the oblique axes. Summary illustration of the Mitchell model . (Adapted with permission of the American Academy of Osteopathy from AAO Yearbook 1965, vol. 2: Mitchell FL "Structural Pelvic Function.")

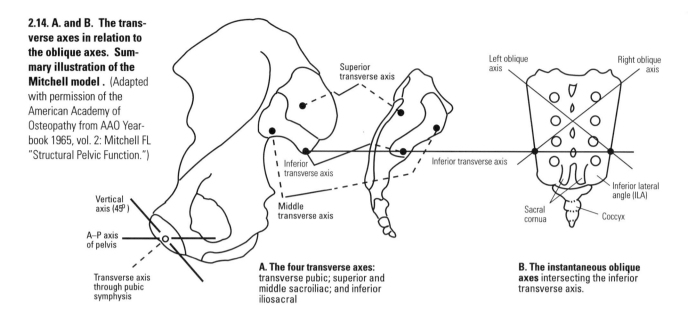

Superior transverse axis

Inferior transverse axis

Middle transverse axis

Vertical axis (45°)

A–P axis of pelvis

Transverse axis through pubic symphysis

A. The four transverse axes: transverse pubic; superior and middle sacroiliac; and inferior iliosacral

Left oblique axis

Right oblique axis

Inferior transverse axis

Inferior lateral angle (ILA)

Sacral cornua

Coccyx

B. The instantaneous oblique axes intersecting the inferior transverse axis.

the weight is equally distributed on both feet, the weight of the trunk is transmitted through the sacroiliac ligaments, which suspend the sacrum between the ilia, and is distributed evenly to both legs. A more stable unilateral load transmission is achieved when the weight of the spine passes through the sacrum directly to the iliac bone on one side at a point where there is articular close-packing between sacrum and ilium and the body weight is supported on one leg. This may occur statically in standing, or dynamically in walking or running.

The close-packed point of load transmission is the pivot point identified as the inferior transverse axis. It is stabilized by the articular geometry of the sacroiliac joint and the tonic contraction of the piriformis muscle.

The load-bearing ilium can rotate anteriorly or posteriorly on this pivot point, while it is engaged (stabilized). As we shall see in Chapter 3, the sacrum may rotate on the same pivot using an oblique axis that intersects the inferior transverse axis. Such is the case in walking or running which integrate sacroiliac and iliosacral functions as they respond to spine, leg, and inertial forces.

Note regarding terminology: The term "rotation," as it is used in other parts of the body, describes movement around a vertical axis. The term "rotation" is uniquely described in the iliac context as movement around a transverse axis. The reader should also be aware that, although apparently similar to the movement designated by the terms flexion and extension, "rotation" was the term FLM, Sr. preferred to describe this movement, and is the term, modified by "anterior" or "posterior," used throughout the book. In referring to rotations of the innominate, the terms anterior and posterior are used to designate the movement of the iliac crest. In addition, when describing the osteokinematics of the pelvis as sacroiliac and iliosacral, we have followed the anatomic convention of naming the moving bone first and the reference bone second. However, as will become more apparent, in complex pelvic kinematics the reference bone is not necessarily stationary.

In walking, the simultaneous counter-rotation of the non-weight-bearing ilium occurs on the pubic transverse axis. This also requires some shearing and twisting at the iliosacral joint, but not on a stable axis.

The iliosacral movements which permit interinnominate rotation may be rotational or translatory. Because the sacroiliac auricular surfaces are not perfectly parallel sagittal planes, the instantaneous pubic axis is rarely perfectly transverse. Its angulation depends on the shape and orientation of the sacral auricular surface(s) and which innominate is moving relative to the sacrum.

While one innominate is rotating on the sacrum, the other innominate may simply stay with the sacrum, or, if it moves relative to the sacrum, as in negative weight-bearing in the gait cycle, may be free to translate in any direction or rotate about a rapidly changing (unstable) instantaneous axis.

Summary of Pelvic Axes

Axes in the Mitchell model are compiled in Figure 2.14.A and B. The three transverse axes of the sacrum (inferior, middle, and superior), the transverse axis of the pubic symphyses, and the two oblique axes are illustrated. The oblique axes (the major topic of Chapter 3) are shown intersecting the inferior transverse axis. At this point, the two instantaneous axes are, in a sense, integrated.

The inferior transverse axis is actually represented by two independent pivot points on each side of the lowest pole of the sacroiliac joint. When an innominate rotates on one of these pivots, the actual axis of its rotation is not a perfectly horizontal transverse axis, but is an instantaneous axis at tight angles to the plane(s) of innominate rotation. It is this (slightly oblique) inferior transverse axis that intersects one of the **sacral oblique axes**, allowing *simultaneous* innominate and sacral rotation on the same pivot when interinnominate rotation occurs at the pubis.

Medio-lateral Displacement of PSISs with Nutation/Counternutation

Some observers have noticed that nutations and counter-nutation of the sacrum can produce medial-lateral displacement of the posterior superior iliac spines bilaterally. When the sacral base moves posteriorly-superiorly on this axis, it pushes the iliac crests apart, and when it moves anteriorly-inferiorly, it allows the iliac crests to move medially toward each other. The distance between the posterior superior iliac spines on the iliac crests can vary as much as 2 millimeters with such flexion and extension movements of the sacrum. Counternutation tends to spread the PSISs apart. This phenomenon occurs inconsistently, but when it does occur, it provides supportive evidence of sacroiliac mobility. When the phenomenon does not occur it does not, however, indicate absence of sacroiliac motion (Figure 2.15).

Voluntary *versus* Involuntary Sacral Motion

In describing the motions of the sacrum on the ilia, various categories or distinctions can be made to describe the nature and make more comprehensible the mechanics of these motions. For example, one distinction that can be made is to differentiate between those motions that are associated with involuntary physiologic processes, and those which are associated voluntary movement. The motions associated with the cranial rhythmic impulse, which results in palpable oscillations of the sacrum, are considered involuntary sacral motions, the nature of which has not been quantified with regards to axes and or range. Unless consciously controlled, another sacral motion which *can* fall under the category of involuntary is the sacral motion associated with respiration. Assuming no abnormalities exist, these motions which accompany respiration are considered to occur about a transverse axis as the sacrum nutates (which is akin to flexion) with exhalation and counter-nutates (which is akin to extension) with inhalation. (see Figure 2.10)

The sacral motions associated with the voluntary movements of flexion and extension of the trunk, are nutation and counternutation (pure sagittal plane motions). Walking and running combine nutation and counternutation with coupled rotation and sidebending.

Regardless of whether the motion is associated with involuntary or voluntary physiologic processes, the movements of the sacrum in relation to the ilia can be described theoretically as rotations occurring about axes, or translations occurring along cardinal planes restrained by the planes of the joint surfaces. The sacrum, as an extension of the vertebral column, will move in relation to forces transmitted through its contact with L_5. The resultant changes in the sacrum's position and orientation will then be reflected in its positional relationships to the ilia, L_5, and to the cardinal planes of the body. Thus, osteokinematically,

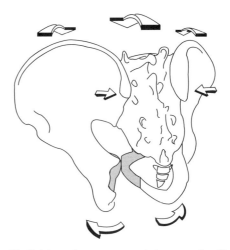

Fig.2.15. Medial-lateral movements of the posterior iliac crests. Nutation of the sacrum allows the iliac crests to fall medially. In some individuals the change in approximation of the posterior superior iliac spines (PSISs) or gluteal tubercles is measurable. Counternutation spreads the PSISs apart.

we can describe the relative orientation of the sacrum in one of two ways: a) in relation to L_5, and b) in relation to the ilium at the sacroiliac joint. However, for diagnostic purposes it is important to bear in mind that a change in the bony relationships at the sacroiliac joint may be the result of movement of the sacrum on the ilia, or movement of an ilium on the sacrum and in relation to the other ilium.

Translatory movements of the sacrum occur incidental to rotations of the sacrum, but are not necessarily coupled to the rotatory movements of the sacrum. The amplitude of translatory motion is surprisingly large in some research reports (Colachis, 1963; Solonen, 1957; Sturesson, 1989).

Causes of Sacroiliac Motion

Muscles do not directly move the sacrum between the ilia. Instead, sacral movement is the result of gravitational, inertial, and elastic forces resulting from spinal movements, which are indeed the result of muscular activity. The role of elasticity is discussed by Dorman (1992). Similarly, muscles do not directly move the innominate bones in relation to each other, or in relation to the sacrum. Again, such movements result from gravitational, inertial, and elastic forces from the legs.

The bones of the pelvis are moved by the elasticity of the connective tissue comprising the pelvic ligaments and fascial continuity of the trunk, pelvis and lower limb.

Craniosacral Motion

Hypothetically, the flexion-extension actions of the cranial Primary Respiratory Mechanism (PRM) described by

Sutherland (1939) include sacral nutations. The sacrum is conceived as coupled to the occiput by the osseous attachments of the spinal dura mater and thus parallels the occipital movements of the cranial rhythmic impulse (CRI). This theory is based on the observations of early anatomists that the dura mater is a very tough *inelastic* membrane, and therefore the sacrum is obliged to follow the occiput like a marionette. Consequently, as the occiput moves into extension (as the term is defined in the craniosacral system), the sacrum moves into flexion (as the term is defined by the Muscle Energy system). However, the dura does have some elasticity.

Two kinds of craniosacral motion in the pelvis have been described in the literature: the inherent cranial rhythmic impulse (CRI) small amplitude movements of the sacrum, and the larger amplitude sacral oscillation, which is a manifestation of cranial dysfunction. It could be postulated that the oscillation is caused by undulatory movements of the spine driven by involuntary coordinated actions of postural muscles acting on the spine. The oscillations usually occur on an oblique axis, but occasionally simulate unilateral sacral flexion.

Amplitude of Craniosacral Motions

The inherent motions of the occiput relative to the other cranial bones is quite small. (Adams, 1992) It is not likely that a point anywhere on the occiput will inherently move more than a millimeter or that rotation of the bone, relative to the sphenoid or the temporal and parietal bones, will exceed 0.5 angular degrees. With deep breathing, however, the cranial bone excursions are enormously amplified – tripled or quadrupled (Johnson, 1966) Sacroiliac breathing movement is similarly much larger than the inherent craniosacral motion of the sacrum, and so is the movement of sacral oscillation.

It is most likely that the small inherent movements of the sacrum, which are palpable irregular oscillations at 6 to 8 cycles per minute (about 0.2 Hz) independent of breathing (normally, a faster rate), are potentially multi-axial with no inherently stable axis.

Some cranial authors have claimed that the sacrum has only one axis of normal motion, transverse through the second segment. Yet, Lippincott (1958, 1965) in an earlier article, distinguished between iliosacral and sacroiliac lesions. Lippincott and others have confused anterior sacral nutation with an upslipped innominate. Sutherland's perinatal "depressed sacrum" (Lippincott's term), capable of causing post-partum psychosis according to Sutherland, was described by him as an anterior nutation on an abnormal axis and labeled "traumatic anterior sacrum." Indirect treatment techniques described by Lippincott can be effective, provided the operator can feel the "abnormal" axis while seeking the position of easy or balanced tension. Lippincott puts the "abnormal" axis at the sacral apex. Such a traumatic dislocation of the sacrum is theoretically possible, but is certainly not as common as the lesion which we call "unilateral sacral flexion" – a one-sided anterior nutation of the sacrum, which displaces the ipsilateral inferior lateral angle about 1 centimeter (±8mm.) caudad and a little posteriorly.

Note: Historically, most research on pelvisacral mobility has focused on movements in the sagittal plane. The sacroiliac joints on the sides of the sacrum are approximately in parasagittal planes. If one wished to investigate sacroiliac motion (assuming there was any motion at all), it was natural to assume that it would occur in the sagittal plane, rather than the transverse or coronal planes. Also, methodologically it was easier for researchers to measure sagittal motion. Sagittal plane rotatory movements are customarily described by identifying the location of the transverse axis around which the object (the sacrum) turns.

Several transverse axes have been proposed and discussed in this chapter. Although most readers will have a clear understanding of the anatomic use of the terms "flexion" and "extension," some ambiguity persists in their meanings. For example, in the craniosacral model their meanings have been reversed because of the emphasis on the Primary Respiratory Mechanism (PRM) where inhalation is coupled with flexion and external rotation, etc.

Some readers may be using the physics definition of flexion – "approximation of two ends of an arc." The physics definition is difficult to apply to pelvisacral mechanics. To avoid misunderstanding, we prefer to use the terms nutation and counternutation as defined in this chapter to describe the sagittal plane rotatory movements of the sacrum, regardless of the location of the transverse axis.

CHAPTER 3

Normal Coupled Motions in the Sacroiliac Joints: Torsion and Unilateral Sacral Flexion

In addition to the symmetrical sagittal plane motions, normal movements of the sacroiliac joints include rotation and sidebending, which are coupled asymmetric motions. This chapter will discuss the ways in which rotation and sidebending are combined in different proportions as the sacrum responds to shifting loads applied to it by the moving spine.

Two different kinds of asymmetrically coupled physiologic sacroiliac movement can be distinguished: **sacral torsion** and **unilateral sacral flexion**. The principal characteristics of each include the following:

The distinguishing features of *sacral torsion* include:
• The sacrum *pivots* on a close-packed bone-to-bone weight transmission point on the ilium;
• Rotation is coupled with contralateral sidebending at the sacral base. In addition, as the sacral base moves forward (or backward) on one ilium, the inferior lateral angle (ILA) on the opposite side of the sacrum simultaneously moves backward (or forward) in relation to the ilium on that side;
• Torsional movement of the sacrum, which occurs about an **oblique axis** (Mitchell model), is in response to *balanced* sidebending of the trunk (Figure 3.1). With balanced trunk sidebending, the load vector on the sacral base shifts to the side *opposite* to the direction of the lumbar sidebend, creating the necessity for torsional movement;
• The *primary* motion at the sacral base is rotation, with contralateral sidebending as the secondary coupled motion.

The distinguishing features of *unilateral sacral flexion* include:
• The mechanism of weight transmission is through the posterior sacroiliac ligaments, and the movement is a *swinging motion* of the suspended sacrum (Figure 3.19);
• One-sided anterior motion of the sacral base occurs with inferior/posterior movement of the ILA *on the same side*;
• Unilateral sacral flexion is a response to loaded (weight bearing) *unbalanced* sidebending of the trunk, which can produce a non-oblique axis sidebend of the sacrum *toward* the side of trunk sidebending. (Figure 3.1)
• The *primary* motion is sidebending, with contralateral rotation secondary.

In this chapter:

■ *Sidebending/rotation coupling in the sacroiliac joints*

■ *Oblique axis (torsion) motions of the sacrum*

■ *Spinal forces and sacral torsion*

■ *The walking cycle and the pelvis*

■ *Effects of balanced and unbalanced sidebending of the spine on sacral movement*

■ *Primary sacral sidebending (unilateral sacral flexion)*

■ *The spine-sacrum connection (lumbosacral mechanics)*

■ *Intrapelvic adaptive mechanisms*

Note: It has been customary to use the same terms for describing both the *physiologic* movements of the sacrum and for describing *somatic dysfunctions* (impaired physiologic function) of the sacrum. This is obviously a potential source of confusion. We propose a remedy already applied to the intervertebral joints: namely – use the gerund endings ["-ing," or "(t)ion"] as in "sidebending," "flexion," or "torsion" for the physiologic motions, and the past tense endings ("sidebent," "flexed," "torsioned") for the somatic dysfunctions. This chapter deals exclusively with the physiologic motions of sacral torsion and unilateral flexion. The common expression, "You have a sacral torsion," clearly means "You have a torsioned sacrum." Minus the article "a" it clearly means, "You have the normal mobility necessary for sacral torsion movement."

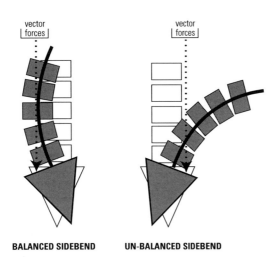

BALANCED SIDEBEND   UN-BALANCED SIDEBEND

Figure 3.1. Balanced right sidebending (associated with sacral torsion) versus unbalanced right sidebending (associated with unilateral sacral flexion) – posterior view. The sacrum is passively sidebent by the lateral shift of the load. With *balanced* sidebending to the right, the sacrum sidebends and rotates out from under the load, and the load force is applied on the side opposite to the sidebend causing anterior motion of the sacral base on the left. With *unbalanced* sidebending to the right, the sidebending load is greater, and applied ipsilateral to the direction of sidebend. All the sidebending motion occurs on the right ilium. The displacement of the ILA on the right is more inferior than posterior.

The reasons for the differing characteristics of the two types of coupled motion, which will be developed in more detail throughout this chapter, include the following:

• Varying load forces and vectors;
• Presence or absence of close-packing forces in one of the sacroiliac joints;
• Anatomic structure of the sacroiliac joints;
• Degrees of lumbar lordosis;
• The effect of different postures (erect, bent, or arched) on the loading of the posterior sacroiliac ligaments, and the persistence of that loading during trunk sidebending;
• Anatomic variations in lumbosacral angle;
• Degree of anatomic declination of the sacral base.

The discussion of coupled motions of the sacrum begins with a description of sacral torsion – focusing on what the sacrum does relative to the left and right iliac crests – followed by an analysis of the walking cycle (which incorporates sacral torsion). The mechanics of unilateral sacral flexion are then described, followed by a discussion of the mechanics of sidebending and rotation between lumbar vertebrae and the sacrum at the lumbosacral joint.

Sacral Torsion and the Oblique Axes

The oblique axis is an **instantaneous axis** (see Note below) which runs from the inferior extremity of the sacroiliac *joint* on one side of the sacrum (the inferior pole of the oblique axis) to the region of the superior posterior sacroiliac *ligaments* (with some variation either inferiorly or superiorly) on the other side of the sacrum. Hence, there are two symmetrical oblique axes as defined by Mitchell Sr.: the **left oblique axis** and the **right oblique axis**. The "left" and "right" qualifiers designate the side of the sacrum where the *superior* pole of the oblique axis crosses. (Figure 3.2)

Rotation in either direction about one of these axes is called **left (or right) sacral torsion**, with the direction of the rotation named for the direction (left or right) the *anterior* surface of the sacrum faces.

In Mitchell Sr.'s theoretical model of pelvic motion, the oblique axes are used solely to describe the torsion movements of the sacrum, and *not* the unilateral sacral flexion movements. It is important to note that, due to the close fit and broadness of the sacroiliac interface, *pure y-axis rotation* is very limited. Because of this anatomic limitation, significant rotation, combined with sidebending to the opposite side, *cannot* occur without an oblique axis.

Recognize that the oblique axis is operant – and considered "stationary" – only when the sacrum is moving *around it,* and that the moving parts of the torsioning sacrum are the quadrants opposite to where the oblique axis intersects the two sacroiliac joints. For example, in the case of the left oblique axis (which passes through the upper left and lower right quadrants), movement of the sacrum will be greatest in the lower left quadrant and the upper right quadrant. The direction and degree of movement of each quadrant is primarily determined by sacroiliac joint anatomy, and by the amount and direction of load.

Rotation on the oblique axis requires movement of the sacrum along the *short* arm of the auricular surface on one side, accompanied by *simultaneous* movement along the *long* arm of the opposite sacroiliac joint. With torsion movements of the sacrum, the sacrum follows the path that the contour of the auricular surfaces provide. This anatomic configuration, which allows for a "twisting" type movement between the innominates, permits more significant rotation at the sacroiliac joints than would otherwise be possible on the *y-axis.*

Sidebending at the sacral base (in relation to the ilia and the spine) is always coupled with contralateral rotation, and rotation is always coupled to contralateral sidebending. Paradoxically, because of the anatomy and orientation of the sacroiliac joints and the curved shape of the sacrum, as the sacral base sidebends one way and

---

Note *regarding instantaneous axis*: An axis is not a physical entity; it is a mathematically based imaginary line used to define the orientation of a rotational motion for a given object. There can be no axis without movement. An *instantaneous* axis is an axis occurring or present at a particular instant for an object involved in rotation; the axis may move to another parallel location or change its orientation when the plane of rotation changes. When rotation motion stops, the axis "disappears." Another axis will "appear" in another location when another kind of rotation occurs. In this sense all axes are instantaneous, depending on rotary motion for their "existence." Pure rotation on a fixed axis is a rare occurrence in the human body.

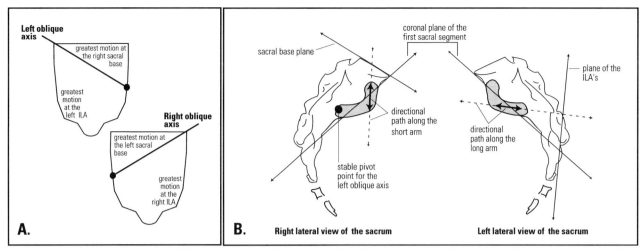

Figure 3.2. A and B. – Figure 3.2. A. The left and right oblique axes. The oblique axes, about which torsion motions occur, run from the inferior extremity of the sacroiliac joint to the region of the sacral sulcus on the opposite side. As the sacrum torsions, movement occurs primarily in the quadrants opposite to where the axis intersects. These oblique axes are instantaneous axes and, as such, only one can be operant at any given time depending on the nature of the torsional motion. **Figure 3.2. B. Sacral torsion relative to the auricular surfaces, and the planes and directions involved.** Displacement of the sacral base results from movement of the sacrum along the short arm of the auricular surface, which is oriented in a mostly inferior and slightly anterior direction; displacement of the ILA results from movement of the sacrum along the long arm of the auricular surface, which is oriented in a mostly posterior and slightly inferior direction. Because of the forward orientation of the sacrum in relation to the coronal plane of the body, and the biconvex shape of the sacrum, the planes referred to in assessing a positional change of the sacral base is different than it is for the ILAs.

rotates the other (about an oblique axis), **the inferior lateral angles (ILAs) of the sacrum will always demonstrate ipsilateral coupling** (i.e., sidebending and rotation to the same side) – *in relation to the cardinal planes of the body.*

One reason for the seeming paradox of contralateral coupling at the sacral base with ipsilateral coupling of the ILA is that **displacement of the *sacral base* is primarily the result of motion along the *short arm* of the auricular surface on one side, and displacement of the *ILA* is primarily the result of movement along the *long arm* on the other side.** (A more detailed discussion of this paradox will be found at the end of this chapter.)

Another reason is that one characteristic of the oblique axis, as defined in the *current* revised Mitchell model, is that the *inferior* pole (of either a left or right oblique axis) is considered the stable pivot point for motion about that oblique axis (whether torsioning left or right) – *but* there can be, however, some slight translocation, or change in orientation, at the less stabilized *superior* pole of an oblique axis. This slight translocation, or "tipping," at the superior pole of the oblique axis, as demonstrated in Figure 3.3., can allow the ILA that is moving posteriorly on one side to also move in a more inferior direction relative to the ILA on the other side, which is stabilized.

If the superior pole of the oblique axis did not "tip," then as one side of the sacral base moved forward and inferior about the oblique axis, the ILA on the other side would move posterior and *superior*. But as the oblique axis tips down in a coronal plane, the ILA shifts inferiorly on the side moving posteriorly.

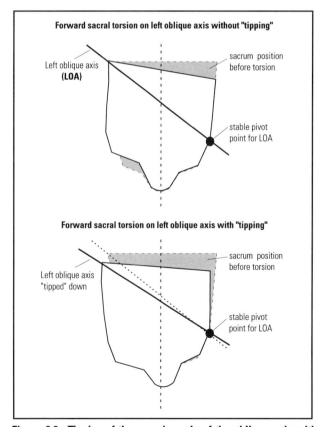

Figure 3.3. Tipping of the superior pole of the oblique axis with sacral torsion. The graphic model of sacral torsion on top demonstrates how the ILA would move superior as it moves posterior if the superior pole of the oblique axis did not "tip." However, with tipping of the superior pole of the oblique axis, the posterior movement of the ILA is guided inferiorly by the long arm of the sacroiliac joint.

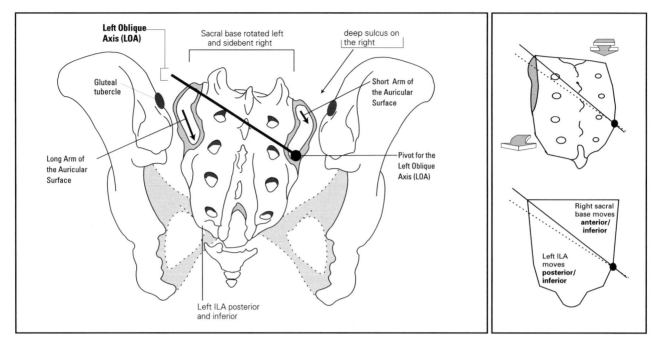

Figure 3.4. Forward torsion on the left oblique axis of the sacrum is also referred to as a "Left-on-Left Torsion," and has the *sacral base* rotating left (and sidebending right) about the left oblique axis. The sacrum is depicted so that both articular surfaces are visible at the same time. In this example, the sacrum turns to face the left side of the body by rotating on the left oblique axis. The right side of the sacral base goes anterior and inferior following the short arm of the right auricular surface. Because of this anterior movement, it is sometimes called "forward torsion to the left." This expression indicates that the sacrum rotated on the left oblique axis. Whereas the sacral base moves mainly on the right side, the inferior portion of the sacrum moves mostly on the left. The left ILA moves posteriorly guided by the sliding motion of the left side of the sacrum on the long arm of the auricular surface. This necessitates that the upper end of the oblique axis is not as stable as its lower end, and must tilt down (dotted line) as the sacrum rotates around it. This is why the oblique axis must be designated an "instantaneous axis," because the left ILA must move a little inferior to go posterior.

The Four Sacral Torsion Movements

Altogether, there are **four possible sacral torsion movements**. Torsional movements about either the left or right oblique axis may be called "backward" torsion or "forward" torsion, referring to the direction of sacral base movement.

Left torsion on the left oblique axis (**Left-on-Left**) occurs as the right side of the sacral base moves anterior about the left oblique axis. *Right torsion on the right oblique axis* (**Right-on-Right**) occurs as the left side of the sacral base moves anterior about the right oblique axis. Both are designated **forward torsions** because the sacral base is moving "forward" on one side. (Figures 3.4 and 3.6)

Left torsion on the right oblique axis (**Left-on-Right**) occurs when the left side of the sacral base moves backward about the right oblique axis. With *right torsion on the left oblique axis* (**Right-on-Left**), the right side of the sacral base is moving backward about the left oblique axis. In these instances (i.e., Left-on-Right or Right-on-Left), both are considered **backward torsions** because the sacral base is moving "backward" on one side. (Figures 3.5 and 3.7)

The description of the four sacral torsion movements just outlined describes torsion motion in terms of the sacral base. This is not only because the sacral torsion motions are initiated by forces *from above*, and the way these forces are transferred from L_5 onto the sacral base, but also because the nomenclature used to distinguish the types of sacral torsion is based on describing the movement of the sacral base. But equally important – and perhaps more important when discussing evaluation of the sacroiliac joint – are the ILA positions associated with the four types of sacral torsion. To briefly summarize, **if the sacrum is torsioning forward** – that is, the sacral base is moving anterior/inferior along the short arm of the SACROILIAC joint on one side – then the ILA on the opposite side will move posterior and inferior as the sacrum moves down the long arm of the auricular surface on that side. **If the sacrum is torsioning backward**, then the side of the sacral base that is moving posterior/superior along the short arm of the SACROILIAC joint – will have the ILA on the opposite side moving anterior and superior as the sacrum moves up the long arm of the auricular surface on that side.

Familiarity with both sacral base and ILA dynamics is important when performing the evaluation procedures. Without this understanding, it will be unclear as to whether an ILA that appears left rotated is left rotated because the upper left quadrant has moved posteriorly, or because the upper right quadrant has moved anteriorly. (Figures 3.4, 3.5, 3.6, and 3.7)

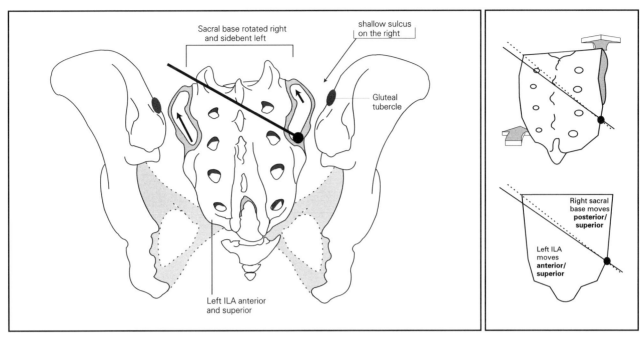

Figure 3.5. Backward torsion on the left oblique axis of the sacrum is also referred to as a "Right-on-Left Torsion." This expression means that the sacrum has turned to face the right side of the body by moving the right side of the sacral base posteriorly. The short arm of the right auricular surface guides the right side of the sacral base posterior and superior (hence, "backward" torsion). The left ILA is guided anterior and slightly superior by the long arm of the left auricular surface.

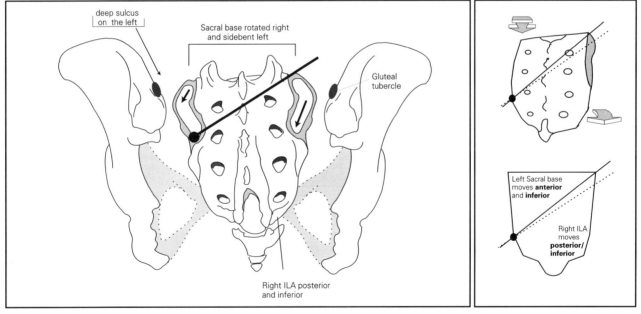

Figure 3.6. Forward torsion on the right oblique axis of the sacrum is also referred to as a "Right-on-Right Torsion." The sacrum turns to face the right by sliding the left base anteriorly along the short arm of the S-I joint, and the right ILA posteriorly along the right long arm.

Spinal Forces and Sacral Torsion

As previously discussed, the lumbar spine applies load forces to the sacral base in different ways, depending on the amount and direction of spinal bend, and gravitational vectors. Torsioning of the sacrum is induced by lateral flexion (i.e., sidebending) of the lumbar spine. However, even though sacral torsion is caused by sidebending of the lumbars, the principal movement at the sacral base is always rotation (which distinguishes torsion from unilateral sacral flexion, where the primary motion of the sacral base is sidebending). Also mentioned was that spinal sidebending may occur as either a *balanced* (causing sacral torsion) or an *unbalanced* (causing unilateral sacral flexion) motion (Figure 3.1). Balanced sidebending may occur standing, sitting, or even recumbent. The term "balanced" refers to equalized distribution of body masses around a central core

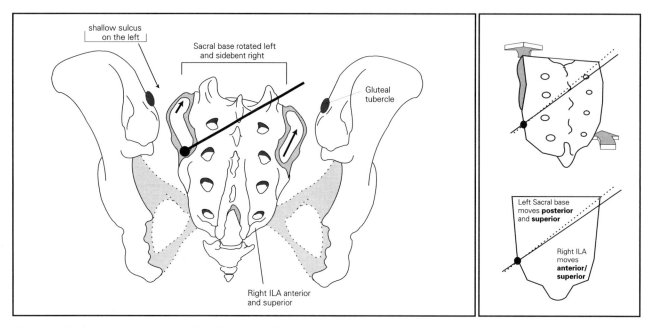

Figure 3.7. Backward torsion on the right oblique axis of the sacrum, is also referred to as a "Left-on-Right Torsion." The sacrum faces left by sliding up the left short arm and anterior on the right long arm of the auricular surfaces.

line – either the net gravity line in the erect posture, or the central line representing the intersection of the sagittal and coronal cardinal planes.

Understanding the influence of sidebending the lumbar spine on the sacrum is complex because sidebending and rotation are coupled motions both in the lumbar vertebral joints *and* in the sacroiliac joints. In the lumbars contralateral and ipsilateral coupling are variable, depending on intervertebral joint loads, and which movements precede, or follow, other movements. When the *initial* primary movement in the lumbar spine is sidebending (and not axial rotation), the coupled rotation of the vertebral segments will be observed in fairly predictable patterns, sometimes called neutral (Type I) motion. In other words, when loaded sidebending – whether balanced or unbalanced – is initiated in lumbar neutral, the vertebral segments tend to follow the neutral law of spinal mechanics (rotation and sidebending contralaterally coupled up to the apex of the neutral group, and ipsilaterally coupled above the apex). {Refer to Volumes 1 and 2 for detailed discussion of this concept.}

Assuming there is no non-neutral dysfunction at L_5, whether the coupled motions occurring with L_5 are reversals of the coupled motions occurring at the sacral base depends on whether the spinal sidebend initiating sidebending at the sacral base is balanced or unbalanced.

With balanced sidebending of the trunk, vector forces are transmitted from L_5 onto the sacral base on the side *oppo-*

site to the direction of the sidebend. The forming convexity shifts the gravitational load onto that side of the sacrum causing it to move so that it becomes a continuation of the convexity. Under these circumstances, the sacrum is most likely to sidebend by rotating on its oblique axis, the movement we have labeled "forward torsion."

In contrast, unbalanced sidebending of the trunk causes the load forces to be transmitted from L_5 to the sacral base *on the same side* as the direction of sidebend. The mechanics of this latter condition, which generates unilateral sacral flexion, will be presented in greater detail later in this chapter.

Forward torsion occurs in response to sidebending, starting with the trunk *erect or slightly extended*, which is either balanced and loaded, or sidebending which is non-weight bearing. **Backward torsion**, on the other hand, is the result of sidebending of the trunk from a *forward bent* position (whether standing, seated, or lateral recumbent).

Mitchell Sr.'s choice of the word "torsion," (which means "twist") to refer to the oblique axis rotations of the sacrum was not arbitrary. But it is somewhat of a "*double entendre*." In one sense it can be understood to mean the twisting movements of the sacrum in relation to the ilia. In another sense it can also be understood to mean the twisting motion at the lumbosacral junction, which is a consequence of the lumbar spine forming a sidebent curve with coupled rotation. It is the formation of this sidebent curve that shifts the load on the sacral base to one side or the other, causing sacral motion between the ilia.

Figure 3.8. Left sacral torsion on the left oblique axis with lumbars sidebending left. Left sacral torsion on the left oblique axis occurs with balanced or unloaded left sidebending of the lumbar spinal column, provided the normal lumbar lordosis is present. The load on the sacral base shifts to the right and forward, driving the sacral base inferior and forward on the right side. As the sacrum moves down the short arm of the right auricular surface, it moves down the long arm of the left auricular surface, bringing the left ILA posterior and a little inferior. The left sidebending lumbars rotate slightly to the right, counteracting the left rotation of the sacral base. This position of the sacrum and lumbars occurs at midstride when the weight is on the right foot. The incumbent weight on the sacral base is transmitted to the right ilium through the close-packed pivot at the lower pole of the right sacroiliac joint.

Neutral spinal biomechanics apply to the sidebending lumbars. If L3 is the apex of the curve, L3, L4, and L5 will sidebend left and rotate right. From L2 up to the cross-over, rotation and sidebending are coupled ipsilaterally.

Figure 3.9. Right sacral torsion on the right oblique axis with lumbars sidebending right. Right sacral torsion on the right oblique axis occurs with balanced or unloaded right sidebending of the lumbar spinal column, provided the normal lumbar lordosis is present. The load on the sacral base shifts to the left and forward, driving the sacral base inferior and forward on the left side. As the sacrum moves down the short arm of the left auricular surface, it moves down the long arm of the right auricular surface, bringing the right ILA posterior and a little anterior. The right sidebending lumbars rotate slightly to the left, as a group, counteracting the right rotation of the sacral base.

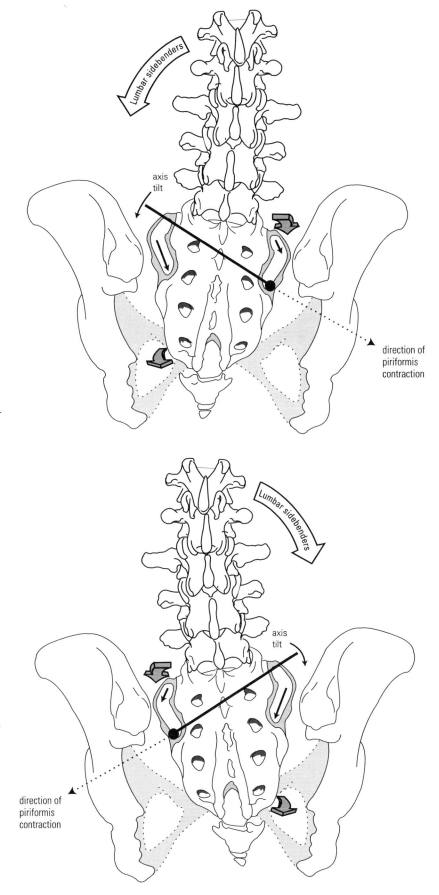

Figure 3.10. Backward torsion on the left oblique axis with lumbars sidebending right. When the lumbars are actively or passively sidebent right while the lumbar lordosis is absent or even kyphotic, the lumbosacral joint may buckle as the load force vector pushes backward on the sacral base and the sacrum becomes the lower end of the left convex curve by sidebending left and rotating right. The left ILA moves more anterior and slightly superior, following the direction of movement along the long arm of the left auricular surface.

In recumbent passive or active right sidebending of the spine the left oblique sacral axis may not be as stable as it is with sidebending that occurs standing or walking. This is because the right inferior pole pivot is not necessarily as close-packed as it would be from reflex *piriformis* contraction. When the muscles relax as they normally do, this movement is physiologic. When the muscles fail to relax, sacroiliac motion is impaired and the sacrum is unable to return to a symmetrical position.

Neutral spinal biomechanics also apply here, even though the lumbar lordosis is diminished.

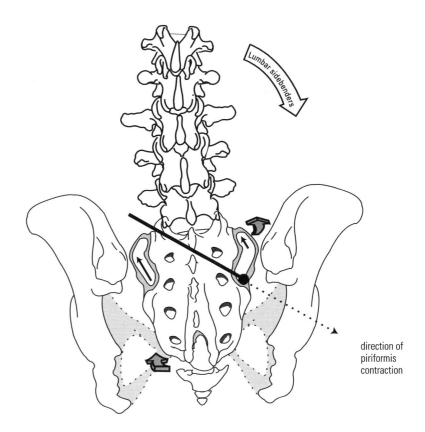

direction of piriformis contraction

Figure 3.11. Backward sacral torsion on the right oblique axis with lumbars sidebending left. Hypothetically, when the lumbars are sidebent left, actively or passively, with the lumbar lordosis lost, or even kyphotic, the lumbosacral joint may buckle as the load vector pushes backward on the sacral base and the sacrum becomes the lower end of the right convex curve by sidebending right and rotating left. The right ILA moves anterior and slightly superior, following the direction of movement along the long arm of the right auricular surface.

In lateral recumbent left sidebending of the spine the right oblique sacral axis may not be as stable as it is in the standing balanced sidebending, because the left inferior pole pivot is not necessarily close-packed.

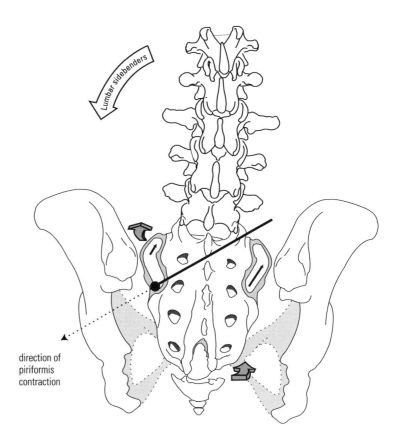

direction of piriformis contraction

The Walking Cycle and the Pelvis

Analyzing the walking cycle makes clear the physiologic need for sacral torsion movements, innominate rotation, and interpubic motion as outlined in the Mitchell model. These pelvic joint movements – which involve movement of the sacrum in relation to the ilia, and movement of the ilia relative to each other and to the sacrum – occur as passive movements. Although a few anatomists as early as the seventeenth century began to speculate that the sacrum might have some independent mobility, not until Mitchell, Sr. described the pelvic walking cycle (1948, 1958) had much been said about the purpose of that mobility except to suggest its role in parturition. The pelvic motions described in the Mitchell model assist in making the task of walking – which is to transport the weight of the body, one leg at a time, through space, while conserving energy and avoiding injury – more efficient. Among the reasons for treating a torsioned sacrum or a rotated innominate dysfunction is that the body has a use for those motions in the gait cycle.

Sacral motions occur as the sacrum is pushed by spinal, inertial, and elastic forces from above in available directions, which are based on joint anatomy and limited by the elastic tensions in the fascias of the spine. In the case of walking, the sacral motions are forward torsions on either the left or right oblique axis, depending on which side the piriformis is contracting to stabilize the inferior pole of the operant axis.

The ilia can be rotated in opposite directions in relation to each other by the elastic fascial tensions of the thigh and hip. These rotations are either anterior or posterior, and occur about the pubic transverse axis. Thus, one ilium may rotate anteriorly, while the other rotates posteriorly simultaneously.

The purpose of this section is to provide a rational theoretical model for the role that sacral torsions and innominate rotations play in the normal gait cycle, and the specific points in the gait cycle when these pelvic motions occur.

Original Walking Cycle as Described by Fred Mitchell, Sr.

From Structural Pelvic Function, Academy of Applied Osteopathy Yearbook (1958):

"The cycle of movement of the pelvis in walking will be described in sequence as though the patient were starting to walk forward by moving the right foot out first.

To permit the body to move forward on the right, trunk torsion in the thoracic area occurs to the left accompanied by lateral flexion to the left in the lumbar with movement of the lumbar vertebrae into the forming convexity to the right. There is a torsional locking at the lumbosacral junction as the body of the sacrum is moving to the left, thus shifting the weight to the left foot to allow lifting of the right foot. The shifting vertical center of gravity moves to the superior pole of the left sacroiliac, locking the mechanism into mechanical position to establish movement of the sacrum on the left oblique axis. This sets the pattern so that the sacrum can torsionally turn to the left, thereby the sacral base moves down on the right to conform to the lumbar C curve that is formed to the right."

Mitchell Sr. believed that the oblique axis reversal occurred at mid-stride, instead of at heel strike. We now believe that axis reversal occurs at heel strike.

"When the right foot moves forward there is a tensing of the quadriceps group of muscles and accumulating tension at the inferior pole of the right sacroiliac at the junction of the left oblique axis and inferior transverse axis. The movement is increased by the backward thrust of the restraining leg when the heel strikes the ground. As the heel contacts the ground, tension on the hamstring begins; as the weight swings upward to the crest of the femoral support, there is a slight posterior movement of the right innominate on the inferior transverse axis. The movement is also increased by the forward thrust of the propelling leg action. This ilial movement is also being influenced, directed and stabilized by the torsional movement on the transverse axis at the symphysis. From the standpoint of total pelvic movement one might consider the symphyseal axis as the postural axis of rotation for the entire pelvis.

As the right heel strikes the ground and trunk torsion and accommodation begin to reverse themselves, and as the left foot passes the right foot and weight passes over the crest of the femoral support, and the accumulating force from above moves to the right, the sacrum changes its axis to the right oblique axis and the sacral base moves forward on the left and torsionally turns to the right."

Note: *Since the walking cycle was described by Fred Mitchell, Sr., in 1958, the concept has undergone considerable metamorphosis and elaboration. The 1958 version of the pelvis model was a drastic departure from the pelvis described in Mitchell's 1948 article, indicating that most of the modern pelvic model developed during that decade. Mitchell's 1958 concept placed the establishment and maintenance of the sacral oblique axis ipsilateral with the stance leg. We will take exception to this and other aspects of that model. Our present working model was formulated in the 1970s and takes into account the evidence of EMG kinesiology of the walking cycle.*

Kinesiology of the Walking Cycle

Walking combines **phasic actions** of *gluteus maximus, biceps femoris, rectus femoris, gastrocnemius* and *tibialis anterior* muscles, with **tonic stabilizing functions** of the *piriformis, gluteus medius, medial hamstrings, vastus medialis* (Patia, 1991), and *peroneus* muscles. The ligaments and fascias of the hips and pelvis participate in the walking cycle both by stabilizing bone relationships in the antigravity chain of skeletal postural support, and also by storing elastic potential energy, which is later released as kinetic energy to assist the movements of locomotion. The sequential firing of the *piriformis* and *quadratus lumborum* muscles in the gait cycle is important in the Mitchell model, and can be extrapolated from the general concept that the muscle firing sequence progresses up the leg, through the pelvis, and into the contralateral lower back (Janda, 1985).

Phases of the Gait Cycle

The gait cycle can be analyzed in terms of its component sequential phases, the names of which are mostly self-explanatory: **heel strike, bipedal support, contralateral toe-off, propellant stance, ballistic stance, mid-stride and contralateral swing,** and **toe-off.** Propellant stance is the first part of the stance period when the *gluteus maximus* muscle acts to pull the pelvis forward. Bipedal support is a small fraction of the total cycle when both feet are on the ground; this phase ends shortly after the onset of propellant stance. Following propellant stance, the pelvis coasts forward by inertia through mid-stride and contralateral swing. Running essentially eliminates the bipedal support phase. The first step taken from a stationary stance is different in several respects from the steps taken after walking is already in progress.

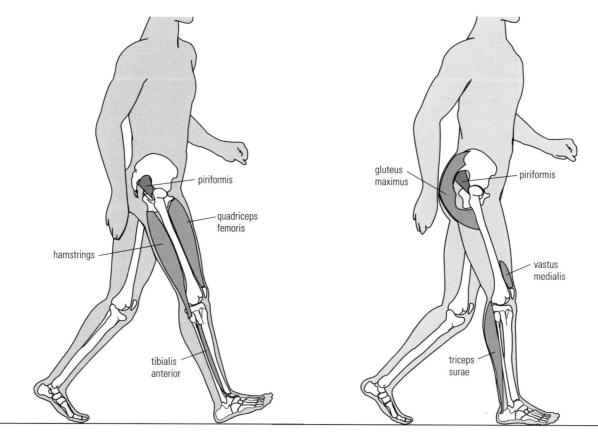

Figure 3.12. Right heel strike. Right *piriformis* tonically contracts reflexly to stabilize the sacrum on the right ilium, thereby establishing the left oblique axis; this in preparation for weight transmission through the sacrum to the right ilium. The sacrum's position, relative to the spine, is straight. The right innominate is completely rotated posteriorly, and the left innominate is almost fully rotated anteriorly. The right *tibialis anterior* fires eccentrically to prevent toe-slap.

Figure 3.13. Propellant stance and contralateral toe-off. Right *piriformis* contraction persists throughout the stance phase, stabilizing the left oblique instantaneous axis while it is in use. Sacral torsion to the left on the left oblique axis commences as the right rotated lumbars begin to sidebend left. The innominates begin to rotate from their extreme positions on the transverse pubic axis. The primary kinesiologic propellant, the right *gluteus maximus*, fires phasically to pull the pelvis forward, and then rests through the ballistic phase. Contralateral toe-off often assists propulsion through *sural* muscle action. The *hamstring, sural,* and *vastus* muscles continue to stabilize the knee.

The following description of the walking cycle begins with right heel strike. At right heel strike, the right innominate is completely posterior, the left innominate is *almost* completely anterior; the sacrum is straight, but the right *piriformis* is stabilizing the inferior pole of the left oblique axis before torsioning commences. At contralateral toe-off, the left innominate reaches maximum anterior rotation. Left swing rotates the left innominate posteriorly. Through left swing, the left *quadratus lumborum* contracts, first concentrically and then eccentrically, reaching its shortest length at mid-swing. The left sidebend of the lumbar caused by *quadratus lumborum* contraction, pushes the sacrum into left torsion on the left oblique axis, which reaches maximum at mid-stride/mid-swing. During the eccentric contraction of *quadratus lumborum*, the sacral torsion gradually straightens, becoming perfectly straight at left heel strike.

Gait studies in the laboratory (Inman, 1981; Rose, 1994)

have established the following partial sequence of muscle actions during the gait cycle. A few milliseconds prior to right heel strike, the phasic right *gluteus maximus* begins its contraction, which persists through the propellant stance phase. The contraction reaches maximum a few milliseconds after heel strike, and relaxes shortly thereafter. Having initiated hip extension to propel the pelvis and body forward with a powerful contraction, *gluteus maximus* rests and allows ballistic inertia to complete the forward pelvic translation during the stance period.

The right *gluteus medius* acts more like a tonic muscle. Having a shorter chronaxie, the *gluteus medius* begins its contraction 2 or 3 milliseconds before *gluteus maximus* and does not reach maximum until mid-stance, after which it begins to relax. Clearly the *gluteus medius* is acting as a hip abductor through right mid-stride, holding the left side of the pelvis up to prevent the swinging left foot from dragging on the ground.

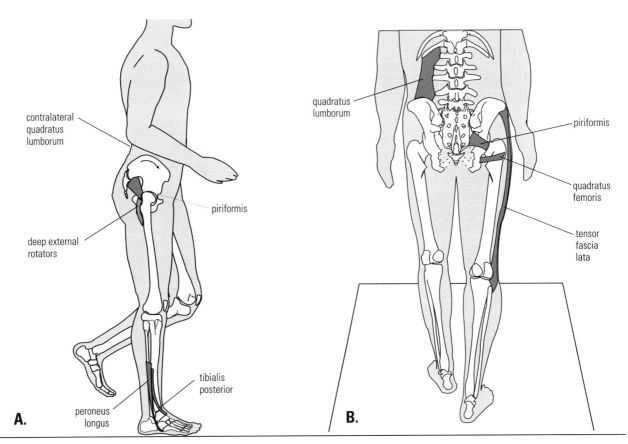

Figure 3.14. Ballistic stance, mid-stride, mid-swing.
A. Stirrup muscles – *tibialis posterior* and *peroneus longus* – fire myotatically in response to plantar stretch. The deep rotators turn the femur externally, stabilizing the acetabular joint, and close packing the knee and tarsal joints.

B. The right *tensor fascia lata*, along with right *gluteus medius* and left *quadratus lumborum* prevent Trendelenburg sagging of the left hip, avoiding stumbling. The *quadratus* sidebends the lumbar spine to the left, generating left sacral torsion on the left oblique axis. The left oblique axis is stabilized by the right *piriformis*, which continues contraction as long as weight is on the right leg.

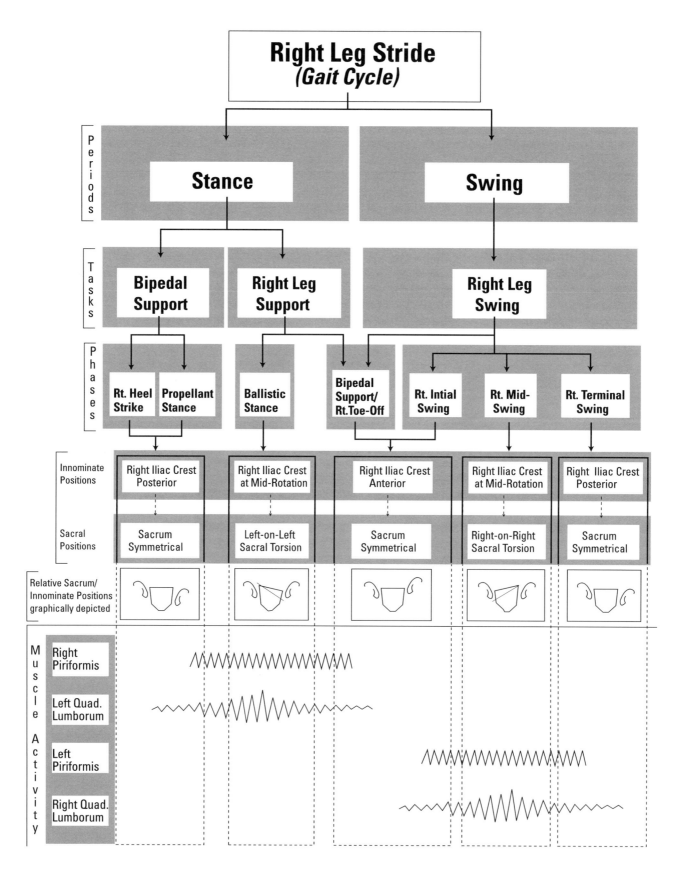

Figure 3.15. Phases of the gait. One full gait cycle is shown from right heel strike through right toe-off to right terminal swing. For the Mitchell model the important features are the activity of the *piriformis, quadratus lumborum,* and *latissimus dorsi* muscles, and the oscillations of the sacrum. Innominate rotations and sacral torsion are 90 degrees out of phase.

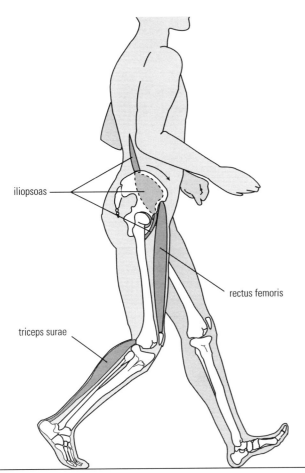

Figure 3.16. Preswing toe-off, left heel strike. The right *piriformis* has relaxed and the left *piriformis* has contracted in response to left heel strike. *Rectus femoris* and *iliopsoas* prepare to swing the femur forward. *Triceps surae* pushes the body forward before the foot leaves the ground.

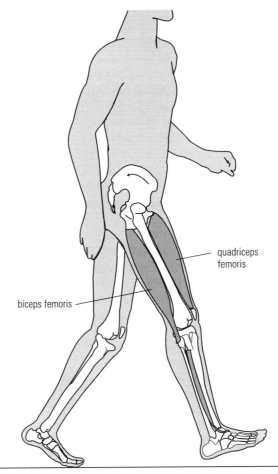

Figure 3.17. Right swing. The right *piriformis* remains relaxed through this ballistic phase of the gait cycle. The swinging leg passively rotates the right innominate posteriorly in relation to the left innominate which has been rotating anteriorly. The tonic *hamstring* and *quadriceps* muscles provide relative stability for the hip and knee, thus transferring the ballistic motion of the leg to the innominate.

Immediately after toe-off, the right *rectus femoris*, a phasic muscle, contracts forcibly to throw the right femur into flexion as the gait cycle proceeds to swing phase. As the right leg gains inertia in the swing phase, the tonus of the muscle gradually reduces in a controlled eccentric isotonic contraction. The inertia of the swinging leg is transmitted to the pelvis through the hamstring, rotating the right innominate crest posteriorly on the transverse pubic axis. The action of the *vastus medialis*, which began at mid-swing to straighten the knee (and persists through heel strike, propellant stance, and mid-stride) is assisted by the dwindling tonus in the *rectus femoris*. Part of the *quadriceps* muscle, *vastus medialis* (Figure 3.13), a weakness-prone muscle, acts to stabilize the straightened knee, and fires strongest after heel strike. *Rectus femoris* fires at the beginning of the swing phase.

Starting in terminal swing phase the right *biceps femoris* and the *medial hamstrings* sustain their contractions through the first half of the stance period (which includes the phases of heel strike, bipedal support, propellant stance,

and mid-stride), with the biceps predominating to assist in the lateral rotation of the tibia as the knee extends. Working together, the knee flexors and extensors stabilize the knee.

Right *tibialis anterior* (Figure 3.12) contracts in anticipation of heel strike and sustains contraction through mid-stride, when it is joined by *tibialis posterior* and *peroneus longus* (Figure 3.14) in a myotatic reflex jerk to close-pack the tarsal arch for increased weight support, while the foot and ankle are inverted by the externally rotating leg.

Extrapolating hypothetically from these data, it is reasonable to assume, at least until proven wrong, that the deep femur external rotators – right *obturators, gemelli, quadratus femoris*, and, especially, the *piriformis* muscles (Figure 3.12) – contract throughout the stance to stabilize the hip and sacroiliac joints. The point of sacroiliac stabilization provided by the right *piriformis* is a pivot on the inferior pole of the right sacroiliac joint. Weight bearing, through a chain of close-packed bones (fifth lumbar, sacrum, ilium), runs through this oblique axis. Anterior rotation of the right ilium on the sacrum, and forward sacral torsion on the left oblique axis (Left-on-Left) between the ilia (a consequence of left lumbar sidebending caused by the *quadratus lumborum* pulling the iliac crest toward the ribs to prevent the swinging foot from dragging on the ground) may all occur simultaneously.

Being a tonic, stabilizer type of muscle, the *piriformis* is prone to abnormal shortness, usually on the right side. Such unilateral shortness may inhibit function of the opposite *piriformis*, rendering the contralateral sacroiliac joint less stable during its stance period. This circumstance has potential for increased nociception from the contralateral sacroiliac joint, which may manifest sciatic pain referred from *gluteal* myofascial trigger points (Travell). When *piriformis* contracture is more extreme, it may compress the sciatic nerve, causing numbness, paresthesia, and/or spasm or atrophy of leg muscles. Sciatic entrapment is more likely to occur in the small percentage of anatomic variants in which the sciatic nerve, or some part of it, pierces the piriformis muscle instead of taking its normal course through the sciatic notch below the *piriformis.*

Thus, at the moment of right heel strike we assume that the right innominate is in a posteriorly rotated position, and the left innominate is anteriorly rotated. The spine and sacrum are straight, although the thoracolumbar spine is axially rotated right and the cervicothoracic spine is rotated left. When the *piriformis* anchors the sacrum to the inferior pole of the right sacroiliac joint at right heel strike, the weight is shifted to the right leg, and the right ilium begins its anterior rotation on the sacrum. The sacrum begins to rotate on its left oblique (diagonal) axis turning its anterior surface to the left by dropping the right side of the sacral base forward and inferior on the short arm of the right sacroiliac joint and bringing the left ILA posterior and inferior on the long arm of the left sacroiliac joint. The sacrum attains maximum torsion to the left on the left oblique axis at mid-stance when the action of the contralateral *quadratus lumborum* is greatest, and then derotates to be straight at left heel strike.

As the right heel strikes the ground, the right toes are being dorsiflexed by the action of *extensor hallucis* and *extensor digitorum* muscles, and the right ankle prior to heel strike has been dorsiflexed by contraction of the *tibialis anterior* muscle. After heel strike, as the pelvis and leg move forward over the right (stance) foot, *tibialis anterior* will perform an eccentric isotonic contraction to slow the rate of contact of the forefoot with the ground, preventing toe slap. After the forefoot has contacted the ground, *tibialis* remains relaxed (electromyographically quiet) until mid-stride.

Just prior to heel strike, *hamstrings* have acted to slow the rotating tibia at the knee, which is straightening. Its tonus persists at heel strike and after, as it stabilizes the knee and the hip.

Role of Striated Muscles in Movements of Passive Pelvic Joints

As already noted in introducing the Mitchell model of the pelvis, the joint between sacrum and ilium is essentially a passive joint, although the *piriformis* muscle, as well as occasional fibers from *gluteus maximus*, crosses the joint. The *piriformis* muscle serves as the stabilizer of the diagonal axis of the sacral torsion motion, but it does not move the sacrum on the ilium. There are no muscles crossing the sacroiliac joint which cause sacral movement on the ilium or ilial movement on the sacrum. With the exception of the pubic symphysis subluxations, which are treated by altering the length and tonus of thigh or abdominal muscles, all treatments of subluxations and somatic dysfunctions of the pelvis are treatments of passive joints, even though the patient's muscles may be used in the treatment.

The joints of the pelvis are stabilized by striated muscles, fascia, and ligaments. These muscles play no direct role in causing movement in the joints of the pelvis. However, when striated muscles move the bones of the spine or lower limbs, the movement of those bones exerts mechanical forces on the sacrum and innominates which result in their movement *relative to each other.* For this reason the joints of the pelvis are spoken of as passive joints. However, these small movements of the pelvic joints are very important in the ergonomic dynamics of the body.

Unilateral Sacral Flexion Movement

With unbalanced sidebending of the trunk, unilateral sacral flexion may occur. Unilateral sacral flexion is inferior movement of the sacrum on one side, with the sacrum following the short and long arms of the same auricular surface. The movement of the sacrum along this arcuate path involves some contralateral rotation of the sacral base.

When the sacrum sidebends in that manner it is able to move farther than it would if it were doing pure sidebending, i.e., rotation about an A-P axis. This arcuate path can be visualized as a swinging of the sacrum on the posterior sacroiliac ligaments with the sacrum twisting around an A-P axis as its base moves inferiorly. (Figures 3.18. A. and B.) The net result is a marked sidebend of the sacrum with superior/inferior asymmetry of the inferior lateral angles of the sacrum on the order of 1-2 centimeters. Inferior displacement of the ILA is always accompanied by some posterior displacement, consistent with the "track" of the long arm of the sacroiliac joint. Such movements are not, strictly speaking, torsion movements; with torsion movements, the rotation component predominates.

For those readers who find it difficult to visualize a unilateral sacral flexion movement, a model resembling a playground swing may be helpful (Fig. 3.19). The seat of the swing is analogous to the sacrum, the ropes represent the axial ligament portion of the posterior sacroiliac ligaments, and the frame represents the innominates.

When the sacrum is hanging on these ligaments, and not

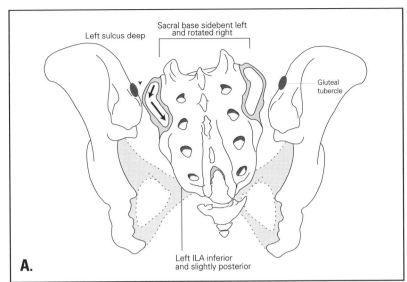
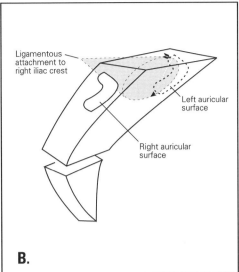

Figure 3.18. A and B. Left unilateral sacral flexion. The left sulcus gets deeper and the left ILA moves more inferior. The sacrum slides on the left auricular surface, but very little on the right surface. Left sacral sidebending can be compared to the sacral nutation which occurs with spinal hyper-extension, except that the nutation occurs on one side only. The motion of the sacrum could be described as rotations around instantaneous axes, all of which pass through a common point located where the posterior sacroiliac ligament attaches to the right iliac crest. The base of the sacrum goes down the short arm of the auricular surface of the left ilium, making the left sacroiliac sulcus deeper as the base of the sacrum sidebends left and rotates right in relation to the ilium. The long arm of the iliac auricular surface is directed inferiorly and posteriorly, and guides the left ILA into a left sidebent, left rotated position in relation to the cardinal planes of the body. (Scale proportions were altered for graphic clarity)

close-packed on an innominate, it is free to nutate by swinging on the ligaments, just like the seat of a swing. Any child knows that swings do not always swing straight; sometimes they twist on the chains as they swing back and forth. The sacrum can also swing with a twist, resulting in one side traveling farther than the other.

The paths for this uneven swinging motion are the sacroiliac auricular surfaces on the innominates, which guide the sides of the sacrum in an arc.

The symmetrical swinging movements of the sacrum can be generically described as sacral flexion or extension on the superior transverse axis. When one side of the sacrum swings through a longer arc than the other side, moving the ILA inferiorly and posteriorly on that side, the sacrum can be said to be unilaterally flexing on that side. This motion is a physiologic response to unbalanced sacral base loading with trunk sidebending.

The superior transverse axis is still operating, in a way, because the sacrum swings on the posterior sacroiliac ligaments. But the mathematical description of the instantaneous axis of the motion would orient the axis more anteroposterior, since the asymmetric position assumed by the sacrum is mainly sidebent (Figure 3.18.B.)

When the sacrum sidebends left by following a longer arc on the left auricular surface, the left side of the sacral base goes anterior as it slides down the short arm of the "L" and the ILA, sliding down the long arm of the "L" is guided slightly posteriorly.

Thus, the sidebending-rotation coupling, as it was described for the sacral torsion motions, is similar for the unilateral flexion motion, in that the sacral base continues to couple sidebending and rotation contralaterally. But the two motions are different quantitatively. **Torsion of the sacrum is more of a rotation; whereas unilateral flexion is more of a sidebending. With torsion, ILA displacement is more posterior and less inferior; with unilateral sacral flexion, ILA displacement is mostly inferior and not much posterior.**

Lumbosacral Mechanics

There is some question as to how L_5 and the sacrum will move at the lumbosacral joint when the sacrum is torsioning or unilaterally flexing. To answer this question, we must be perfectly clear whether normal physiologic motion or abnormal dysfunctional motion (or motion restriction) is being described.

Generally, the rotation of the sacral base is opposite to the direction of rotation in a sidebending lumbar group; hence, the twist. This principle is equally true for both sacral torsion motion and unilateral sacral flexion motion. However, the fifth lumbar may, at times, act like a mobile segment of the sacrum, and rotate with the sacrum, sidebending ipsilaterally. In this case the twist occurs at the next vertebral segment above.

In normal physiologic movements, the lumbosacral joint has a greater repertoire of rotation-sidebending coupling than it has in lumbosacral dysfunction. There is some research evidence that rotation-sidebending of the lum-

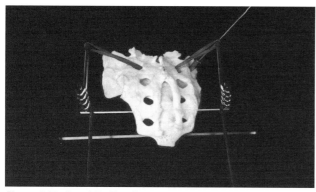 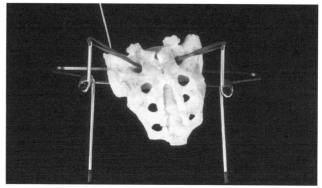

Figure 3.19. A and B. The above pictures have the sacrum suspended by a rubber band and attached to a metal frame through the posterior foramen between S_1 and S_2. The rubber band serves to mimic the function and support of the Ligament of Zaglas, which suspends the sacrum like a "swing." **The picture on the left demonstrates left torsion on the left oblique axis**; the sacral base rotated left and sidebent right, and the left ILA is posterior and a little inferior. **The picture on the right demonstrates left unilateral flexion**; the sacral base is sidebent left and a little right rotated, and the left ILA inferior and a little posterior.

bosacral joint is consistently ipsilateral, similar to a cervical intervertebral joint (Bogduk, 1991). This data is based on axial rotation as the *initial* movement; so far, coupled motions with initiated sidebending have not been researched. If Bogduk's postulate is borne out by future research, only a slight adjustment of the sacral torsion model will be necessary.

For now, let us assume that L_5 is normally capable of neutral (Type I) motion, (i.e., a small amount of contralateral rotation), in response to initiated sidebending. Thus, with loaded *balanced* neutral sidebending of the lumbar spine to the right, forming a group curve convex to the left, the left side of the sacral base is pushed inferior and anterior. The sacral base, then, is sidebent left and rotated right (right on right torsion).

In this example, there are two possible scenarios for how the fifth lumbar moves relative to the sacrum, each of them consistent with clinical observations: sidebending and rotation may be coupled contralaterally, or ipsilaterally.

In the first scenario, the fifth lumbar acts like the lowest segment of a group curve and counter-rotates toward the convexity, i.e., in the opposite direction from sacral base rotation. Thus, the fifth lumbar can be said to have reversed every aspect of sacral base motion – rotation, sidebending, and flexion (nutation). Sidebending and rotation are reversed by the fifth lumbar by simply following the law of neutral sidebending of groups of vertebrae. Because the sacral base moved forward, the fifth lumbar (and usually other lumbar segments) bend backward increasing lordosis, in order to maintain postural balance.

The amount of fifth lumbar counterrotation varies relative to the sacrum and relative to the amount of sidebending, depending to some extent on the orientation of the zygapophyseal joints. Such rotation is favored by intermediate or coronal facet orientation. The counterrotation may involve several adjacent lumbar segments up to the apex of the group curve, where derotation commences. In this case, the fifth lumbar, compared to the coronal plane

of the body, may appear to be slightly rotated in the same direction as the sacral base.

In the second scenario, the fifth lumbar left rotates (with the right sidebending group) and left sidebends as it bends backwards. To date, no anatomic basis for ipsilateral sidebending-rotation coupling has been proposed; it has simply been observed in experiments where the initial movement was axial rotation of the spine. Such ipsilateral coupling is analogous to the ipsilateral rotation-sidebending which normally occurs above the apex of an adaptive group curve. In this case, the lumbosacral junction is the apex of the lumbosacral group curve. A group curve with the apex at the lumbosacral junction is not constituted the way normal group curves are since it includes the sacrum as the lower half of the curve. This mechanism may have a brief existence, even when the balanced sidebending is an adaptation to leg length asymmetry, since the ipsilateral rotation/sidebending is predisposed to convert to non-neutral dysfunction. (see Volume 1).

Loaded, unbalanced, neutral sidebending of the lumbar spine will push the sacral base down on the same side as the sidebend. If, in response, the sidebending at the sacral base were to occur as an oblique axis torsion, it would be sidebending and rotating in the same directions as the lumbar segments. {**Note:** This is a physiologic possibility. But when this combination is seen with sacroiliac dysfunction, it means that a Type II lumbosacral dysfunction exists concurrently.}

Normally, unbalanced lumbar sidebending to the right causes the sacrum to sidebend on only one sacroiliac joint, the joint ipsilateral to the direction of the sidebend. Such movement may be characterized as "unilateral sacral flexion on the right" in contrast to sacral torsion. As the sacrum adapts to the lumbar load shift to the right, the sacrum slides down the arc of the entire right sacroiliac auricular surface. This will occur if the load on the sacrum is supported by the posterior sacroiliac ligaments instead of on the left iliac bone at the inferior pole of the left auricular

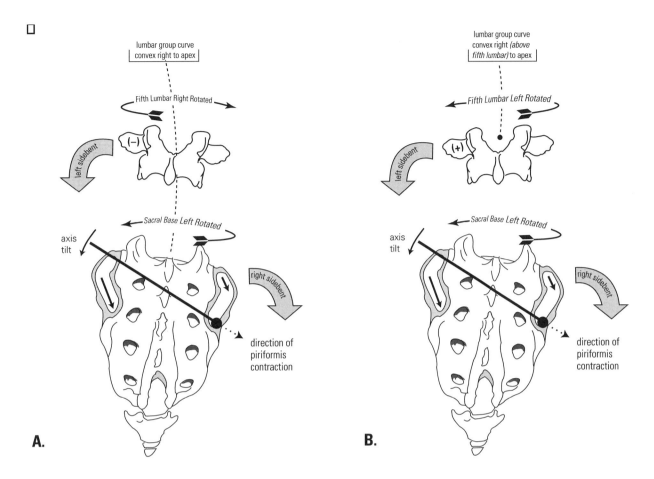

A.

B.

Figure 3.20. A and B. A. With Left-on-Left sacral torsion, the fifth lumbar normally twists in opposite directions from the sacral base, in effect tightening the lumbosacral joint. Sometimes the fifth lumbar mainly sidebends opposite the sacral base and rotates as if it were a segment above the apex of a scoliotic curve (not Type 2 mechanics). Spinal compensation for sacral base rotation occurs higher up, in that case.

surface, as it is with balanced right sidebending. The right sidebending L_5 normally rotates to the left, the same direction as the sacral rotation with right sacral flexion. So far, this describes a physiologic event, which will reverse itself when the spine straightens. If, however, in the process of sidebending and straightening the trunk, a sacroiliac dysfunction is produced (i.e., sacrum flexed on the right), the straightened spine is obliged to adapt to the sacral base asymmetry by forming a right convex curve. This requires L_5 to sidebend left and rotate right.

When lumbar sidebending occurs from a flexed position, standing or sitting, there is a tendency for the sacrum to move into backward torsion, because of the cephalad traction of the erector spinae muscles on one side of the sacrum. Thus, flexed right sidebending may produce sacral torsion to the left on the right oblique axis.

Sidebending the lumbar spine from a hyperextended position, on the other hand, may produce unilateral sacral flexion on either side, depending on whether the load on the sacral base shifts to the right or the left. Hyperextended lateral flexion may be balanced or unbalanced, in other words.

Recumbent lateral flexion of the lumbar spine, i.e.,

unloaded, is more likely to produce a forward torsion movement of the sacrum, unless the lumbosacral joint is flexed. Flexed unloaded sidebending can produce a backward torsion movement.

As pointed out earlier, sacroiliac joint anatomy limits sacral axial rotation to a miniscule movement. If the sacrum is obliged to passively follow axial rotation of the fifth lumbar, it tends to do it with a forward torsion movement, the only way sacral rotation is reasonably free. Thus, left axial rotation should produce left-on-left sacral torsion, automatically converting axial rotation of the lumbar spine to contralaterally coupled rotation/sidebending of the sacrum.

Intrapelvic Adaptive Mechanics

Given that the descriptions of unilateral sacral flexion and sacral torsion have been derived from observed asymmetries due to somatic dysfunction, and not based on radiogrammetry, it is important to note that in the presence of sacroiliac dysfunction there is *automatic* adaptive interinnominate displacement. This innominate adaptation typically displaces the anterior superior spines' symmetry one to two centimeters. Because of the inter-innominate displacement, which changes the relationship of the left innominate relative to the right, a system of coordinates based on iliac landmarks will not correspond to the cardinal planes and x, y, z axes of the body.

The Sacral Base/ILA Paradox Revisited

Earlier in the chapter, the paradox of how the sacral base can exhibit contralaterally coupled rotation and sidebending while – simultaneously – the ILA exhibits ipsilateral coupling was addressed. The mechanics of this paradox were partly explained in terms of the sacrum tracking the auricular surfaces of the sacroiliac joints, and the "tipping" of the superior pole of the oblique axis. But even armed with that explanation, it is not uncommon for clinicians to experience some confusion when, in the course of practice, they encounter a sacrum *positioned* with the sacral base contralaterally sidebent and rotated, while the ILA is ipsilaterally sidebent and rotated.

Remember that in applying Muscle Energy clinically, we evaluate joint function by assessing the static position of bony landmarks, before and after movement or, in some cases, treatment. The observed sacral positions can only be understood, and an accurate diagnosis rendered, by relating the findings from physical examination to the Mitchell model of pelvic biomechanics. For example, a determination that the sacral base is in a sidebent position is not made from a directly observable phenomenon, i.e., it is not *visually* apparent in physical examination. Rather, it is determined by relating the *felt* sulcus depth to a model of sacroiliac arthrokinematics. If the sulcus is deeper on one side as compared to the other, then, based on the Mitchell model, it can be inferred that either the sacral base has slid down the short arm on that side, or slid up the short arm on the other side. Either way, the sacral base is rotated away and sidebent towards the side with the deeper sulcus.

In point of fact, the Mitchell model of pelvic mechanics was originally developed by Mitchell, Sr. to explain the paradoxical findings he encountered in practice, and then later was further refined by Mitchell, Jr., after years of teaching and clinical application, as well as relevant research findings (his own and others) that came to light after Mitchell, Sr. died in 1974.

To better explain and clarify, in a rational way, how this paradoxical positioning is possible, involves considering two things: the unique anatomy of the sacrum and the reference points employed by the evaluation methodology. A uniquely different set of coordinates is used when assessing the position and movement of the sacral base (based on innominate bone landmarks) versus the ILAs, (which are compared to the standard cardinal planes of the body). The reason that these two landmarks – the sacral base and the ILAs – are evaluated within two different frames of reference has to do with the biconvex shape of the posterior sacrum and its orientation relative to the iliac crests and the cardinal planes of the body.

The sacrum's orientation to the cardinal planes is difficult to describe because of its curved shape. Its base is sharply tipped forward, yet a plane tangent to the sacro-coccygeal curve at its most posterior point would be approximately parallel to the coronal plane, i.e., because of the curvature of the bone, the fifth sacral segment posterior surface faces almost straight back. Furthermore, even though anatomic illustrations depict the sacrum as if it were flat and in a coronal plane with its posterior surface facing straight backward, the first sacral segment is normally tipped forward 41±1 degrees (modified Ferguson's angle).

When the sacral base is evaluated *clinically*, its position is determined in relation to the iliac crests. The procedure relies on the felt depth of the sacral sulci in relation to the left and right iliac crests, which are palpated simultaneously – by pressing the two thumbs just medial to the iliac crests at the level of S_1 – on a prone patient. By examining the patient in the prone position, the ASISs and pubis are stabilized by the surface of the examination table, making the left and right iliac crests more reliable points of reference for determining sulcus depth. The determination should be entirely a palpatory experience, and not at all visual. Palpating the sacral base without touching the iliac crests leads to visual comparison with the cardinal planes of the body – *which is not recommended*.

Often, because of the examiner's perspective, the deeper sulcus is interpreted as the sacral base being "anterior" on that side. However, we must be careful when using the terms "anterior" and "posterior" to describe the sacral base because the "anterior" surface of S_1 does not face straight anteriorly; it faces infero-anteriorly, almost as much inferior as anterior. When we say that the sacral base, one or both sides, is "anterior," it really is inferior-anterior; hence, the sacral base is sidebent (i.e., inferior) one way and rotated the other as a result of the anterior displacement. The short arm of the sacroiliac auricular surface tracks movement in this direction, or its reverse. The wideness of the joint track apparently provides enough slack to permit the movement of torsion and unilateral flexion as they are described.

The deepness of the sulcus is due almost as much to inferior displacement of the sacral base as to its anterior displacement. Since the sacrum adapts its position to the relative innominate positions as they rotate in relation to each other, the position of the sacral base relative to the cardinal planes of the body is not a good indicator of sacroiliac motion, which is movement of the sacrum *in relation to the innominates*. Thus, the sacral base should be compared to points on the iliac crests, and not to the cardinal planes of the body.

By comparison, the portion of the curved sacrum where the ILAs are found lies in a plane which is more or less consistent with the coronal plane of the body. Additionally, because of the shallow location of the ILA under the skin, the ILA is a more reliable landmark for visual assessment of the sacroiliac joint, and more amenable to describing its position relative to the cardinal planes of the body.

CHAPTER 4

Overview of Manipulable Disorders of the Pelvis

S ix types of manipulable disorders of the pelvis can be distinguished: **subluxations, sacroiliac dysfunctions, iliosacral dysfunctions, breathing movement impairments, visceral dysfunctions and malpositions, and craniosacral dysfunction.** Of these six, the first three can be classified as *locomotor dysfunctions*. Although sacroiliac and iliosacral both refer to the same joint anatomically, they are classified separately because sacroiliac dysfunctions are caused by spinal forces, whereas iliosacral dysfunctions are caused by forces from the lower limbs. The term **pelvic dysfunction** is generic and may refer to any of the above except subluxation.

Subluxation is defined as an incomplete dislocation, or minor dislocation. Normal movement functions are lost when joints dislocate or subluxate, putting a bone anatomically out of place. A **somatic dysfunction (joint dysfunction) is a loss of normal movement function,** *without any dislocation* **of the joint.** Historically, subluxations and dysfunctions were indiscriminately called "lesions," without attempting to distinguish between them.

Pelvic subluxations include:
• **pubic symphyseal dislocation (subluxation) of the pubic bones**— also described as a **vertical shear** of the pubic symphysis or **pubic subluxation;**
• **upslipped innominate,** which can be described as an **inferior shear of the sacrum on the ilium**, not to be confused with unilateral anterior nutation of the sacrum – a somatic dysfunction;
• **innominate inflare** (rhomboid pelvis), which is manifested by a lateral asymmetry of the ASIS (in the transverse plane) toward midline (i.e. umbilicus);
• **innominate outflare** (rhomboid pelvis), which is manifested by a lateral asymmetry of the ASIS (in the transverse plane) away from the midline.

Note: Flare lesions may be reliably diagnosed only after innominate rotation has been successfully treated.

Subluxations are fairly common in the pelvic joints, and, when present, may stress the whole body. Pelvic subluxations may be caused by persistent stabilizer muscle imbalance, as is the case with pubic subluxation; or by physical trauma, as with upslipped

In this chapter:

■ *Subluxations of the pelvis*
  • *Pubic subluxations*
  • *Upslipped innominate*
  • *Innominate flared lesions*

■ *Sacroiliac dysfunctions*
  • *Flexed sacrum*
  • *Forward torsioned sacrum*
  • *Backward torsioned sacrum*

■ *Iliosacral dysfunctions*
  • *Anterior and posterior innominate dysfunction*

■ *Manipulable muscle imbalance*

■ *Respiratory sacroiliac dysfunction*

■ *Oscillating sacrum*

Table 4.A.

The Six Types of Manipulable Pelvic Disorders, and Possible Variants for Each:

1. **Subluxations** – *caused by trauma or muscle imbalance*:
   a. Pubic symphyseal dislocation or subluxation (designated either up or down on the left or right side);
   b. Upslipped innominate (generally manifest on the left *or* right side – but can be bilateral);
   c. Rhomboid pelvis (designated as flared in or out on either the left or right side).

2. **Sacroiliac Dysfunction** – *caused by spinal forces from above, altering ligamentous-articular mobility of the sacrum*:
   a. Unilaterally flexed sacrum (designated left or right for the side the dysfunction is present – *or* may be bilateral);
   b. Torsioned sacrum (designated as left or right torsioned about either the left or right oblique axis).

3. **Iliosacral Dysfunction** – *caused by abnormal movements of the lower limbs, altering osseous-articular mobility of one ilium*:
   a. Anteriorly rotated innominate (designated left or right for the side the dysfunction is present);
   b. Posteriorly rotated innominate (designated left or right for the side the dysfunction is present).

4. **Breathing movement impairments** – *caused by pelvic edema or compression of the sacroiliac joint*:
   Sacroiliac respiratory restriction (designated left or right for the side the dysfunction is present – *or* may be bilateral).

5. **Craniosacral dysfunction** – *caused by cranial dysfunction*:
   Sacral oscillation (either of a rotary or lateral flexion type, or some combination of both). Each oscillation cycle is approximately 10 seconds long.

6. **Pelvic visceral dysfunction** – *caused by trauma or faulty postural statics*. See Woodall (1926), and for a less mechanical perspective, Barral and Mercier (1988).

For those in clinical practice, the following provides the ICD 9 CM codes for the diagnoses listed above:

1.a. Pubic symphyseal dislocation [839.69]	2.a. & b. Sacroiliac dysfunction [739.4]	4. Breathing movement impairments [739.4]
1.b. Upslipped innominate [839.42 or 718.35]	3.a. & b. Anteriorly/posteriorly rotated	5. Craniosacral dysfunction [739.0]
1.c. Rhomboid pelvis [718.25]	innominate [739.5]	

---

innominate lesions. The traumatic subluxation is distinguished from pelvic dislocation only as a matter of degree. It is possible that many "subluxations" may have microscopic tissue avulsion, but this fact is not easily ascertained clinically. Both dislocation and subluxation produce joint hypermobility.

In addition, subluxations impair the physiologic movement functions of the pelvic joints, sometimes bizarrely displacing the bony landmarks used to detect the presence of somatic dysfunction in the pelvis. Subluxation disrupts some of the axes for physiologic motion, preventing effective treatment for somatic dysfunction. For these reasons *subluxations are looked for and treated, if necessary, before attempting to diagnose or treat somatic dysfunctions of the pelvis*.

Sacroiliac dysfunction is caused by excessive or persistent abnormal loading of the sacral base by the spine from faulty lifting or muscle imbalance. Additionally, scoliosis, spinal segmental dysfunctions, spine trauma, even head/neck trauma produces abnormal asymmetric spinal forces. The sacrum adapts its position to these forces, and, over time, may lose the ability to assume other positions. Many of the principles and mechanics of the physiologic motions of torsion and unilateral sacral flexion, as described in Chapter 3, can also be used to describe the sacroiliac dysfunctions herein denoted as a *torsioned* or unilaterally *flexed* sacrum. As the past tense would indicate, a sacrum that presents such dysfunctions is one which has become static or restricted somewhere, and to some degree, in the range of the normal physiologic motions discussed in Chapters 2 and 3.

Iliosacral dysfunction is initiated by myofascial tension

imbalance in the hips and legs; as it becomes more chronic, the movement restriction may be maintained by shortened sacroiliac ligaments.

Of the two non-locomotor disorders, one type affects **breathing movements** (also known as respiratory restriction). The cause of impaired sacroiliac breathing movement is pelvic edema, which may cause synovial gelosis in the sacroiliac joint. The second type of disorder is an oscillatory movement phenomenon of the sacrum caused by osseous-articular dysfunction of cranial sutures. The corrective treatment for this **craniosacral dysfunction** is applied to the cranium, not to the pelvis.

Both sacroiliac or iliosacral dysfunction, as well as respiratory and craniosacral dysfunction, can result in the presentation of a wide range of symptoms, or in some cases may even be temporarily asymptomatic. The purpose of this chapter is to outline the different varieties of pelvic dysfunction, presenting an account of the mechanics of these dysfunctions sufficient to interpret clinical findings and to understand the rationale for treatment.

This overview of manipulable disorders of the pelvis will begin with the possible subluxations of the pelvis, i.e., pubic symphyseal subluxation, upslipped innominate and ilial inflare/outflare (also known as rhomboid pelvis). From there, we will examine the two varieties of sacroiliac dysfunction (the unilaterally flexed sacrum and the torsioned sacrum), followed by the iliosacral dysfunctions (anteriorly rotated and posteriorly rotated innominate), a brief discussion of muscle imbalance, and concluding with a discussion of the non-locomotor dysfunctions of the pelvis: respiratory restriction and craniosacral dysfunction.

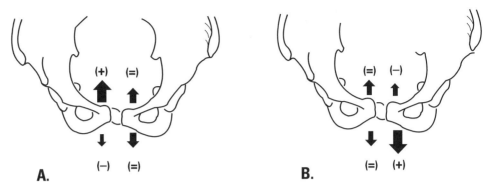

Figure 4.1. Pubic subluxation may be up on one side **(A)**, *or* down on the other side **(B)**, depending on which side has muscle imbalance. The size of the down and up arrows on either side of the symphysis indicate muscle balance (same size – "=" signs) or imbalance (disparate size – "+" or "-" signs).

A.

B.

Subluxations of the Pelvis
Pubic Symphyseal Dislocation or Subluxation

The most common subluxations of the pelvis are inferior or superior pubic shears. Without the aponeurotic extensions of the *transversus, obliquus, rectus abdominis,* and the adductor muscles of the hip, the pubic symphysis would permit 3 to 6 millimeters of vertical shear without avulsion. Based on clinical observation, the symphysis appears to have no *intrinsic* stabilizing structures to hold the pubic bones firmly in place, and in symmetrical relationship with each other. The diagnosis is made by precise palpatory location of the pubic crests while observing for superior/inferior asymmetry. When such asymmetry exists, one side is normal and the other side is subluxated. **The subluxated side consistently has impaired (restricted) movement in the ipsilateral sacroiliac joint, which can be detected by a standing flexion mobility test.**

Positional stability of the pubic symphysis is provided by the abdominal and thigh muscles whose motor nerves originate in the lower thoracic and upper lumbar segments. Thus, when the integrity of this myotonic stabilizing mechanism is compromised, it is no surprise that one frequently finds dysfunction and stress affecting the thoracolumbar region. The altered muscle tonus that accompanies a pubic subluxation is sometimes palpable in the abdomen or thighs. MET consistently restores the integrity of the myotonic stabilizing system (at least temporarily), even when the spinal dysfunction is still present. MET applied to the normal side will simply have no effect.

Impairment of movement functions in the pelvis or sacroiliac joint significantly stress postural adaptive mechanisms, locomotor functions, and circulatory dynamics, as well as trophic and regulatory nervous system functions. Pubic subluxation may be accompanied by dysuria, urinary frequency, hesitancy, incontinence, or suprapubic pain or discomfort, leading to a clinical diagnosis of cystitis. However, in such cases, the urine cultures frequently grow no pathogens.

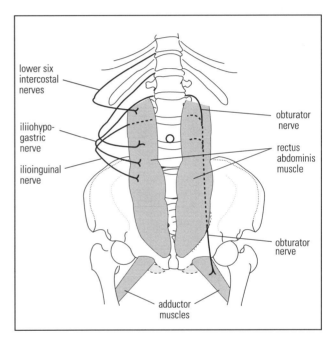

lower six intercostal nerves

iliohypo-gastric nerve

ilioinguinal nerve

obturator nerve

rectus abdominis muscle

obturator nerve

adductor muscles

Figure 4.2. Muscular stability of the pubic symphysis. The muscles which stabilize the relationship of the pubic bones to each other, prinicipally the rectus abdominis and the thigh adductors are innervated by nerves from the lower thoracic and upper three lumbar segments. Quite obviously, maintaining this stable relationship in various circumstances of locomotion requires a lot of trans-segmental interneuron activity. This finely tuned neural activity may be disrupted by somatic dysfunction anywhere in the lower back, resulting in abnormal positioning of a pubic bone – a pubic subluxation.

Summary of Diagnostic Criteria for Pubic Subluxation:
■ Superior or inferior pubic crest malalignment;

■ Positive standing flexion test on the side of the lesion;

■ Suprapubic and ilioinguinal tenderness is variable;

■ Thigh and abdominal muscle imbalance is sometimes palpable.

MET Principles for Treatment of Pubic Subluxation:
■ Co-contraction of imbalanced muscles or their antagonists resets the interneuron reflexes.

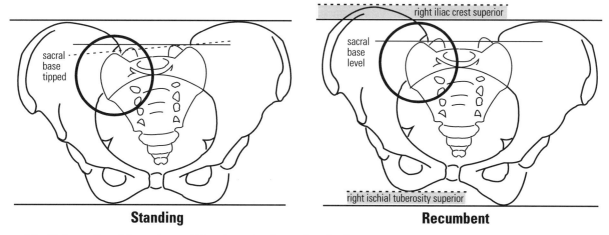

Figure 4.3. Right upslipped innominate. When the patient is standing, the iliac crests look level; the sacrum is sheared down on the ilium. When the patient lies down, the sacrum becomes straight with the spine, and the right innominate is displaced superiorly. The horizontal line on top of the left illustration represents equal iliac crest heights with the subject standing. The two horizontal lines on the right illustration show a level sacral base with the body supine, and cephalad displacement of the right ischial tuberosity.

Upslipped Innominate

The second most common pelvic subluxation (based on clinical observation) is the "**upslipped innominate.**" Originally described by Fryette (1914) with several complicating variations, **this lesion is essentially a vertical shear between the sacrum and ilium which shortens the distance between the sacrococcygeal attachment of the sacrotuberous ligament and its ischial tuberosity attachment**. The lesion is typically found on one side only, but can be bilateral. The acute injury can be easily and quickly reduced, and the reduction is stable about half the time. Such short-lived conditions which remain stable after reduction are classified as **sacroiliac subluxation**. If the joint does not stay in place after the reduction, the condition is classified as **unstable sacroiliac joint**, which requires orthopedic stabilization (usually in the form of a sacroiliac belt) for two or three months while the sacroiliac ligaments heal.

One common misconception is that an upslipped innominate causes the iliac crest to become superior *in the standing position* as well as in the recumbent positions. However, in order for this to be so, the person afflicted with the upslipped innominate would need to be standing on one leg! The reason for this is that an upslipped innominate does not change the length of the leg, the size of the innominate, or the relationship between the femur and the acetabulum. All that changes is the relationship between the sacrum and the innominate. In the recumbent non-weight-bearing position, the lesioned innominate assumes a superior position relative to the sacrum, which is in its normal position relative to the other innominate and to the spine. The sacrum's position on the lesioned side, on the other hand, is in an inferior position relative to the ilium on that side. In the standing position the sacrum will assume an *inferior* position relative to the innominate, but the innominate's distance from the floor remains unchanged.

Fryette's variations tended to muddle the subluxation concept, mainly because in 1914 the distinctions between dysfunction and subluxation were not regarded as important; the distinction is still blurred for some. Thus, superior vertical shear was discussed in combination with anterior or posterior rotation of the iliac crest, without considering the possibility that the iliac rotations might be adaptive to the dislocation, or produced independently, and not a part of the lesion mechanism *per se*.

In the Mitchell model, rotations of the ilium are not considered subluxations, but are viewed as restrictions of physiologic functions – somatic dysfunctions. **A subluxation is commonly viewed as "a bone out of place," a minor dislocation, whereas a restriction of physiologic function (somatic dysfunction) refers to a joint whose normal range of motion is limited, whether due to traumatic injury or as the result of biomechanical adaptation.** In the Mitchell model, the distinction is considered important.

Pratfalls (falls on the buttock) are probably the most frequent cause of iliac dislocations, which are diagnosed by observing the prone patient's superiorly displaced *ischial tuberosity* on one side and palpating the comparative laxity of the corresponding ipsilateral *sacrotuberous ligament*. Clinical observations of 10 +/-5 mm. superior displacements of the ischial tuberosity in the prone position are typical. It is estimated that 5-15% of the asymptomatic population has an upslipped innominate. Reduction with longitudinal distraction of the involved hip is usually easy (see task analysis technique descriptions). Such reductions are stable to weight bearing about half the time.

Downslipped innominate lesions have been reported despite the obvious curative effects of gravity, but it is rare enough to have eluded the author.

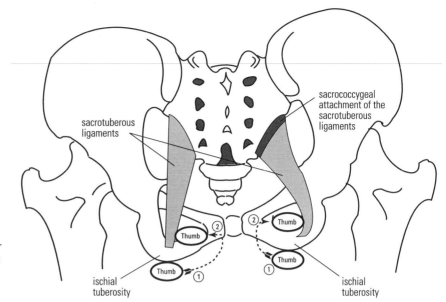

Figure 4.4. Right upslipped innominate, posterior view. The superior displacement of the right ischial tuberosity is detected visually by precise placement of the thumbs. The sacrotuberous ligament on the right is also slack.

Varieties of upslipped innominate include:

1. **Acute sacroiliac dislocation or subluxation** [ICD9CM 839.42].
   This is diagnosed within a few days after a slip-and-fall pratfall, or similar trauma.

2. **Chronic upslipped innominate** [ICD9CM 718.25].
   This is sometimes discovered in nonsymptomatic patients. The incidence in the nonsymptomatic population is probably 5–15%. It is a backache or a headache waiting to happen. The vertical displacement is one centimeter or less. This condition is the easiest to manage, because the joint stays in place once the subluxation is reduced.

3. **Recurrent sacroiliac dislocation or subluxation** [ICD9CM 718.35].
   This is equivalent to sacroiliac instability [ICD9CM 718.85]. These lesions are too unstable to stay in place after reduction. Management is much more complex. They may be due to sacroiliac sprain, acute [ICD9CM 846.1] or chronic [ICD9CM 724.6].

4. **Congenital sacroiliac dislocation** [ICD9CM 755.69].
   The sacroiliac joint maybe dislocated *in utero*. These are rarely discovered by pediatricians or obstetricians and may persist throughout life.

Summary of Diagnostic Criteria for Upslipped Innominate:
- Superior displacement of an ischial tuberosity with the patient prone;
- Slack sacrotuberous ligament on the same side;
- Dynamic leg length test shows hypermobility on the same side;
- The standing flexion test is variable.

MET Principles for Treatment of Upslipped Innominate:
- With the patient in the prone position, a quick traction tug on the leg (ipsilateral to the side with upslip) is applied in line with the plane of the sacroiliac joint simultaneous with the patient's cough (the cough helps stabilize the sacrum and spine).

Rhomboid Pelvis

The least common of the pelvic subluxations are the **inflare and outflare lesions**, labeled "dished in" and "dished out" by Fryette (1914). Flare lesions are dislocations occurring primarily at the sacroiliac joint, and secondarily at the pubic symphysis. A rare form of pelvic subluxation, it is presumed to occur only at the sacroiliac joint whose sacral auricular surface is convex in shape. A muscle imbalance of the *obliquus* and *transversus abdominis* muscles probably plays a role in distracting the ilia from its normal relationship with the sacrum, but only in combination with a sacroiliac joint that is inherently unstable due to an anatomic anomaly (i.e., the convex auricular surface).

Inflare lesions involve an anterior arcuate shearing of the ilium at the sacroiliac joint, which is accompanied by a slight posterior/medial shearing at the pubic symphysis. The anterior arcuate shear of the ilium results in displacement or asymmetry of pelvic landmarks; the ASIS of the lesioned side being more proximal to the midline of the abdomen (i.e., the umbilicus), and the pubic crest on the lesioned side being more posterior.

Outflare lesions involve posterior arcuate shearing of the ilium at the sacroiliac joint, which is accompanied by a slight anterior/lateral shearing at the pubic symphysis. In contrast to inflare, the posterior arcuate shear of the ilium associated with outflare results in the ASIS of the lesioned side being more distal to the midline of the abdomen (the umbilicus), and the pubic crest on the lesioned side being more anterior.

Do not confuse this lesion with the "pelvic distortion" lesion described by Cramer (1965), the common pattern of which appears to be a combination of a left unilaterally flexed sacrum – Lewit (1999) describes it as a "one-sided nutation" – and a right innominate rotated anteriorly on a transverse pubic axis. This combination occurs so frequently one suspects a mechanical compensation mechanism to be the cause. Innominate rotation alters the umbilicus-ASIS distance and can be misinterpreted as iliac flare. For this reason, iliac rotation is usually treated before making a diagnostic decision about iliac flare. This misinterpretation could account for the high incidence of iliac flares in some clinicians' practices.

In treating the flare lesion, the patient's flexed femur can be used as a lever, and the hip adductor and abductor muscles can be contracted to assist reduction of the flare isotonically.

When instability persists, as indicated by recurring dislocations, either upslipped innominate or flare, a sacroiliac belt may be required for external stabilization following the reduction of the dislocation.

Pelvic flare (**ICD9CM 839.42**) – whether inflare/outflare, left or right – is not to be confused with pelvic obliquity (**ICD9CM 738.6**), which is a manifestation of anatomic (congenital) short leg (**ICD9CM 755.30**).

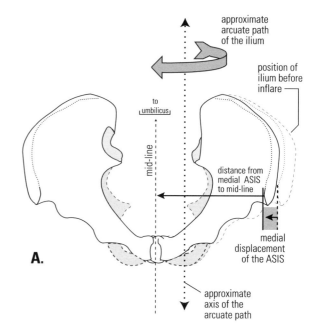

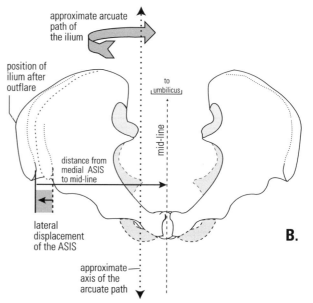

Figure 4.5. Asymmetries of the anterior superior iliac spines due to flaring subluxation of the innominate. Outflared right or inflared left ilium. The side of the lesion is lateralized by a standing or seated flexion test. To make the visual comparison of the ASIS positions relative to the midline, the thumbs are placed against the medial slopes of the landmarks.

Summary of Diagnostic Criteria for Inflared/Outflared Innominate:

■ ASIS closer to/farther from the midline than ASIS on the normal side;

■ Innominate rotation dysfunction has been successfully treated to restore superior/inferior alignment of ASISs;

■ Standing flexion test positive on involved side.

MET Principles for Treatment of Inflared/Outflared Innominate:

■ Femur is used for articulatory leverage.

■ Hip muscle contractions are used to increase sacroiliac joint play.

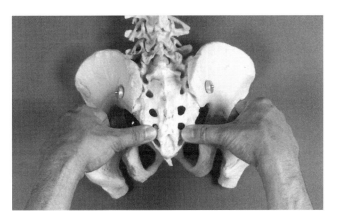

Figure 4.6.A. Palpating the posterior surface of the inferior lateral angles of the sacrum.

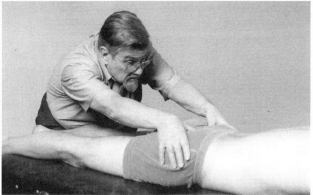

Figure 4.6.B. Palpating the posterior surface of the inferior lateral angles of the sacrum. To assess for rotation, operator must sight parallel to the coronal plane of the posterior ILA.

Sacroiliac Dysfunctions

According to the Mitchell model, there are two types of sacroiliac dysfunction: unilaterally flexed sacrum and torsioned sacrum. Such dysfunctions can result from faulty lifting, muscle imbalance, trauma, or perhaps may begin as an adaptive response to dysfunction somewhere in the spine or cranium, and eventually mature into a primary or established dysfunction of its own. The principles and mechanics of the physiologic motions of torsion and unilateral sacral flexion, as described in Chapter 3, can be used to describe the sacroiliac dysfunctions denoted as a *torsioned* or unilaterally *flexed* sacrum.

Either the unilaterally flexed sacrum or the torsioned sacrum can be conceived of as physiologic motion which has been abnormally arrested. Thus, the torsioned sacrum is one whose movement became restricted somewhere within the range of normal sacral torsion; the sacrum that is unilaterally flexed is one which is stuck in unilateral flexion. **Either is indicated when asymmetric displacement of the sacral inferior lateral angles (ILAs) is present.** Unilateral sacral extension dysfunction is a theoretical possibility, but has not been documented in the author's experience. The ILAs are the most significant and most reliable of the sacroiliac diagnostic criteria. If they are symmetrical, there is no sacroiliac dysfunction. They therefore constitute a quick screen for sacroiliac dysfunction.

Evaluating for sacroiliac dysfunction is performed only after the subluxations have been ruled out or eliminated by appropriate treatment. Here the application of physiological reasoning (as opposed to the "bone out of place" theory of pelvic dynamics) led Mitchell, Sr. (1965) to formulate a unified theoretical model of sacroiliac motion physiology and dysfunctions. The model offers the clearest explanation of observable phenomena and the greatest power to predict outcomes of intervention.

Note: All sacral asymmetries are not necessarily lesions. The sacrum can adapt, just as the spine can adapt. It is not uncommon to find that treatment of lumbar or lower thoracic segmental dysfunction spontaneously "heals" the sacral malposition. This is analogous to adaptive spinal curves straightening after the primary lesion is treated.

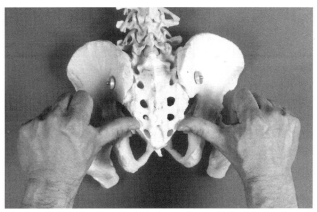

Figure 4.6.C. Palpating the inferior surface of the inferior lateral angles of the sacrum.

Figure 4.6.D. Palpating the inferior surface of the inferior lateral angles of the sacrum. To assess sidebending, operator must sight tangent to the transverse plane of the inferior ILA.

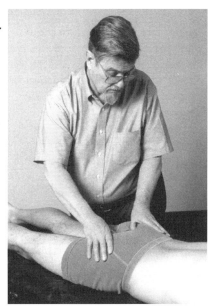

Unilaterally Flexed Sacrum

A sacrum that is unilaterally flexed has become fixed *positionally* in a manner consistent with the physiologic motion of unilateral flexion. The sacral base and ILA are sidebent to the same side. For example, with a left unilaterally flexed sacrum the sacrum is sidebent to the left, with the left ILA typically about a centimeter closer to the feet than the right ILA. This is the result of the left side of the sacral base having moved along the short arm of the auricular surface inferiorly and anteriorly in relation to the left iliac crest, without corresponding movement on the right. At the same time the sacral base moved down the short arm of the auricular surface, the sacrum also moved (on the same side) along the long arm of the auricular surface posteriorly and inferiorly, resulting in the left sidebent position of the ILA (Figure 4.7).

Assessing the sacral base position is done through palpation of the sacral sulci for depth (see Chapter 1 for landmark palpation, and Chapter 8 for evaluation protocol). Differences in sulcus depths, however, are often too subtle to judge reliably. Much more reliable indicators are the ILA positions.

Supplemental landmark tests, such as prone leg length, the seated flexion test, or assessing ILA displacement against two planes (horizontal and coronal), may be necessary to confirm the diagnosis of *left unilaterally flexed sacrum*. For example, flexion tests can be used to confirm the side of restricted pelvic joint motion. The reason is that, as the trunk bends forward the sacrum is pulled cephalad between the ilia. If the sacrum encounters a restriction at a sacroiliac joint on the left side, then the sacrum will become "stuck" in an anteriorly nutated position on the left ilium. After meeting the restriction, as forward trunk bending increases, the sacrum will pull the left ilium along with it, moving the left gluteal tubercle, or PSIS, more superiorly on the left than on the right. Thus, for a unilaterally flexed sacrum on the left, one would expect the seated flexion test to be positive on the left, because that is the side with the restricted pelvic joint motion.

The lesion is named and described positionally. But it could also be described in terms of restricted movement of the sacrum, i.e., *unilateral restricted counternutation of the sacrum on the left (or right)*.

As mentioned in Chapter 3, unilateral movement of the sacrum along the short and long arm of the auricular surface is arcuate. In the case of the unilaterally flexed sacrum, the sacrum has become wedged in the pelvis at the extreme end of this arcuate movement, and is unable to return back up the arc.

Note: This arcuate movement distinguishes a unilaterally flexed sacrum from an upslipped innominate, which is a straight vertical translation (Figure 4.8.).

The superior transverse axis is probably involved in bilateral and unilaterally flexed sacral lesions, in which the inferior lateral angles of the sacrum may be displaced as much as 1 or 2 centimeters. This is based on the assumption that

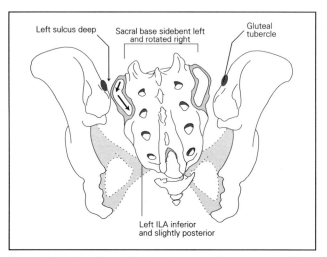

Figure 4.7. Left unilaterally flexed sacrum. The movement of the left sacroiliac auricular surface is arcuate, and consists of inferior-anterior displacement along the short arm (short arrow) and inferior-posterior displacement along the long arm (long arrow).

such lesions are acquired when ligamentous strains resulting from extreme truncal forces, such as those resulting from motor vehicle accidents and overhead lifting strains, are induced.

When the sacral base declines to the left, the normal lumbar adaptation is a neutral (without facet engagement) left convexity created by contraction of spinal right sidebender muscles. This usually has the effect of shortening the right leg in the prone position. In the straight prone position, leg length discrepancy is detected by observing the heel pads, preferably with the feet off the end of the examining table. Anatomic differences in leg length must be taken into account when implementing this procedure. For example, if the standing left iliac crest height is one centimeter inferior to the right crest, indicating anatomic shortness of the left leg, and the prone position makes the heel pads symmetrical, one must assume the right leg to be functionally shorter by one centimeter due to dysfunction and adaptation in the pelvis and lumbar regions.

The following lists the diagnostic criteria for unilaterally flexed sacrum on the left, any two of which is sufficient for diagnosis:

Summary of Diagnostic Criteria for Sacrum Flexed Left (SFL):
- A positive seated flexion test (++), and a positive standing flexion test (+);
- ILA inferior and slightly posterior on the left;
- Sacral sulcus deeper on the left;
- Prone leg length longer on the left (if L_5 is free to rotate left and sidebend right).

MET Principles for Treatment of Sacrum Flexed Left (SFL):
- Muscle Energy treatment of unilateral sacral flexion dysfunction utilizes careful positioning of the prone patient to loose-pack the sacroiliac joint, focused sustained operator pressure against the S_5 segment tangent to the arc of the joint, and deep inhaling efforts by the patient.

Mechanism of Injury in Sacral Flexion

Sudden unilateral compressive forces without coordinated muscle activity – such as occur in rear-end automobile collisions (Figure 4.9.), or suddenly attempting to lift a weight from an unbalanced sidebent position – produce a sidebend of the sacrum causing it to slide down the auricular surface on that side, where it may get stuck.

Catching or supporting a weight overhead, as in storing luggage in an overhead compartment on an airplane, while it may conceivably flex the sacrum bilaterally because of the lordotic lumbar load, most often has a greater wedging effect on one side, usually the left side. That wedged side may remain flexed after normal posture is assumed, and the free side (right) returns to a relatively extended position consistent with normal lordosis. Under such circumstances, the base of the sacrum must go, and remain, slightly anterior on the wedged side because of the *short* arm of the auricular surface; the apex of the sacrum moves inferiorly along the *long* arm of the joint, which guides it slightly posteriorly. Thus the sacrum rotates (in an anatomic sense) slightly toward the side opposite the sidebend.

If the sacrum becomes fixed in this position, it is referred to as "**unilaterally flexed sacrum**," a pelvic somatic dysfunction. This borders on subluxation, but it *must* be distinguished from the more dramatic subluxation – or dislocation – of the sacroiliac joint, the "**upslipped innominate**." Inasmuch as the unilaterally flexed sacral dysfunc-

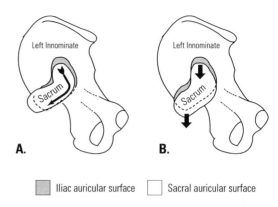

Figure 4.8. Comparison of left unilaterally flexed sacrum and left upslipped innominate. **A.** Left unilaterally flexed sacrum, medial view. **B.** Left upslipped innominate subluxation, medial view.

tion is a change in sacral position *along the physiologic path of the sacroiliac joint*, it should not be referred to as a subluxation. The upslipped innominate, on the other hand, is a subluxation, or even a luxation (dislocation) of the sacroiliac joint. The difference is that the dislocated, or subluxated, sacrum does not follow the *physiologic* path of the joint; it simply shears in a vertical translation.

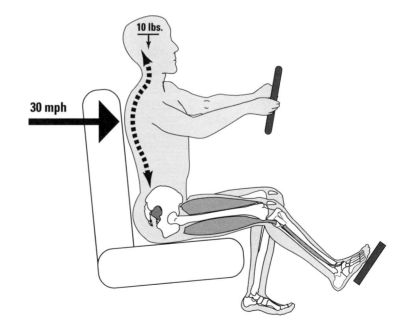

Figure 4.9. Mechanisms of injury in flexed sacrum dysfunction associated with "whiplash." The victim typically is waiting at a stop light, foot on the brake, head forward waiting for the light to change. Suddenly, his car is hit from behind. The ten pound inertia of the head resists acceleration, but the seat back suddenly moves forward at 30 m.p.h.. Straightening of the spinal A-P curves against the inertia of the head causes a great compressive force up against the base of the skull and down against the sacrum. "Whiplash" is usually more than a neck injury. Patients who are significantly injured invariably have a unilaterally flexed sacrum. Failure to treat the sacroiliac dysfunction will prolong recovery from the neck injury.

Figure 4.10. Four varieties of torsioned sacrum.

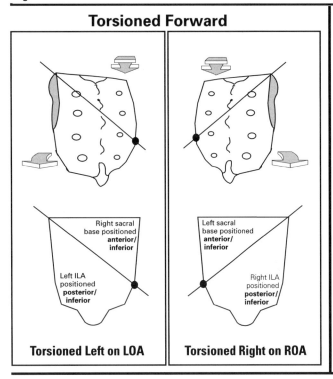

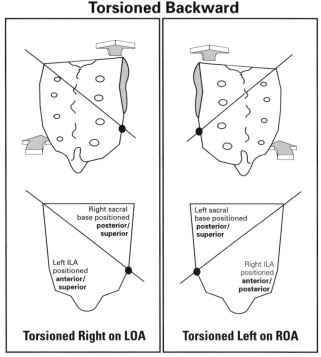

Torsioned Sacrum
Forward and Backward Sacral Torsions

There are two types of torsioned sacrum: sacrum torsioned forward and sacrum torsioned backward, each of which can be torsioned to the left or to the right. Thus, of the four possible ways in which a sacrum may become torsioned, two are **forward** – *torsioned left on the left oblique axis (LOA) and torsioned right on the right oblique axis (ROA)*, and two are **backward** – *torsioned left on the right oblique axis and torsioned right on the left oblique axis.* (Figure 4.10.)

In Chapters 2 and 3 it was demonstrated how unilateral spinal compressive forces on the base of the sacrum tend to produce either rotation-sidebending (torsion) or sidebending-rotation (unilateral flexion) of the sacrum, depending on the tonus of the erector spinae and iliopsoas muscles, and that in walking or marching in place, the alternating unilateral compressive forces of the spine on the sacral base produce rotation movements (called torsion) of the sacrum about either of the oblique (diagonal) axes. However, under certain conditions the sacrum may, in the process of performing the otherwise normal sacral torsion, become arrested somewhere in the range of the movement, and lose its normal physiologic function.

In the relationship between the sacrum and the spine, mechanical coupling at the lumbosacral junction predisposes the sacrum to move opposite the movements of the fifth lumbar with balanced sidebending/rotation. Thus, if the lumbars sidebend left and form a right convexity, the sacrum tends to sidebend right by lowering the right side of its base. If the lumbar lordosis increases by bending the spine backwards, the base of the sacrum tips forward. Just as the lumbars couple left sidebending with right rotation, the sacrum couples left rotation with right sidebending. It is this torquing mechanism of the lumbosacral joint which led to calling the oblique axis rotation of the sacrum "sacral torsion," referring to the torque between the fifth lumbar and the sacrum. Once torqued, the joint becomes relatively rigid.

Based on what is known about normal physiologic pelvic motion, as well as from clinical experience, we can articulate a mechanism for how a sacrum could become torsioned forward or backward.

Two factors are the determinants: 1) the side and direction of the lumbosacral load, and 2) the side of sustained *piriformis* contraction. The asymmetric lumbosacral load must be persistent to maintain the torsioned sacrum lesion. The lumbosacral load may be directed anteriorly by a lordotic lumbar spine or posteriorly by a kyphotic, or forward bent, one. A persistently laterally bent lumbar spine, due to sustained *quadratus lumborum* tightness, shifts the lumbosacral load to the side of spinal convexity, unless the sidebend is unbalanced. The side of piriformis contraction is determined by which ilium supports the load of the trunk. Persistent tightness of *quadratus* and *piriformis* can be attributed to altered interneuron firing sequence programs.

Forward sacral torsion motions, according to the Mitchell model, occur normally during walking to accommodate the lateral shifts of the spine. It is likely that the forward torsioned sacrum is caused by an abnormal alter-

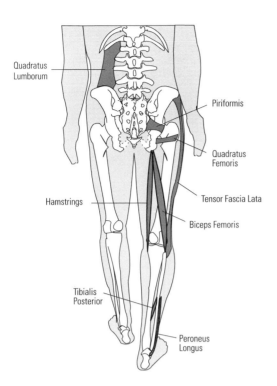

Quadratus
Lumborum

Piriformis

Quadratus
Femoris

Tensor Fascia Lata

Hamstrings

Biceps Femoris

Tibialis
Posterior

Peroneus
Longus

Figure 4.11. Posterior view of right stance mid-stride. *Quadratus lumborum* slowly contracts and relaxes, becoming shortest at mid-swing. *Piriformis* remains contracted throughout stance, stabilizing the inferior pole of the sacroiliac joint for both weight transmission and for normal pelvic arthrokinematics. The short external rotators of the femur (*quadratus femoris, et al.*) hold the femur head snugly in the acetabulum while the whole pelvis ballistically rotates on a *y-axis*. *Tensor fascia lata* assists *quadratus lumborum* in preventing pelvic sag. *Hamstrings* and *quadriceps* stabilize the knee. *Tibialis posterior* and *peroneus longus* stabilize the transverse arch of the foot at mid-stride.

ation of muscle firing sequences in the gait cycle. Normal firing sequences, organized by cord interneurons, include tonic *piriformis* contraction followed immediately by ipsilateral phasic *gluteus maximus* contraction, followed by a slowly recruited contralateral *quadratus lumborum* contraction in two phases – first concentric, then eccentric isotonic. A slight proprioceptive change may disable *quadratus* and *piriformis* relaxation, the last part of the sequence. As long as these two muscles cannot relax, the sacrum remains forward torsioned.

Forward torsioned sacrum to the left on the left oblique axis (Figure 4.12) probably occurs when the *latissimus dorsi/quadratus lumborum* fires prematurely simultaneous with the beginning of contralateral *piriformis* contraction. Proprioceptive cues to trigger gradual relaxation during its eccentric isotonic phase in the gait cycle are either absent or misread, and the *quadratus* fails to relax. Such sequential misfiring is common in the muscle imbalance syndrome described by Janda (1996). Persistence of *piriformis* contraction may also be attributed to altered proprioceptive cues. Probably a neural feedback loop reverberates in the pattern corresponding to mid-stride on the right foot,

Figure 4.12. Left-on-Left Torsion. The term "torsion" describes the state of the lumbosacral joint, where the trunk and the sacrum are rotating, sidebending, and nutating in opposite directions. The fifth lumbar probably rotates only to the point of zygapophyseal impaction, i.e., less than 3 degrees (average).

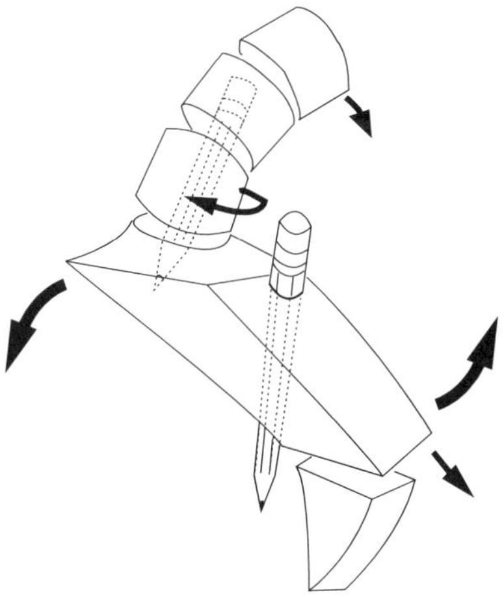

maintaining left-on-left torsioned sacrum. (Figure 4.11.)

In forward torsioned lesions, the *quadratus lumborum* and *piriformis* are co-contracted contralaterally. In backward torsioned lesions the co-contraction is ipsilateral.

In the case of the sacrum that is torsioned backward, "unnatural" movements of the body can result in ipsilateral co-contraction of lumbar sidebenders and hip external rotators, forcing the sacrum to rotate its base backward on the oblique axis (Figure 4.13). These circumstances frequently produce acute low back pain and an antalgic position indistinguishable from that of psoas muscle spasm. In the typical clinical case, the patient gives a history of straightening his back from a right sidebent anteflexed position with a heavy burden in the right hand while simultaneously stepping off onto the left leg. This activity produces a co-contraction of left piriformis and left lumbar sidebenders (*quadratus lumborum*), resulting in sacral torsion to the left on the right oblique axis (Figure 4.14).

Note: Forward torsions straighten with backward bending of the trunk (the "Sphinx" position). Backward torsions become maximally rotated with backward bending of the trunk and straighten with forward bending. **Thus, the prone Sphinx position differentiates forward from backward torsions.**

Effects of Sacral Torsion Dysfunction

When sacral torsion dysfunction occurs, the effect is as if the sacrum loses the use of one oblique axis. Normally the sacrum can rotate in either direction on either oblique axis. **All left sacrum torsioned dysfunctions have a deeper right sacral sulcus (or a shallower left sulcus). All left torsions have a short left leg, prone – except when the fifth lumbar has segmental dysfunction and cannot participate in the normal right convex adaptive pattern which goes with sacrum torsioned left.** However, only the forward torsions (to the left on the left axis or to the right on the right axis) occur in natural walking movements.

Left torsioned on the left oblique axis (forward torsion

Summary of Diagnostic Criteria for Torsioned Sacrum:
A redundant list of criteria for the diagnosis of sacral torsion to the left on the left diagonal axis includes the following:

1.a. Positive seated flexion (++) on the right;
 b. Positive standing flexion (+) on the right;
2. ILA posterior and slightly inferior on the left;
3. Sacral sulcus deeper on the right;
4. Prone leg length shorter on the left (if L5 is free to rotate right and sidebend left);
5. Disappearance of the torsion in the Sphinx position.

Note: The inferior displacement of the left ILA is counterintuitive. It results from the posterior movement of the left inferior ala along the long arm of the iliac auricular surface, which guides the sacrum inferior as it goes inferior. Thus, it appears that the upper end of the oblique axis is obliged to be a little wobbly, whereas the lower end of the axis is a stable pivot. Recall that the diagonal axis is created by contraction of one of the piriformis muscles. This pulls the sacrum obliquely downward against the lower pole of the sacroiliac joint, securing it in that position, and creating a pivot point. This provides an oblique axis, the superior end of which is not fixed. The lack of superior fixation is what allows the inferior lateral angle opposite to the pivot point to displace inferiorly as it rotates posteriorly.

MET Principles for Treatment of Torsioned Sacrum:
■ The treatment of torsions employs reciprocal inhibition of co-contracting antagonist muscles to relax the affected piriformis and lumbar muscles. Sacral torsion to the left on the left oblique axis is maintained by hypertonus of the lumbar left sidebenders and the right piriformis (an external rotator of the femur). By having the patient strongly contract (after appropriate positioning) the muscle groups which are their antagonists, the offending muscles are caused to relax, and the sacrum is freed from its restraints.

Figure 4.13. Backward sacral torsion to the left on the right oblique axis. As the sacral base moves backward, the lumbar lordosis must decrease or even become kyphotic.

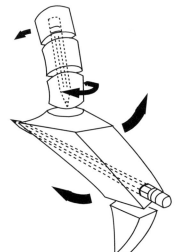

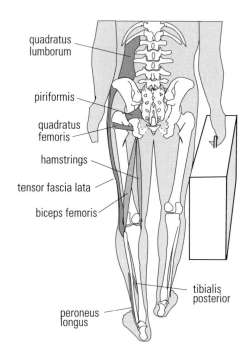

Figure 4.14. Production of Backward Left-on-Right Torsion. In the above example, the soon-to-be-patient reaches down for the suitcase handle during right mid-stride. Straightening the back and lifting the suitcase simultaneous with left heel strike, triggering left *piriformis* contraction simultaneous with left *quadratus lumborum* contraction to straighten the back and lift the load.

lesion) represents the majority of sacroiliac dysfunctions. It often occurs in the absence of pain or disability. In those rare instances when pain is a concomitant complaint, the pain is not confined to the sacral area but often presents as low back pain in the lumbar region. In forward torsion lesion, the patient tends to walk stiffly erect and lists toward the axis of involvement, but these signs are quite subtle. In backward torsions, the patient is stooped and lists away from axis of involvement. This sign is often much more dramatic and presents the clinical picture resembling acute psoas spasm, frequently mislabeled "slipped disc."

Comparison of a Unilaterally Flexed Sacrum on the Left and a Torsioned Sacrum to the Left
The left ILA is prominent in both left sacral flexion and sacral torsions to the left. Left sacral flexion primarily sidebends the sacrum to the left, displacing the left ILA mostly inferiorly (6-10 mm.) and only slightly posteriorly (3-5 mm.). Left sacral torsions have less sidebending effect, and typically displace the left ILA more posteriorly (6-10 mm.) than inferiorly (3-5 mm.). When such comparisons are unambiguous, the differential diagnosis can be made with confidence. When posteriority approximately equals inferiority, supplementary information is required, i.e., sulcus depths, prone leg lengths, flexion (or other mobility) tests, to distinguish between sacral flexion and sacral torsion.

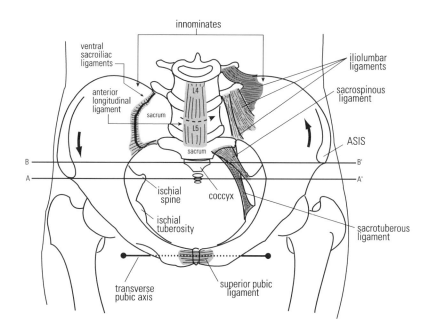

Figure 4.15. Anterior innominate right (AIR) or posterior innominate left (PIL). The asymmetry of the anterior superior iliac spines (ASISs) is indicated by the two horizontal lines drawn across the inferior slopes of the landmarks. The iliolumbar ligaments are not as strong a connection as they appear to be. Much of the time, significant movement can occur without obligatory rotation of the fourth and fifth lumbars. The iliolumbar ligament may have little to do with causing or maintaining iliosacral dysfunction, compared with trunk and leg fascias. The side of the lesion is lateralized by performing the standing flexion test.

Iliosacral Dysfunctions
Anteriorly or Posteriorly Rotated Innominate

Malalignment of the anterior superior iliac spines (ASIS) in the supine position, following successful treatment of pelvic subluxations and sacroiliac dysfunctions, is the best indicator of iliosacral dysfunction. They are best identified and located using palmar stereognosis; for mensuration the pads of the thumbs may be placed against the medial, inferior, or anterior surfaces of the ASIS. In the supine position inferior displacement of the ASIS on the side of a positive standing flexion test (relative to the contralateral ASIS) indicates an anteriorly rotated innominate on that side, and not a posterior innominate on the other side, which has a relatively superior ASIS. Anterior rotation of the innominate also slightly displaces the posterior superior iliac spine (PSIS) superiorly (in the prone position), and moves the pubic crest very slightly anteriorly (not palpable), *but not inferiorly.*

A common mistake is assuming that the pubic symphysis must shear vertically in order for one innominate to rotate on a transverse axis in relation to the other innominate. This would be true if the transverse axis were anywhere other than where it is – through the pubic bones. Such innominate rotations obviously require sacroiliac joint movement; and the logical location of the sacroiliac pivot for such motion (at least on the side of the stance leg in gait) is at the inferior pole of the sacroiliac joint where weight is being transmitted from the spine through the sacrum to the hip.

Throughout the entire stance phase of the walking cycle the iliac crest rotates anteriorly, pivoting at the same point on the diagonal axis where the sacrum torsions. The opposite iliac crest in swing phase rotates in the reverse direction, turning around a transverse axis through the symphysis pubis. **A loss of anterior and/or posterior ilial rota-**tion produces iliosacral dysfunction — right or left "rotated innominate" with the ASIS positioned anteriorly or posteriorly.**

Assessment of the ASISs for innominate rotation dysfunction should be deferred until (1) pelvic subluxations and (2) sacroiliac dysfunctions have been ruled out or treated successfully. If such conditions are present, adaptive shifts of the ASIS landmarks will occur, often resembling anterior or posterior rotation of an innominate.

Successful treatment is predicated on first treating subluxations and sacroiliac dysfunctions to restore alignment to the iliosacral axis. Muscle contractions produce transarticular forces which create compression or shear at the sacroiliac joint. With relaxation of the contraction, the joint is more loosely packed than it was, and the rotation range may be increased by using the femur for leverage.

Summary of Diagnostic Criteria for Anterior Innominate Right (AIR):
1. ASIS asymmetry with the right ASIS more inferior than the left 3-15 millimeters. The right ASIS will also be slightly more anterior than the left.
2. Absence of pubic subluxation, upslipped innominate subluxation, or sacroiliac dysfunction.
3. Positive standing flexion test on the right. This can often be deductively inferred from other pelvic dysfunction findings, obviating the need for repeating the flexion tests.
4. The right leg will be lengthened in the supine position, when the medial malleoli are compared.

Note: Posterior innominate on the left (PIL) looks exactly the same, except that the flexion test would be positive on the left instead of the right.

MET Principles for Treatment of Anterior Innominate Right (AIR):
■ Contraction of the hip muscles against operator resistance increases sacroiliac joint play, facilitating passive rotatory articular release.

Manipulable Muscle Imbalance
Functional Relationship between Weakness-Prone and Tightness-Prone Muscles

Having mentioned the role of muscle imbalance in producing and maintaining pelvic dysfunction, a brief discussion of the concept of muscle tightness and weakness is appropriate here. The spectrum of MET applications includes procedures for relaxing and lengthening tight muscles and strengthening weak ones. Most of these concepts and procedures will be presented in detail in a future volume dealing with the limbs. When muscle imbalance appears to be profound, it should be suspected of playing a primary role in producing and maintaining pelvic dysfunction.

Vladimir Janda (1996) has described two types of muscles in the motor system: weakness-prone (inhibited, phasic) and shortness-prone (strong, tight, postural, facilitated, stabilizer, tonic) muscles. Increasing tightness and shortness in the postural muscles increasingly inhibits and weakens the phasic muscles with which they are paired. A common example is weakened abdominal muscles, which are paired with tight short lumbosacral extensor muscles (*multifidi*). Janda has shown with surface electromyography (EMG) that all variations of situp isotonic exercise elicit more EMG activity in lumbosacral and lumbar extensors than in the *rectus abdominis* when the lumbosacral extensors are tight and short. It is clear that situps without prestretching the lumbosacral extensors may worsen the muscle imbalance, rather than correct the muscle weakness (Figure 4.16).

Table 4.B. lists some of the tightness-prone postural or tonic muscles and their associated weakness-prone phasic muscles. The relationship between a tightness-prone muscle and its weakness-prone "partner" is a one-way street. As the tightness-prone muscle gets tighter and stronger, its inhibition of the weakness-prone muscle also gets stronger. There is no reciprocal feedback from the weaker muscle. Strengthening it will not make the tight muscle get looser or weaker. In fact, exercising it to make it stronger will fail, in most cases, because of co-contraction of the tightness-prone muscle, which will benefit more from the exercise than the weak muscle does. The tightness-prone muscle gets stronger and tighter as a result of the exercise. The remedy is to stretch and elongate the tight muscle.

The postural muscles are paired with the phasic muscles which they most inhibit. Notice that, for the most part, they are not arranged in agonist/antagonist pairs, but are arranged in somewhat vertical tiers. There are many other examples of tightness-prone muscles inhibiting weakness prone muscles. Their arrangement into alternating tiers of tight and weak muscles is an important concept – tight hamstrings, weak *glutei*, tight lumbar *erector spinae*, weak *lower trapezius*, tight *upper trapezius*. Whether a muscle is tightness- or weakness-prone is closely related to its phylogenetic history. Muscles which have developed late (e.g., *vastus medialis*) or become larger (e.g., *gluteus maximus*) in evo-

Table 4.B.

Postural versus Phasic Muscles – a Partial List

Muscles prone to tightness (Postural)		Muscles prone to weakness (Phasic)
Gastrocnemeus/Soleus	*Inhibits*	Peroneus
Tibialis posterior	*Inhibits*	Tibialis anterior
Rectus femoris	*Inhibits*	Vastus medialis and lateralis
Hamstrings and Piriformis	*Inhibit*	Gluteus maximus, medius, and minimus
Tensor fascia lata	*Inhibits*	Gluteus maximus, medius, and minimus
Iliopsoas	*Inhibits*	Abdominal muscles, Glutei
Short hip adductors	*Inhibits*	Long hip adductors
Lumbar erector spinae	*Inhibits*	Rectus abdominis, Thoracic erectors
Quadratus lumborum	*Inhibits*	Thoracoabdominal diaphragm
Latissimus dorsi	*Inhibits*	Serratus anterior
Pectoralis major	*Inhibits*	Rhomboids
Upper trapezius	*Inhibits*	Lower trapezius
Sternocleidomastoid	*Inhibits*	Short cervical flexors
Levator scapuli and scalenes	*Inhibit*	Short cervical flexors
Cervical erector spinae	*Inhibit*	Short cervical flexors, Thoracic erectors
Flexors of the upper limb	*Inhibit*	Extensors of the upper limb
Temporalis	*Inhibits*	Digastric, Short cervical flexors

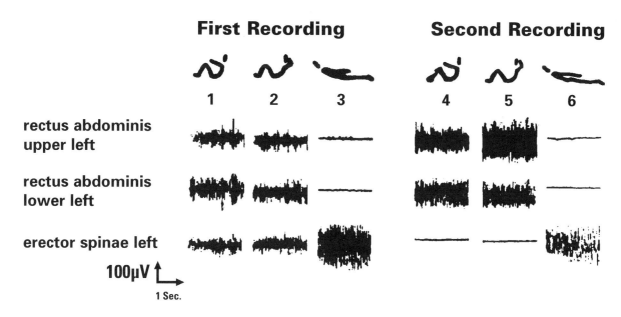

First Recording   **Second Recording**

1   2   3   4   5   6

rectus abdominis
upper left

rectus abdominis
lower left

erector spinae left

100µV

1 Sec.

Figure 4.16. The inhibitory effect of tight *erector spinae* muscles on abdominal muscles' ability to contract when performing a sit-back (a reverse sit-up). exercise. After the *erector spinae* were stretched – second recording – there is no longer co-contraction of lumbar muscles, and abdominal contraction is greater. Even the *erector spinae* firing with prone back extension decreases after it is stretched during post-isometric relaxation. Clearly, the exercise value of sit-ups (or sit-backs) for strengthening weak abdominal muscles is seriously compromised in the presence of tight lumbosacral *erector spinae* muscles. (after Janda V, in Korr IM, Ed. *The Neurobiologic Mechanisms in Manipulative Therapy.* New York and London, Plenum Press. 1978).

lution are weakness prone; those which have become smaller (e.g., *temporalis*) are tightness prone. The functional relationship between muscles is, of course, much more complex than the tier model, as we can see in Table 4.B. – for example, *psoas*-inhibiting abdominals. The same tonic-inhibiting-phasic relationship pertains to the deep tonic and superficial phasic layers of the paraspinal muscles.

Janda's concept pertains to myofascial continuity. As one progresses up the muscle spiral, one finds an alternation of weakness- and shortness-prone muscles. Thus the anterior muscles of the lower leg and the arch of the foot are prone to weakness, the hamstring muscles are prone to shortness, the gluteus muscles are prone to weakness, and the lumbo-sacral extensor muscles are prone to shortness. The muscles of the trunk are also arranged in alternating tiers of weak and short muscle. Overuse and fatigue tends to evoke these muscles' characteristic responses. The relation of these muscles to each other can produce a vicious cycle in which the tight muscles inhibit the weak muscles and make them weaker. When weakness-prone muscles are being inhibited, they fatigue quickly under sustained load. The fatigue is manifested by the onset of gross clonic fasciculations. Exercises that elicit such clonus should be avoided. This model suggests that effective therapy to restore function should commence with stretching the tight muscles before attempting to strengthen the inhibited weak muscles.

Liebenson (1996) examines the role of muscle imbalance in the broader context of rehabilitation from a clinically useful perspective.

Breathing Movement Impairments
Sacroiliac Respiratory Restriction

As previously mentioned, the normal sacroiliac permits almost two angular degrees of sacral nutation with deep respiration (Mitchell Jr. and Pruzzo, 1971). The motion of the sacrum is caused by the straightening lumbar spine pushing it. Restriction of this motion can add significantly to the work of breathing, since the average person takes about 23,000 breaths a day. When the sacroiliac breathing motion is restricted, each breath must move an entire hip the amount normally moved by the sacrum alone. The cause of restriction could be postural, craniosacral, or due to adapted breathing patterns. Pelvic edema may be the mechanism of restriction.

Impairment of this breathing motion is easy to detect and treat. However, it has a variable effect on the standing flexion test. Restoration of breathing mobility to the sacroiliac joint can profoundly improve respiratory and circulatory dynamics of the entire body, even though the movement is relatively small.

Craniosacral Dysfunction

It has been a maxim in the osteopathic cranial community that the sacrum and the cranium mutually influence each other.

"Sacral lesions prevent permanent correction of occipito-atlantal lesions and vice versa, there being a definite interrelation between the two areas." (Magoun, 1951)

Functional Relationship of the Pelvis to the Cranium

The overriding primacy of the postural-vestibular reflex system dictates that the suboccipital muscles be immediately activated to level the eyes and semicircular canals whenever the sacral base of spinal support becomes asymmetric or threatens to disturb postural balance. This head leveling action may initiate the formation of patterns of adaptive spinal curves from the occiput down to the pelvis, or even through the legs. In a 1966 study of children and adolescents, Lewit reported (1999) that of 80 children ages 14 to 41 months, 11 had pelvic distortion. In the 3-6 year age group of 181 children, there were 81 instances of pelvic distortion, and in 459 children ages 9-15, there were 199 pelvic distortions. Some degree of scoliotic deformity was found in 38 percent of the older children, 8 percent of the nursery school children, and less than 2 percent of the infants. In a later study (1982) of 75 nursery school children (ages 3-6 years), pelvic distortion was found in 24, of whom 23 had movement restriction at the occipito-atlantal joint. In 12 of these, atlas-occiput manipulation was carried out, with the result that in every case the pelvic distortion disappeared spontaneously! Lewit concluded that most of the children with pelvic distortion probably had occipito-atlantal dysfunction, the primary cause of their pelvic distortion (Schildt, 1975).

Fulford (1996) has suggested that the common patterns of fascial and articular movement blockages can be attributed to the usual right occiput anterior presentation of fetuses and the traumatic effects of labor on the left occipital condyle and the left shoulder being forced against the mother's pubic bone. Probably, the common pattern of pelvic distortion in pregnant women partly accounts for the high incidence of right occiput anterior presentations. Lewit's findings imply that the common patterns of dysfunction are acquired. Many agree that dysfunctions at the top end of the spine can generate dysfunctions at the lower end. Jirout (1974, 1990) demonstrated the dynamic influence of craniocervical motion impairment on lower spinal segments.

Conversely, the presence of somatic dysfunction of the sacrum is presumptive evidence of spinal adaptation up to, and including, the occipito-atlantal joint. Such adaptation is not necessarily spontaneously reversible and may require manipulative intervention to restore normal function, after sacral base symmetry is restored.

Tightness of the suboccipital muscles, in response to vestibular righting reflexes, may compress or lock movable components of the skull, thereby altering the pattern of inherent motility of the cranium. Of the shortness-prone muscles attaching to the skull, the trapezius and sternocleidomastoid muscles are major influences, and when they are tight they may lock the occipitomastoid suture or distort the condylar parts of the occipital bone, usually on one side. Impairments of cranial motility may affect the function of one or more cranial nerves.

Inherent motility of the central nervous system produces very slight mechanical movements of the sacrum, rocking it gently but continuously between the ilia. It is thought that the spinal dura, extending from the foramen magnum to the sacrum, imparts this rocking motion to the passive sacrum as the foramen magnum tips back and forth slightly in the pattern of the cranial rhythmic impulse. It appears that the craniosacral system can usually tolerate and adapt to sacroiliac dysfunctions without pathophysiologic evidence of stress, as can be manifested in cranial nerve malfunctions.

Sacral Oscillation

Sutural mobility impairments of the cranial base, especially in the posterior fossa, often produce a startling phenomenon: *sacral oscillation*. Oscillatory movements of the sacrum can be observed in a prone patient by keeping the thumbs in firm contact with the sacral alae at the level of S_5 (the Inferior Lateral Angle – ILA), and visually watching the alternating unilateral anterior and posterior thumb movements for at least 10 seconds. The movement is very slow, about 5 or 6 cycles per minute. Usually the oscillation is of a rotatory nature, but occasionally the oscillatory movement of the sacrum is a side-to-side tipping. Amazingly, the amplitude of the thumb movement anterior to posterior is usually on the order of 3 to 10 millimeters. This is much bigger than the movements attributable to the cranial rhythmic impulse, even though it occurs at approximately the same rate. This phenomenon is a reliable general sign of cranial somatic dysfunction, and should probably not be ignored. It does not signify somatic dysfunction in the pelvis. But one may be led into misdiagnosis by hasty judgment. When the cranial dysfunction is successfully treated, the oscillation stops.

The author speculates that the mechanism of sacral oscillation is involuntary activity of lumbar postural muscles – *multifidi*, etc. – in response to *incoherent* vestibular-proprioceptive reflexes. Cranial somatic dysfunction which positions the temporal bones asymmetrically alters sensory input from the bony labyrinthes in the temporal bones to the vestibular nucleus. The vestibular nucleus provides the central nervous system (CNS) with information about the position of the head in relation to gravity. The deep suboccipital muscles provide proprioceptive information to the CNS about the position of the head in relation to the neck. There is also ocular input of head position in relation to the environment integrated into the head posture control system.

That the human body has such complex redundant information input into the head posture control system is testimony to the physiologic imperative of head posture control. Alexander (1997) recognized this important biological principle and incorporated it into his static and dynamic posture retraining programs.

The head posture control system regulates the activity of all the postural muscles of the spine, including the lumbar spine. With part of the system receiving misinformation from the labyrinthes, postural muscle reflex activities become confused. Called upon to do something about the position of the head, but unclear about what needs to be done, the spinal effector circuits in the lumbar field commence alternating left to right contract-relax cycles. These cycles are very slow, about 0.1Hz., presumably because the altered spatial orientation of the labyrinthes makes them sensitive to the movements of the Primary Respiratory Mechanism (Sutherland, 1939) which has a frequency of 0.1Hz.

It is difficult to assign a stable axis to the very subtle and low amplitude motions of the sacrum which are manifestations of the cranial **primary respiratory mechanism (PRM)**. These low amplitude movements are *often out of phase with the cranial rhythmic impulse (CRI) palpated at the head*, although the *rate* of sacral oscillation is usually synchronous with the cranium. Sometimes the motion feels as if the sacrum is rocking on the middle transverse axis. However, there are times when the oscillating motion of the sacrum feels more like a translation in the coronal plane, or occasionally in a transverse plane moving anterior to posterior. Rotational small amplitude oscillations can sometimes be felt, usually on an oblique axis, but occasionally on the *y*-axis (superior-inferior). Some clinicians believe these variations have diagnostic implications relative to the PRM.

CHAPTER 5

Introduction to Evaluation and Treatment of the Pelvis and Sacrum

Dysfunctions of the pelvis can adversely affect many parts of the body. Impairment of movement functions in the pelvis can significantly stress postural adaptive mechanisms, locomotor functions, and circulatory dynamics, as well as trophic and regulatory nervous system functions. Patients with symptoms elsewhere in the body may have somatic dysfunction of the pelvis as their primary manipulable problem. Regardless of the patient's history and symptoms, a screening evaluation of the pelvis should be done routinely. In general, symptoms, signs, and most screening test results are generated by the body's necessary *adaptations* to function failure.

The body's adaptive repertoire is too large to predict precisely which symptoms may be generated. Deductive reasoning, however, can at times point to a probable relationship between subjective symptoms, history, and objective physical examination findings. In addition, symptoms or pathologies which are seemingly beyond the scope of musculoskeletal evaluation (e.g., urogenital, obstetrical, gastrointestinal, etc.) may in fact be a direct result of pelvisacral dysfunction, and not at all related to the types of pathologies they appear to represent or imitate.

Furthermore, findings which appear upon initial evaluation to indicate the presence of primary pelvisacral dysfunction, in some cases, turn out to be secondary to, or caused by, viscerosomatic reflexes induced by pathologies in the organs, cranial dysfunction, muscle and/or postural imbalances, thoracolumbar dysfunction, etc. For this reason, and because the pelvic girdle is the crossroads for so many structural and functional bodily processes, a systematic approach to the evaluation and treatment of the pelvis, with consideration of possible causal relationships, is critical to realizing the best outcome from treatment.

The patient history can play an important role in sorting through the myriad of possibilities, and treating the primary lesion or pathology first. Some frequently occurring types of manipulable pelvic disorders tend to correlate with characteristic *events* or *mechanisms of injury*, and can alert the clinician to the possibility of specific types of dysfunction or subluxation. For example, a high percentage of patients who have been the victims of rear-end automobile collisions have unilateral sacral flexion lesions. Pratfalls and improper landing from high jumps raise suspicion of upslipped innominate subluxation, unilateral or bilateral. A sudden backache resulting from lifting and turning from a trunk rotated position with the weight on one foot suggests the possibility of backward sacral torsion.

Circumstances of aggravation or relief of *symptoms* can also be significant. Patients with chronic unilateral sacral flexion frequently experience a stiff sore backache upon getting out of bed in the morning, which gradually eases within a few hours. The pain of unilaterally flexed sacrum is usually diffuse, and often occurs on the contralateral side in the *gluteus maximus* muscle or as referred sciatica. A patient with a unilaterally flexed sacrum dysfunction tends to exhibit increased lordosis, visceroptosis, and morning stiffness. Lumbago patients who are more comfortable while bending forward probably have a backward sacral torsion. A patient with an upslipped innominate will find that walking worsens lower back pain, especially when the injury is fresh. Patients experiencing symptoms of cystitis – dysuria, frequency, suprapubic pain – or other distal urinary tract symptoms, yet no infection can be demonstrated by culture, often have pubic subluxation.

One contributing factor to consider, especially in patients with recurrent or persistent pelvic dysfunction, is *tightness-weakness muscle imbalance*. Muscle imbalance, when present, can affect static posture or functional mobility/coordination in ways that can stress the pelvis by producing pathognomonic gait and posture patterns (Lewit, 1996) which predispose to pelvic dysfunction. In general, altered gait patterns are usually due to spinal or hip muscle adaptation to pelvic somatic dysfunction or anatomic anomaly, and are rarely directly caused by the small range-of-motion mechanical impairments of pelvic somatic dysfunction or subluxation. Although gait abnormalities are not reliable for determining lateralization of dysfunction in the pelvis, they can strongly suggest the presence of pelvic dysfunction.

Observations of correlations between gait abnormalities and pelvic dysfunction include the following:

• The patient walks bent forward, often clutching the lower back with one hand on the side he is leaning away from, to avoid pain. This is frequently associated with backward torsion dysfunction;

• Asymmetric hip sway from side-to-side can signal forward sacral torsion, or can be a manifestation of lumbosacral zygapophyseal trophism;

• A shorter stride length on one side can be indicative of innominate rotation;

• The patient with anterior innominate rotation tends to externally rotate that leg for its stance phase (just as the long leg is externally rotated in leg length asymmetry).

Lordosis plays an etiologic role in sacral flexion and forward torsion. Kyphosis predisposes to backward torsion. Gluteus weakness leads to contralateral quadratus lumborum tightness, altering trunk undulation to the point of nociception and tending to generate sacral torsion. Leg length inequality with scoliosis (adaptive or compensatory) can lead to sacroiliac dysfunction.

Note: The student, as they become more proficient in applying the evaluation and treatment techniques described in the following chapters, is encouraged to search for the "key lesion" – both within the context of the Muscle Energy paradigm, but within other paradigms as well. In the MET model a "key lesion," or primary dysfunction, is an abnormal finding, the normalization of which results in spontaneous normalization of the physical findings of (secondary) dysfunction elsewhere in the body. Other paradigms define it differently. Ultimately, the search for the key, in addition to analyzing biomechanical relationships, involves taking a systems approach, which draws on clinical judgement in relation to a variety of disciplines.

Lesions of the pelvis, like lesions in other parts of the body, are often the result of postural or locomotor adaptations to dysfunctions elsewhere in the body. Cervical dysfunctions and even the very subtle dysfunctions of the cranial suture joints may be primary to secondary pelvic dysfunctions. The oscillating sacrum phenomenon, which is a primary cranial dysfunction and not a pelvic lesion, can cause backache and even sciatica.

MET and the Evaluation and Treatment of Pelvic Dysfunction

As the beginning of this chapter makes clear, the pelvis is a very dynamic piece in the puzzle of the human body, and has many structural and functional relationships to consider. For this reason, interpreting symptoms and evaluating for functional impairments can draw from a variety of disciplines, and can refer to a range of paradigms or techniques in the course of treatment. The primary focus in the Muscle Energy paradigm is evaluating for functional and/or articular dysfunctions, and applying Muscle Energy principles toward the treatment of such dysfunctions when

present. Clinical experience has demonstrated, many times, that through applying the Muscle Energy paradigm in addressing these functional/articular dysfunctions, an array of seemingly unrelated symptoms are resolved. It must be stressed, however, that effective evaluation of the pelvis is not performed in a conceptual vacuum; we must consider it within a larger, more holistic, framework. General screening examinations can help with this.

As Figure 5.1 shows, there are many steps which precede a more detailed evaluation for specific dysfunctions of the pelvis. Many of these, with the exception of addressing cranial dysfunction, are the subject of Volume 1 (i.e., The Ten-Step Screening examination, and evaluation and treatment of cervical dysfunction) and Volume 2 (i.e., evaluation and treatment of thoracolumbar dysfunctions) of this series.

Ideally, any cervical and/or thoracolumbar dysfunctions (and cranial dysfunctions as well*) have been treated before evaluation of structural or articular dysfunction in the pelvis begins. The rationale for this part of the sequence is that dysfunction of the cervical, thoracic, or lumbar spine can effect adaptive mechanisms in the pelvis, the results of which can mimic signs of primary dysfunction in the pelvis. Unless those dysfunctions are addressed first, we risk treating neutral adaptations in the pelvis as if they were non-neutral dysfunction, a practice which can stress the patient.

Screening examinations which may have been performed at the beginning (i.e., before thoracolumbar evaluation, etc.), may be performed again after segmental spinal dysfunctions have been treated and/or ruled out. One aspect of physical examination of the musculoskeletal system is gait analysis, which may involve no more than noticing whether the patient walks with a limp. Postural statics (addressed in Chapter 6) are then considered, noting the presence of scoliosis, anatomic leg length asymmetry, etc.

The first pelvic screening tests performed , most routinely, are the standing and seated flexion tests (see Chapter 6) for asymmetric pelvic joint mobility; the test indicates whether or not there is a problem, and which side of the pelvis is restricted (lateralizes the problem). The results of the standing and seated flexion tests will either confirm the side of lateralization or, on occasion, may indicate complex dysfunction(s), as when the side of lateralization changes.

Note: Many versions of the forward bend test are extant, but they are not interchangeable. Diagnosis in the Mitchell model of the pelvis depends on changes in the static positions of precise bony landmarks. Although soft tissue changes may be considered essential data in other modalities, in MET they are considered irrelevant distractions.

After examining and treating the **thoracolumbar spine**, but before evaluating for specific sacroiliac dysfunction, the next immediate concern is to find and treat pelvic **subluxations** (the subject of Chapter 7). The rationale for addressing subluxations/dislocations before addressing sacroiliac/iliosacral dysfunctions is that they disrupt the axes about which these dysfunctions occur, making it

Table 5.A. Flow Chart for MET Evaluation and Treatment Sequence of Manipulable Pelvic Disorders.

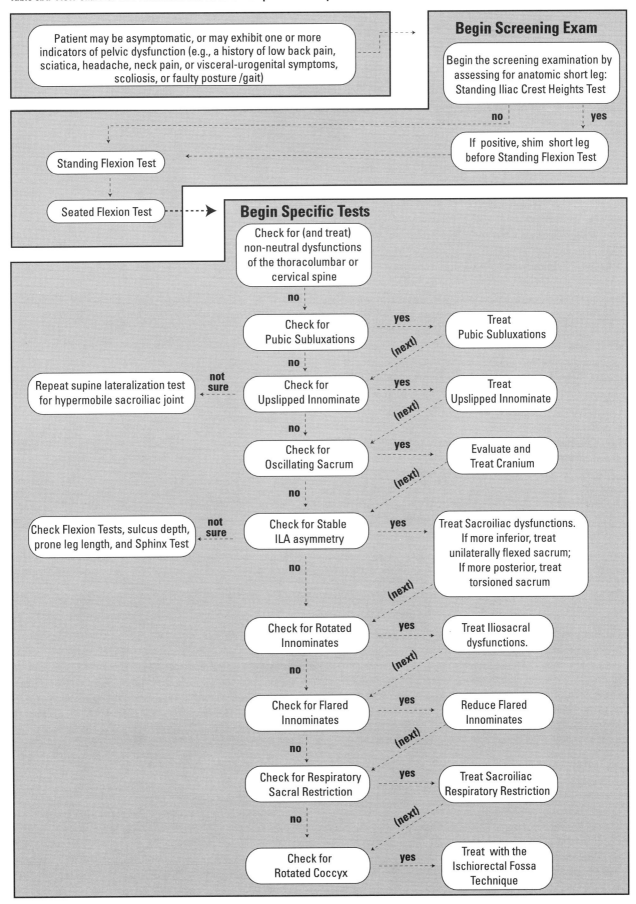

impossible to accurately assess physiologic function. **Pubic subluxations** – being the most frequently occurring non-physiologic pelvic lesions – are addressed first; then **upslipped innominate** (vertical shear) and finally (ideally) **flares**.

Evaluating and treating **sacroiliac dysfunctions** is the next order of business (Chapter 8), because they must be corrected in order to restore articular pivots on which the ilia move in relation to the sacrum.

The **thoracolumbar spine** is addressed again right after sacroiliac diagnosis, to take into account the position of the sacral base.

Finally, the **anterior** or **posterior rotated innominates** (iliosacral dysfunctions) are addressed. Anterior innominate is usually found on the right and posterior innominate on the left. After the pelvis is balanced, there are some other things which must be taken care of promptly. The craniocervical junction (occiput, atlas, axis) should be reevaluated to be sure the automatic re-compensation of the posture will be a change toward normal. Treating the craniocervical region before examining the pelvis is always a good idea, because of its potential influence on lower back mechanisms.* In addition, muscle imbalances arising from the lower limbs should be treated. Specific range-of-motion scanning tests for length/strength of hip muscles will be covered in a future volume.

***Note:** Cranial treatment should be performed only by those trained in Sutherland techniques.

CHAPTER 6

Screening and Lateralization Tests for the Pelvis

Lateralization is determining which side of the pelvis has restricted articular motion. Determining lateralization is useful in evaluation because different dysfunctions of the pelvis can produce similar displacements of pelvic bony landmarks. Lateralization tests can help to distinguish one type of dysfunction from another.

Performing a lateralization test is the equivalent of performing a screening test. A test which does not show one-sided articular motion restriction indicates that there is either no joint dysfunction in the pelvis, or there is bilaterally symmetrical joint restriction. Although not necessarily used on all patients, the following are basic screening and lateralization tools:

Methods used to determine lateralization include:

■ **Checking for anatomic leg length differences using iliac crest heights measurement**; not a lateralization evaluation *per se*, but is a necessary pre-condition for performing an accurate **standing flexion test** to determine the side of restriction.

■ **Seated flexion test.** In addition to lateralizing the problem, this test can also help distinguish sacroiliac from iliosacral dysfunction.

■ **Supine dynamic leg length test** can detect both hypermobility and articular motion restriction in the pelvis.

■ **Supine pelvic rocking tests** *and* **prone springing tests.** Although these tests are widely used, the author considers them too subjective to be reliable indicators.

■ **Inferior lateral angle (ILA) observation for positional asymmetry** can be used as a general screen for sacroiliac dysfunction.

Before describing the tests for lateralization and screening, material on the clinical significance of anatomic leg length differences, the accurate way to measure leg length, and trunk adaptations to sacral base asymmetry will be presented. Extreme leg length asymmetry can introduce specious error into the standing flexion test, but not into the seated flexion test.

In this chapter:

■ *Anatomic leg length and pelvic inequalities*

■ *Iliac crest heights measurement*

■ *Standing and seated flexion tests*

■ *Prone and supine functional leg length tests*

■ *Stork tests*

■ *Hip drop test*

■ *Recumbent pelvic mobility tests*

Relative Leg Length

Comparative leg length differences are a concern in musculoskeletal evaluation of the pelvis. When considering differences, one must discriminate between *anatomic* leg length and *functional* leg length. Anatomic leg length inequality is due to either dysgenesis (failure of the bone(s) to grow at equal rates) or results from fracture of any of the lower limb bones, from the innominate to the toes. Although anatomic leg length is a significant consideration

in terms of evaluation, it is not a condition directly treatable with manual therapy. Functional leg length asymmetry, however, is correctable and reversible once the manipulable disorder – subluxation, iliosacral dysfunction, or sacroiliac dysfunction – responsible for the inequality has been addressed. *{Note: Healing a fracture of a long bone often lengthens the bone.}*

Table 6.A.

Summary of Lateralization and Screening Evaluation Tests for the Pelvis

Test	Type of Test/Patient position/ Landmark(s) used for the Test	Purpose and indication of positive findings
Iliac Crest Leg Length Test	**Static Test performed with the patient standing:** Superior border of the left and right iliac crests	To determine the presence of an anatomically short leg.
Seated Iliac Crest Heights	**Static Test performed with the patient seated:** Superior border of the left and right iliac crests	To determine the presence of innominate dysgenesis.
Observing Paravertebral Symmetry	**Static Test performed with the patient seated and flexed:** Paravertebral muscle mass to the left and right of the lumbar spinous processes.	To determine the presence of rotoscoliotic adaptation to lumbar or thoracic ERS segmental dysfunction. (Refer to Volumes 1 and 2.)
Standing Flexion Test	**Static/Dynamic Test performed with the patient standing:** PSISs or gluteal tubercle on the left and right innominates.	To determine asymmetric iliosacral/sacroiliac joint motion restriction for screening or lateralization purposes.
Seated Flexion Test	**Static/Dynamic Test performed with the patient seated:** PSISs or gluteal tubercle (PIPs) on the left and right innominates.	To determine asymmetric sacroiliac/iliosacral joint motion restriction for screening or lateralization purposes.
Fowler (Stork) Test	**Dynamic/Active Test performed with the patient standing:** median crest of the sacrum and gluteal tubercle (PIPs).	To determine asymmetric iliosacral/sacroiliac joint motion restriction for screening or lateralization purposes.
Hip Drop Test	**Dynamic/Active Test performed with the patient standing:** Iliac crests and median furrow of the spine.	To compare left with right lumbosacral sidebending mobility.
Springing Articulatory Tests	**Dynamic/Passive Test performed with the patient prone or supine:** Iliac crest, ischial tuberosity, sacral base, sacral apex (left or right).	To compare left with right pelvic joint play mobility.
Functional Leg Length Test	**Static Test performed with the patient supine:** Medial malleoli.	To confirm specific iliosacral dysfunction diagnosis.
Functional Leg Length Test	**Static Test performed with the patient prone:** Heel pads.	To confirm specific sacroiliac dysfunction diagnosis.
Dynamic Leg Length Test	**Dynamic/functional Test performed with the patient supine:** Medial malleoli.	To determine the presence of asymmetric sacroiliac/iliosacral joint motion restriction or hypermobility to confirm upslipped innominate diagnosis.

Measuring Anatomic Leg Length. Anatomic leg length inequalities can be measured either through physical examination or radiogrammetrically. Discovering anatomic leg length inequality in a patient is of immediate concern because:

■ Any measurable degree of anatomic leg length inequality can influence the validity and interpretation of information gathered from other tests;

■ Use of functional leg length tests to confirm a diagnosis of manipulable pelvic lesions presumes that any discrepancy in anatomic leg length has been taken into account;

■ If the difference in leg lengths is greater than 10 millimeters, the shorter leg should be shimmed to make the pelvis approximately level before performing a standing flexion test. The flexion test could be performed without shimming the short leg; however, the results might be different, thereby affecting the accuracy of the diagnostic interpretation.

■ The clinician should consider the possibility that prescribing an orthotic heel or shoe lift might be advisable. Such decisions must not be made in haste, however, since it is possible that an inappropriately applied lift might increase mechanical-postural stresses more than relieve them.

Anatomic leg length asymmetry can be seen (though not necessarily measured) with the patient in both standing and recumbent positions. For review, the landmarks that correspond to each of the patient positions are as follows: a) the iliac crests for the standing position; b) the medial malleoli for the supine position; and c) the calcaneous tuberosities (i.e., heel pads) for the prone position.

In contrast to anatomic asymmetry, **functional asymmetries can *only* be discovered with the patient lying recumbent.** Because functional asymmetries are not due to differences in the length or shape of the bones, they are *not* seen in the standing position.

Of the three patient positions, **the only physical examination procedure which will allow for valid *measurement* of anatomic leg length is the *standing* iliac crest heights test.** Leg length asymmetry observed with the standing iliac crest heights test more accurately represents true anatomic length, because functional leg length asymmetry does not influence leg length in the standing position.

For normal posture of the spine and pelvis, the two iliac crest apices should be equidistant from the floor when a person is sitting or standing with bipedal support. If one iliac crest is lower than the other *in the seated position*, it is an indication that one hip bone is not as tall as the other. If the seated iliac crest heights are level, then a low iliac crest *in the standing position* is indicative of anatomic shortness of the leg on that side. Making the determination of levelness of the iliac crests – if done carefully enough – can be valid and accurate to within 2 mm. and does not require special instrumentation.

In the standing position, the position of the feet and legs has an effect on leg length. Externally rotating the leg and pronating the foot tends to lower the height of the femur head. Standing with the feet too close together can allow the pelvis to sway in an arc whose radius comes from a point between the heels. Inaccuracies in determining leg length due to pelvic sway can be obviated by placing the heels the same distance apart as the femur heads. The distance between the heels should be approximately four or five inches (or approximately the width of the examiner's shoe).

To use the iliac crests as landmarks, the examiner positions the palmar aspects of the index and middle fingers onto the superior apex of the iliac crests. This positioning is best achieved by pressing against the side of the iliac crests and pushing medially and superiorly, so that there is little adipose tissue between the examiners fingers and the bone, until the hands are resting on the apex of the iliac crests. Once the examiner's hands are properly positioned, visual assessment is made – with the eyes in the same transverse plane as the hands – of the comparative distance of the apices of the iliac crests from the floor. However, one

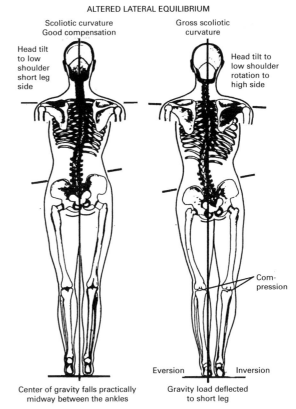

ALTERED LATERAL EQUILIBRIUM

Scoliotic curvature
Good compensation

Gross scoliotic curvature

Head tilt to low shoulder short leg side

Head tilt to low shoulder rotation to high side

Compression

Eversion   Inversion

Center of gravity falls practically midway between the ankles

Gravity load deflected to short leg

Figure 6.1. Anatomic short leg compensations.
One way to judge the appropriateness of postural compensation is to look at the distribution of body masses in relation to gravity. Both illustrations show an "S" curve scoliosis, but in the right hand drawing the gravity load is shifted off-center. The left hand drawing is a better compensation because the body masses are centered between the feet and the body masses are as close as possible to the mid-gravitational line. (Reprinted with permission of the American Academy of Osteopathy from AAO YEARBOOK, 1949, Ellis, WA, "Osteopathic Structural Diagnosis.")

must bear in mind that *if the innominates are rotated in relation to each other, the apex may be moved forward or backward, introducing a source of error in crest height comparison.*

Discrepancies in the iliac crest heights larger than three or four millimeters may be more difficult to quantify visually than making the decision, "level" or "not level." Use of a temporary shim of known thickness is recommended when estimating the amount of discrepancy between the left and right leg. Most leg length inequalities are less than $1/4$ inch (6mm.). Based on visual assessment, estimate the thickness of shim that would be required to make the iliac crests heights level, and then insert the shim under the foot corresponding to the inferior iliac crest. If upon reexamination the iliac crest heights look symmetrical, the examiner knows that the leg length discrepancy is equal to the thickness of the shim. If the estimated shim thickness is within 2 millimeters of the actual anatomic shortness of the leg in question, the iliac crests should appear level as near as the untrained eye can determine.

Such painstaking measurement of anatomic leg length

differences in physical examination is important. Comparison of leg length in recumbent positions provides data relevant to the diagnosis of dysfunctions and subluxations of the pelvic joints. If the patient has a known anatomic difference in leg length of one centimeter, recumbent measurement comparisons of leg length using the medial malleoli or heel pads which do not exactly equal one centimeter are indicators of asymmetric positions of the pelvic bones or lower back.

Trunk adaptations to sacral base asymmetry. An anatomically short leg, or a lateral tilt of the sacral base due to sacroiliac dysfunction, requires scoliotic adaptation. Normal adaptation to an unlevel sacral base is rotoscoliosis convex to the lower side and its absence is pathological, especially if the thoracolumbar junction does not stand directly above the sacrum. The base of spine support is not always the sacrum; occasionally it is the fifth, or even the fourth, lumbar. Some anomalies may be permanent, as in sacralization of the lumbar vertebra, or may represent manipulable disorders.

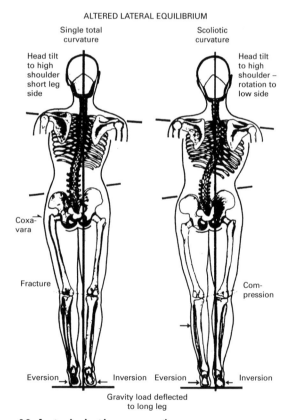

Figure 6.2. Anatomic short leg compensations.
With a left convex "C" curve, the mass of the trunk is shifted to the left of the line of gravity, contributing to body movement inefficiency.

(Reprinted with permission of the American Academy of Osteopathy from AAO YEARBOOK, 1949, Ellis, WA, "Osteopathic Structural Diagnosis.")

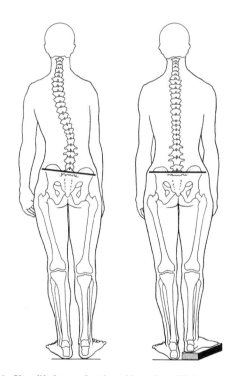

Figure 6.3. Shoe lift therapy for altered lateral equilibrium.
Most authorities are agreed that the goal of shoe lift therapy is to correct postural imbalance in the frontal plane by leveling the sacral base. The success of this therapy depends on many factors: chronicity of the scoliotic compensation, anatomic spinal or sacral anomalies, age of the patient, patient compliance, and so on. Even when the outcome looks as perfect as it does in the illustration, there may be no corresponding symptomatic improvement.

[Reprinted with permission from Neumann, HD. Introduction to Manual Medicine, Springer-Verlag, 4th ed. 1994; 5th ed.(German) 1999.]

Variance in scoliotic patterns is to be expected as the developing scoliosis goes through *stages* of compensation. In Volume 2, the stages were outlined as follows:

Stage I – a long "C" curve convex on the side of the short leg (or the side to which the sacral base tilts), with a contralateral sidebend in the upper cervicals to level the eyes and vestibular apparatus. The sacral base plane is consistent with the leg length asymmetry.

Stage II – the sacral base plane changes by tipping down on one side, probably depending on the side carrying the greatest postural load. If the load increases on the side of the scoliotic convexity, the sacrum may tip down on that side, increasing the compensatory scoliosis.

Stage III – with the increase of imbalance of body masses, "S" curves are formed to rearrange the body masses in more balanced relationship relative to the center line of gravity. This sometimes results in reversal of the lumbar compensatory scoliosis . Non-neutral dysfunctions tend to develop at the base or the crossovers of the "S" curves.

Knowledge of the stages of postural compensation for anatomic short leg helps with planning the sequence of treatment. For example, sometimes treatment outcomes are more beneficial if Stage III adaptations are addressed before Stage II, and Stage II before Stage I; to, in effect, work through the stages in reverse before prescribing a short leg shim, or correcting a sacroiliac dysfunction. Leg length asymmetry may cause muscle imbalance with altered firing sequences of the *latissimus dorsi, quadratus lumborum, erector spinae, iliopsoas, gluteus*, and hamstring muscles. Before beginning the treatment for muscle imbalance, it is important to correct the non-neutral and nonadaptive spinal and sacroiliac dysfunctions (Janda, 1996).

Note regarding postural X-rays. For effective management of anatomic short leg and sacral base asymmetry in the coronal plane, postural X-rays are sometimes necessary, and thus a brief word on the subject is appropriate here. For an excellent discussion on the technique for postural X-ray studies, refer to Lewit (1999).

Radiogrammetry can be used to determine the direction and degree of sacral base declination in the coronal plane. It can also be used to both verify the presence of any leg length inequality, and to measure the discrepancy in leg length for the purpose of prescribing an orthotic heel lift.

Experience and research have demonstrated that there are ways to increase the clarity of the image, as well as produce an image which is better suited for accurate measurement of asymmetries. For the purposes of measurement, establishing a vertical reference line is absolutely necessary and can be accomplished in one of two ways: by suspending a plumb line between the cathode ray and the film; or by taping a vertical line directly to the film (Lewit, 1999). By drawing lines perpendicular to the vertical reference line, asymmetries or declinations in the coronal plane can be measured. With an A-P film, a line drawn across the sacral base can be compared with a line drawn between the iliac crests, and to a line drawn between the tops of the femur heads.

Accurate reading of radiogrammetric images is influenced by the clarity of the image, and by knowing the direction the image was taken rel-

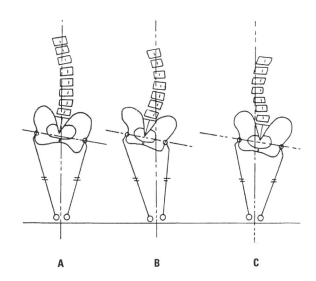

Figure 6.4. Three stages of spinal adaptation to an anatomically short leg.
The Beilke/Grant model of the progression of spinal compensations to anatomic leg length inequality. Fig. 6.4.A shows the first stage, a long "C" curve convex on the short leg side with compensatory tilting of the head and neck to level the eyes and labyrinth. Over time the trunk mass shift to the right often drives the sacrum down on the short leg side producing the effect seen in Figure 6.4.B, increased lumbar scoliosis and pelvic shift toward the long leg side. To bring body masses closer to the mid-line of gravity, and, thereby conserve energy, the vestibular-cerebellar postural control system creates more alternating curves in the spine (Figure 6.4.C). Often the first crossover occurs in a lower lumbar segment with a non-neutral dysfunction harmonic with a similar dysfunction in the upper cervical region and pelvic shift to the short leg side.
(Reprinted with permission of the American Academy of Osteopathy from AAO YEARBOOK, 1966: Larson, N. "Sacroiliac and postural changes from anatomic short lower extremity")

ative to the patient. A lead (Pb) marker can be taped to the patient's buttock which indicates the left or right side (this because of the high incidence of left/right confusion when sides are not identified). To improve the clarity of the image, for both the A-P and lateral films the center beam of the cathode should be aimed horizontally across the sacral base, i.e., in a plane midway between the iliac crests and the greater trochanters. Turning the cathode sideways will allow utilization of the anode heel effect (Pruzzo, 1971) to maximize penetration through the pelvic bones while avoiding overexposure of the lumbars. The cathode should be as far from the film as possible to minimize distortion, ideally 2 meters. Obviously the plumb line must not move when the patient presses against the film cassette. This is why Lewit advises taping the line to the cassette.

As has been pointed out in this chapter and elsewhere, in addition to anatomic short leg, declinations of the sacral base in the coronal plane can be attributed to a variety of conditions, eg. pelvic dysfunctions, subluxations, or anatomic anomalies. When these latter influences are concomitant with anatomic short leg, the plane across the sacral base is often not parallel with the planes resting on top of the iliac crests or the femur heads. For measuring leg length, as well as for other diagnostic purposes, these paradoxes may be avoided by manipulating the pelvis before the X-rays are taken.

Fig. 6.5. Locating the iliac crests.
To position the hands on the apex of the iliac crests requires pushing the soft tissues out of the way to avoid trapping subcutaneous fat between the iliac crest and the hand.

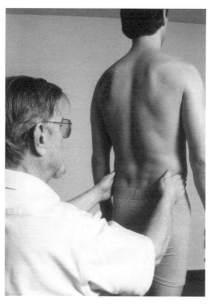

Fig. 6.6. Visual comparison of iliac crest heights.
Tip the palms to face caudad as the index fingers rest on top of the iliac crest apices. Observer's eyes should be level with the hands. By placing a shim under the short leg the iliac crests can be made approximately level in preparation for the standing flexion test.

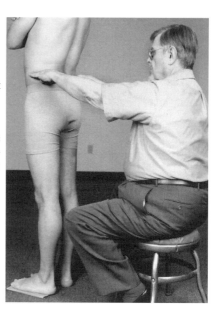

Iliac Crest Heights Tests

Standing Iliac Crest Heights Test

In preparation for performing the Standing Iliac Crest Heights Test, the examiner should preferably be seated behind the patient, with the eyes positioned so that visual assessment is made in the same transverse plane as the iliac crests. The patient should stand with their heels approximately 4 to 5 inches apart, taking care not to externally or internally rotate one leg more than the other. The feet should be pointing straight ahead.

Procedure Task Analysis

1. With the patient standing in front with their back to you, place your hands on the sides of the pelvis and use palmar stereognosis to find the lateral portions of the ilia.

2. To avoid varying thickness of soft tissue between hands and crests, hands are first placed laterally below the iliac crests, pulling the skin down from the waist (Figure 6.5). Position the palmar surface of the index and middle fingers near the apices of the iliac crests and press medially until pressed against the bone of the ilia.

3. Flesh is then pushed superior-mediad until the index fingers top the crest (Figure 6.6). While continuing to press medially against the ilia, push superiorly up to above the apices of the crests, then pronate the arms so that the palmar surfaces are facing the floor. This maneuver avoids trapping adipose tissue.

4. Make the visual comparison between the left and right iliac crest heights relative to a horizontal plane. Be sure to position your line of sight in the same transverse plane as your hands, and your eyes at arm's length from your hands to get both hands in your central visual field.

5. If a difference in crest heights is noted, place shims under the foot on the low side until the crests look level with the horizontal plane.

6. Measure the thickness of the shim. It will be within 2 mm. of the actual difference in anatomic leg lengths.

Note regarding heel lift therapy. The clinical method of visually estimating comparative anatomic leg lengths by observing the standing iliac crests is usually quite reliable. Even untrained eyes can discern differences in heights as small as 2 millimeters (Mitchell Jr., 1976). But various pelvic distortions due to dysfunction, subluxation, or bony dysgeneses may compromise the validity of the test. Adaptations to sacroiliac dysfunctions frequently displace the apices of the iliac crests, introducing a potential error in the measurement of their heights.

The criteria for heel lift therapy are somewhat arbitrary, hence, controversial. The goal of heel lift therapy is to reduce stress on the postural mechanisms, which in turn may stress other systems. Some practitioners introduce heel shims in small increments, hoping to "sneak up on the body" and change it without stressing it. The author's practice has been to make measurements on the X-ray, and then prescribe about 3 millimeters less than what appears to be required by the X-ray, to take into account the magnification factor and the standard error of reproducibility of the X-ray technique.

Since we are unable to predict how much change constitutes unacceptable stress for a given patient, it may be sensible to consider that perhaps one episode of stress would be better instead of multiple episodes. Shims thicker than 6 millimeters usually require some undercut beveling of the back of the heel to avoid toe slapping, whether the shim is inside or outside the shoe. Shims thicker than 9 millimeters cannot be practically worn inside the shoe or boot and should be added to the heel and preferably the entire sole of the shoe, to avoid stressing the ankle.

Evaluating the effectiveness of heel lift therapy cannot be done by X-ray alone. There are probably as many ways to evaluate heel lift therapy as there are clinicians who believe it is important for health care. Each clinician has specific criteria, mostly related to postural balance and locomotor efficiency. The patient's subjective assessment should be given high priority. If the patient feels worse, the shim should probably be changed or eliminated. A successful shim should put the body of the twelfth thoracic vertebra in the mid-sagittal plane (Lewit, 1999).

Seated Iliac Crest Heights Test

Old pelvic fractures or dysgenesis of the pelvis can make the hipbone sizes unequal. The resulting asymmetry of the seated posture can be stressful enough to cause symptoms anywhere in the body. Shimming the small side of the pelvis with a magazine or book to level the iliac crests should be done in these cases, in order to observe the effect on spinal curvatures. This anatomic asymmetry may have effects similar to those of an anatomic short leg. Shimming the small side of the pelvis can be an important part of therapy. The patient can carry along his own shim to sit on.

Note: Asymmetry of the size of the os coxae (hip bone, a part of the lower limb) occurs rarely, but can be ruled out by comparing the heights of the iliac crests with the patient in the seated position.

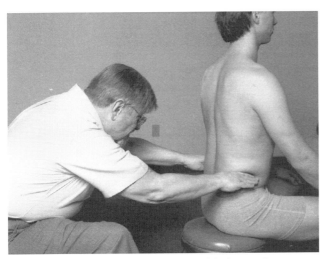

Figure 6.7 Seated iliac crest heights test for pelvic dysgenesis.
The seated spinal posture can be stressed by unequal hip bone size (due to pelvic dysgenesis or old pelvis fracture). Such patients can benefit by carrying their own shim to sit on. The examiner's eyes must be level with the hands in order to compare iliac crests.

Interpreting Crest Heights Tests

Anatomic short leg (ICD9CM 755.30) is very likely to produce a scoliotic spinal adaptation. However, this does not always occur. A sacroiliac dysfunction, a contralateral innominate dysgenesis, or even a subluxation, may entirely compensate for the short leg, obviating the need for spinal adaptation. The only goal of heel lift therapy is to reduce postural stress on the spine. Clearly, there are some circumstances of anatomic short leg for which heel lift therapy is contraindicated.

Pelvic dysgenesis (ICD9CM 755.60) comes in many forms. Only those dysgenetic asymmetries which cause sacral base imbalance may require shimming to reduce spinal postural stress.

These bony anomalies may occur on the same side, or on opposite sides. It is best to delay interpreting the crest heights tests until both standing and seated tests have been performed.

Flexion Tests for Pelvisacral Mobility

The purpose of the flexion tests is to determine whether there is movement restriction of a sacroiliac joint on one side. Fortunately, bilateral symmetrical restriction is rare. Flexion tests are performed by monitoring either the PSISs or PIPs from behind the seated or standing patient as they move with trunk and hip flexion. Normally, when the trunk goes into flexion, the entire pelvis rotates anteriorly on the acetabular axis, and the sacrum moves independently *between* the ilia (either nutates or counternutates). While the sacrum is flexing between the ilia there is simultaneous tilting forward of the innominates on the acetabular axis. As the pelvic tilt nears its limits, superior/anterior motion of the PSISs slows and stops, but the sacrum continues to nutate, or possibly counternutate.

It is crucial to understand that forward bending of the spine is always accompanied by anterior nutation of the sacrum (sacral base tipping forward), at least at the beginning of flexion. At extreme trunk forward bending, the phenomenon of sacral counter-nutation may occur, as explained in Chapter 2. Sacral counter-nutation with trunk hyperflexion probably occurs in less than fifty percent of cases.

Note: For some the idea that the sacrum nutates in response to flexion of the trunk has been a source of confusion. This confusion has stemmed, in part, from the overgeneralized rule that, in the case of sacroiliac dysfunction, L_5 *always* moves opposite to the movement of the sacral base, in all three planes. Thus, if the sacral base was flexed, sidebent right, and rotated left, then L_5 was expected to be extended, sidebent left and rotated right. Two problems arise from too rigid adherence to this rule: 1) empirical evidence has shown that the fifth lumbar does not follow this rule in all cases; and 2) there has been a tendency to assume that if the fifth lumbar always moves opposite to movements of the sacral base, then the sacral base must also always move opposite to the movements of the fifth lumbar. Thus, many students beginning to learn the Flexion Tests have been misguided by the preconception that the sacrum always counternutates when the trunk forward bends. This preconception would make it difficult or impossible to correctly interpret Flexion Test results.

When the spine bends forward or backward, the sacrum moves in the *same* direction as L_5 from the beginning of the bend. If both sacroiliac joints have normal freedom, then, even though the ilia are rotating anteriorly as well, the sacrum will nutate (on the middle transverse axis) an additional 6 to 8 degrees independent of the ilia.

However, if the sacrum is adhered to the ilium on one side – the right side, for example – there will be a difference in the movement pattern of the normal (left) ilium *versus* the restricted (right) one. When the sacrum engages the restriction on the right ilium, as the sacrum continues to nutate, moving freely and independently relative to the left ilium (the normal side), it will carry the right ilium farther for those last few degrees of trunk flexion. *Thus the PSIS side that is moving all by itself near the end of the bend is the restricted side, i.e., the PSIS with the greatest (longest) excur-*

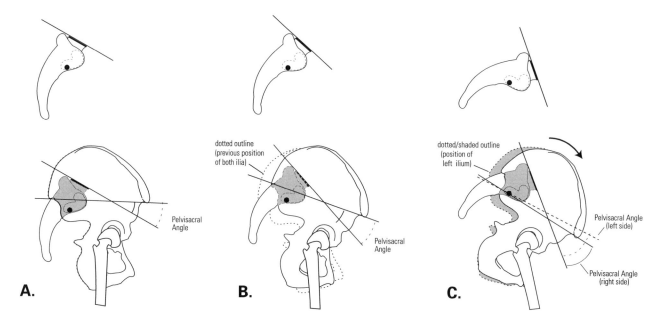

A.

B.

C.

Figure 6.8.A. Prior to trunk flexion. In the neutral erect position, the sacral base is in a somewhat nutated position, oriented anteriorly and inferiorly. As trunk flexion continues in the midrange, the sacral base nutates further about the middle transverse axis as the vertebral body of L5 directs load vectors onto the anterior portion of the sacral base. At some point in hyperflexion, the sacrum may counternutate (see Chapter 2). For now, what is important to recognize is that the sacrum will nutate in response to the flexion of L5. Prior to encountering restriction, even though the ilia will rotate anteriorly about the acetabular axis, nutation of the sacrum occurs independently and in addition to rotation of the innominates, increasing the pelvisacral angle.

Figure 6.8.B. Initial phase of trunk flexion. In the initial phase of trunk flexion, as the sacrum begins nutation in response to trunk flexion, the ilia will rotate anteriorly (and symmetrically) about the acetabular transverse axis. This rotation is represented in the above illustration; the solid outline of the ilia represents the anteriorly rotated left and right ilium, the dotted outline represents the position of the ilia before trunk flexion was initiated. In addition, by comparing the pelvisacral angles, we can see that the sacrum has nutated in the same direction as the ilia, and there is little change in the pelvisacral angle.

Figure 6.8.C. Phase of trunk flexion after restriction is encountered at the right sacroiliac joint. Toward the end of the initial phase of trunk flexion, the ilia will reach a point where they no longer are symmetrically rotating anteriorly. The illustration above depicts what occurs after the initial phase of trunk flexion, and after restriction is engaged at the right sacroiliac/iliosacral joint. The shaded outlined ilium represents the left ilium, which has reached the end of its normal range of anterior rotation about the acetabular axis. In the presence of SI/IS restriction on the right, flexion beyond this point will result in the right ilium (which is tethered to the sacrum) being carried further into anterior rotation than the left ilium, as the sacrum continues to nutate further relative to the left ilium.

sion is considered the abnormal ("positive") side. The path of PSIS movement on the positive side will be inferior to superior on the way down, and superior to inferior on the way back up. Because of the occasional counternutation of the sacrum, the path is sometimes altered: anterior to posterior going down, and posterior to anterior coming back up. The range of "positive" movement varies from a barely perceptible 1 millimeter to a more noticeable 20 millimeters (about an inch). The ilium that moves farther does so because it is adhered to, and therefore must follow, the sacrum.

When there is dysfunction involving the sacroiliac-iliosacral joint, the sacrum and ilium become compressed against each other and the sacrum cannot complete its movement without taking the ilium on the side of the restriction with it as it continues to move on the unrestricted side. It does not matter if it is the sacrum compressed against the ilium, or the ilium compressed against the sacrum; the result is the same. **The goal of the flex-**

ion test is solely to identify (lateralize) the side of dysfunction. A more definitive diagnosis requires more detailed evaluation procedures.

Why is lateralization necessary? Why is not lateralization sufficient to make a diagnosis? Is it not enough to know that the sacrum and right ilium are stuck together, for example? If the lateralization test shows right side restriction, any one of eleven different manipulable lesions of the pelvis could account for that restriction – namely, right superior pubic subluxation, right inferior pubic subluxation, right upslipped innominate, right outflared innominate, right inflared innominate, flexed sacrum on the right, left torsioned sacrum on the left oblique axis, right torsioned sacrum on the left oblique axis, right sacroiliac respiratory restriction, right innominate rotated anteriorly, or right innominate rotated posteriorly. Combinations of two or more of the twenty-two possible pelvic dysfunctions are common. Additionally, sacral adaptations to spinal dysfunction or scoliosis can also cause flexion test positives.

However, even though the flexion tests do not permit a definitive diagnosis, let us consider the ways some specific manipulable disorders of the pelvis can affect the flexion tests, and the mechanism/nature of those specific types of restriction. When there is sacroiliac dysfunction present (whether unilaterally flexed or torsioned), the sacrum is blocked on the ilium; the sacrum is compressed – its movement restricted osteoarticularly – *against the ilium.*

In the case of the torsioned sacrum, whether forward or backward, the sacrum has an osteoarticular block at the pivot point where the inferior pole of the oblique axis intersects the ilium. This compression or blockage is maintained by the contraction of the piriformis on the side where the oblique axis is stabilized. Thus, for a sacrum that is torsioned on the left oblique axis, the blockage is on the right, because the left oblique axis is stabilized by the right piriformis. In this case, because the sacrum is blocked on the right, as the patient goes into trunk flexion the PSIS/PIP on the right will move superior as the sacrum continues to nutate. Likewise, a sacrum that is torsioned about the right oblique axis will be blocked on the left, because the left piriformis is what is causing the sacrum to be compressed on the ilium. As one would suspect, a sacrum torsioned on the right oblique axis will yield a positive flexion test result on the left.

In the case of the unilaterally flexed sacrum, the blockage is on the same side that the sacrum is flexed. The mechanism of intraarticular blockage in unilateral sacral flexion is probably joint compression due to increased tension on the anterior sacroiliac ligaments. If the sacrum is unilaterally flexed on the left, then the osteoarticular blockage is on the left. If the blockage is on the left, then the flexion test will yield a positive finding on the left; *vice versa* for a right unilaterally flexed sacrum.

With either the anterior or posterior rotated innominate, the restriction is on the same side as the lesion. In this case, it is the ilium which has become compressed against the sacrum. Because the restriction is on the side of the lesion, the *standing* flexion test will yield a positive finding on that same side, and probably the seated flexion test, as well, but to a lesser degree.

It is important to note that there are some mechanical differences between the flexion test performed with the patient standing, and the one performed with the patient seated.

In the standing flexion test the ilium, which is compressed on (stuck to) the sacrum, is free to follow the sacrum by tipping forward on the femur, resisted only by the *gluteus* and *fascia lata.* In seated flexion the innominates are resting on the seat, and are somewhat braced by the horizontal femurs in the acetabula. If the sacrum is stuck to one innominate, that innominate rocks forward on the ischial tuberosity as the sacrum pulls the ilium forward and superior.

These slight differences in standing and seated flexion mechanics gives the iliosacral dysfunction slightly more influence in the standing flexion test, and sacroiliac dysfunctions relatively more influence in the seated flexion test. The difference in influence is slight, however.

The Standing Flexion Test

The Standing Flexion Test is mostly a test for *iliosacral* motion, i.e., how the ilia move on the sacrum. However, *sacroiliac* dysfunctions can also effect on the standing flexion test, though probably to a lesser degree. Because of this carried over effect, the standing and seated flexion tests are rated + or ++, whenever possible. Other tests will allow you to diagnose the *type* of iliosacral lesion, but the *Standing Flexion Test* determines the *side* of the lesion. The iliosacral dysfunctions manifested by a positive standing flexion test are, in order of frequency of occurrence:

1. Right anterior innominate rotation
2. Left posterior innominate rotation
3. Left anterior innominate rotation
4. Right posterior innominate rotation

When performing the standing flexion test, the patient's feet should be positioned parallel and approximately acetabular distance apart. After the patient has bent forward, place the thumbs firmly against the *inferior slopes* of the bony prominences in order to follow the movement of the iliac crests (bone, not skin) as the patient bends forward and backward. Firm placement of the thumbs against the PSISs/PIPs is necessary in order to minimize the tendency of the soft tissues to pull the thumbs off of the landmark as the skin and fascia of the back tighten. To maintain firm contact on the landmark without pushing the patient off balance, one's fingertips may grasp the *gluteus* muscle mass to help pull the thumbs in on the inferior slope of the point of bone. Additionally, while the patient is forward bent, or bending forward, the examiner must not push forward, but rather allow the patient's pelvis to come back.

The standing flexion test as originally taught by Mitchell, Sr., had the examiner following the PSISs/PIPs *while* the patient was bending forward from an erect position. One of the problems with this older method of doing the tests was the frequent occurrence of spurious movements and palpable tissue changes accompanying the initial phases of trunk flexion. Those who expected to see the positive test movement phenomenon at the beginning of flexion tended to misinterpret these spurious movements and tissue changes.

An important improvement in the flexion tests was later developed by Mitchell, Jr. Instead of observing the landmarks while the patient was bending forward, the examiner observes the movements of their thumbs *during the first few degrees of straightening, after the patient has bent all the way forward*. The *positive* side will move alone, before the normal side begins moving. This part of the action can be observed repeatedly by having the patient flex and extend within this narrow range. If the test is even slightly positive, there will be unilateral movement in some part of this range.

This modified version of the flexion tests increases the sensitivity and reliability of the test so significantly that *it is the preferred way to do it – especially for beginners*. Instead of following the PSISs/PIPs during the forward bend, have the patient flex first and then follow the PSISs/PIPs for the first moments of straightening.

Occasionally, at the extreme of flexion, posterior motion of the PIP or PSIS occurs in addition to superior motion. The explanation is that the sacrum, at the extreme end of the trunk flexion, counternutates on the non-restricted side of the pelvis, and pulls the restricted innominate with it. This anterior-posterior motion of the PIP can be interpreted as equivalent to the superior (cephalic) and inferior (caudal) movement of a positive test result.

Theoretically, contralateral hamstring tightness can cause a false positive result by restraining hip joint flexion. Strangely, this almost never happens. While the patient is flexed, the hamstrings can be palpated for tightness, but the best test for hamstring tightness is the supine straight leg raise. The hamstring and *fascia lata* influence is eliminated when the patient sits down.

Prior to Performing the Standing Flexion Test

Leveling the Pelvis with a Shim. *It is always a good practice to begin the evaluation of the pelvis with the comparison of standing iliac crest heights*. If the results of the standing and seated iliac crest heights tests indicate that one leg is anatomically short, and the discrepancy is greater than one centimeter, then to enhance reliability of the standing flexion test, a shim the same thickness as the discrepancy in leg length should be placed under the short leg. If possible, measure the thickness of the shim, and write it down. If the iliac crests are not leveled with a shim before performing the standing flexion test, then the landmarks used to monitor the pelvisacral motion will not be in the same transverse and coronal plane at the start of the test. Although a determination can be made under such circumstance as to whether one side is moving more than the other, it makes it more difficult to visually quantify the degree of discrepancy, i.e., whether it is positive + or ++.

Locating the PSISs/PIPs. A prerequisite to performing the flexion tests is locating the PSISs or posterior iliac prominences (PIPs) on the patient. Either the PSIS or the PIP may be used to perform standing or seated flexion tests, since each is a landmark on the same bone. The visual and stereognostic methods of finding the PIPs have already been described in Chapter 1. When performing the test, one's thumbs should maintain constant contact with the inferior slopes of the landmarks during the act of bending forward *and straightening up.*

Before doing the flexion test, the bilateral symmetry of these prominences may be assessed. Apparent static asymmetry could be the result of having the thumbs on different points. If, after leveling the crests with a shim and making sure the thumbs are on analogous landmarks, the landmark is inferior on one side compared with the other side, it suggests either posterior innominate rotation on the inferior side, or anterior rotation of the other innominate. Such rotation is not necessarily an iliosacral somatic dysfunction. Most of the time it represents a shift of the pelvic bones to adapt to sacroiliac dysfunction. If the asymmetry is anterior-posterior, there is probably hip rotator muscle imbalance causing the whole pelvis to rotate on the legs.

Task Analysis for Finding the PIPs

1. Sit or stand behind the standing patient

2. Place the flats of three finger pads on the area of the back where the dimple is, or should be.

3. With the other hand stabilizing the pelvis from in front, move the skin under the finger pads in a circle with firm inward pressure (Figure 6.10.).

4. Feel for knots, and select the hardest, most stable, one. *Note:* If more than one knot is felt, the extra knots are usually fibrolipomata, benign subcutaneous tumors composed of encapsulated fat, which are somewhat softer than bone and more movable, but are sometimes rather firmly attached to the periosteum of the bone and cannot be easily pushed aside.

5. If both PIP and PSIS are discerned, choose the best one to follow.

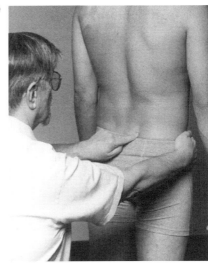

Figure 6.9. Locating the gluteal tubercle (PIP). The dimple of Michaelis.

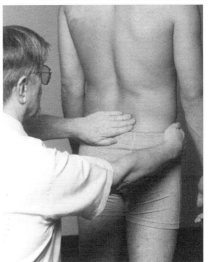

Figure 6.10. Locating the gluteal tubercle (PIP). Using circular motion stereognosis to locate the gluteal tubercle deep to the dimple of Michaelis, which is sometimes not visible. After the patient has fully flexed, the gluteal tubercle can be located with the same circular motion.

The Standing Flexion/Extension Test
Protocol Task Analysis

1. The patient is barefooted and stands, or attempts to stand, erect. If the iliac crests were not level, a temporary shim should be in place.

2. The feet are apart so that the heels are directly under the acetabula. The toes should point straight ahead. The weight should be evenly distributed on both feet. The arms hang freely at the sides.

3. Stand or sit directly behind the patient so that your eyes are above the level of the patient's pelvis.

4. Instruct the patient to keep the knees straight and bend forward as far as possible, as if attempting to touch the toes.

5. Find the *inferior slopes* of the gluteal tubercle (PIP) on both sides and place your thumbs firmly on them.

6. Instruct the patient to straighten (extend the back) a little, "about a foot," and to stop in that position. Watch your thumbs closely for any asymmetry of *inferior (and/or anterior)* movement of the gluteal tuberosities or PSISs, i.e., one side moving and the other side not moving. Repeat the flexion and extension movements in this small range if you are not sure of the results.

7. Make the comparison. Be sure to note the *linear distance* of the positive side motion for later comparison with the seated flexion test.

Note: This new variation of the Standing Flexion Test has been taught in Muscle Energy Tutorials and in classrooms since about 1985. The previous version had the examiner trying to follow the iliac crest landmark while the patient bent forward. To keep from pushing the patient off balance, it was necessary to grasp the gluteus muscle mass with the fingertips to pull the thumbs firmly into contact with the same points and keep them there as the patient bent all the way forward at the hips, keeping the knees straight. This method often presented difficulty because of the increasing tension in the skin and fascia, which not only tended to pull the thumbs off the landmark, but was frequently misinterpreted by students as a positive finding. Of those who continue to use the previous version, many became skillful at it and obtain valid and reliable results in spite of its disadvantages.

As noted above, a common error is allowing the thumbs to be pulled superiorly by the soft tissue tensions generated by the forward bend. This is more likely to happen at the beginning of the forward bend. Keeping firm thumb contact on the inferior slope of the landmark may prevent this error. However, it is difficult to maintain precise contact. Even more problematic is the tendency of the observer to be seduced by palpable changes in the soft tissues and to misread those changes as linear movements of the bony landmarks. Following the advice of steps 5 and 6 will help prevent this problem. Renaming these procedures the "Standing Extension Test" and the "Seated Extension Test" was considered, but it was decided that the names would introduce more confusion than clarity. Instead they were tentatively renamed "Standing Flexion/Extension Test" and "Seated Flexion/Extension Test." However, we never broke the habit of calling them "flexion tests."

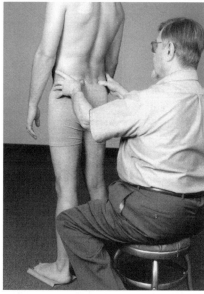

Fig. 6.11. Standing flexion test – conventional starting position.
Placement of the thumbs on the inferior slopes of the gluteal tubercles. Note the fingers gripping the gluteal muscles to pull the thumbs firmly against the landmark without pushing the patient off-balance.
The eyes are level with the hands. The patient is standing erect.

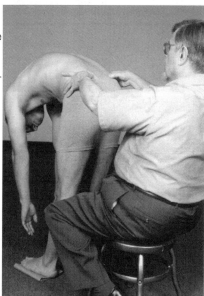

Fig. 6.12. The new standing flexion test.
Step 1. After first having the patient do a full forward bend, the thumbs are placed firmly on the inferior slopes of the gluteal tubercles. As the patient bends forward, allow the hips to move posterior in relation to placement of their feet.

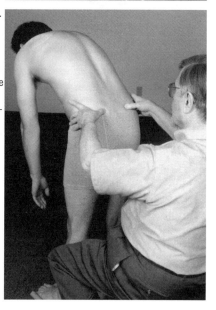

Fig. 6.13. The new standing flexion test.
Step 2. The patient is instructed to "Come up a foot and stop." The thumbs follow the movements of the gluteal tubercles, the eyes watch the thumbs for unilateral movement, indicating restricted iliosacral mobility on the moving side. This method will improve detection of the more subtle asymmetries.

Interpretation of Results

■ The bilateral PIP (or PSIS) should be pulled superiorly in equal amount all the way to the completion of the forward bend, if both sides are normal. Readers familiar with the "overtake phenomenon" taught in various parts of the world should make special note of the differences in concepts of the forward bending tests. Some of the initial movement of the sacrum in relation to the ilium is presumed to be relatively free. But after sacroiliac mobility reaches its limit, the ilium is obliged to follow the sacrum. Therefore, it is rare to see unilateral movement of an iliac crest landmark such as the PIP at the *beginning* of the forward bend. If it does occur at the beginning, it signifies that sacroiliac mobility of that side is nearly absent, an uncommon condition. If there is slight restriction of a sacroiliac joint, the evidence will appear *near the completion of the forward bend*.

■ **A positive test is demonstrated when one PSIS (or PIP) is pulled (or pushed) farther after its mate has stopped moving; the side demonstrating motion, which is followed by your thumb, is the restricted (lesioned) side.** It is only superficially paradoxical that the side which moves more is the restricted side. The bone moves because it is unable to allow the sacrum to move freely on it. Other tests will make the definitive diagnosis; the Standing Flexion Test has merely indicated the side with the restriction.

■ *Carryover effect.* The two flexion tests for the pelvis, standing and sitting, do not completely separate iliosacral from sacroiliac functions. The sitting and standing tests overlap a lot. Only by *comparing* the results of the Standing and Seated Flexion Tests can iliosacral be separated from sacroiliac dysfunctions (without the usual follow-up evaluation of pelvic landmarks). Often the linear distance of the positive test movement is nearly the same standing and sitting, giving no basis for distinguishing sacroiliac from iliosacral dysfunction other than examining the rest of the pelvic landmarks, which you expect to do, anyway, especially if there is screening evidence of pelvic dysfunction.

If pelvic landmark asymmetry is found in the absence of flexion test positive findings, it is reasonable to assume that the flexion test was symmetrically, or bilaterally, positive. In this case, there would be a strong possibility of a contralateral lesion, also.

■ **One to two centimeters difference in superior-inferior PIP excursion constitutes a strongly positive test result.** One-half to one centimeter is weakly positive. If there is a noticeable difference between standing and sitting tests, the weaker positive can usually be regarded as "carried over" from the stronger positive test, and can be accounted for by a single dysfunction, unless, of course, the positive result switches sides. The strength of the "carried over" effect varies greatly, and a single dysfunction may cause standing and seated test results of equal magnitude.

With complex lesions (more than one dysfunction simultaneously), bilateral positives are possible.

■ *False positive.* If the difference in inferior/superior position of the PSISs was marked in Seated Flexion and only mild in Standing, you are likely seeing carryover from the Seated Test (sacroiliac) to Standing (iliosacral); there may be no iliosacral lesion.

■ *False negative.* If a difference in inferior/superior position of the PSISs was marked in Seated Flexion, but was not present in the Standing Flexion Test, suspect a false negative on the other side. There should always be some carryover from sitting to standing. Symmetrical results can conceal bilateral lesions with equal restrictive effects. A bilateral positive looks like a negative (normal)!

■ Occasionally, when the PIP is pulled superiorly by the flexing sacrum, a seemingly paradoxical *posterior* motion of the PIP may be seen. In this newer version of the test, the straightening of the spine from the hyperflexed position may cause *anterior* movement of the PIP. This is due to the counternutation of the sacrum which occurs after the flexing sacrum changes its flexion axis from the middle transverse to the superior transverse axis. In order to move superiorly with the flexing spine, the sacral base must follow the path of the short arm of the sacroiliac joint. This may occur on one side only, the other side having become locked on the sacrum. These paradoxical movements can be considered the equivalent of superior-inferior movement and can be added to the linear distance for standing-sitting comparison.

This counternutation reversal phenomenon may be important in the interpretation of standing and seated flexion tests. It could account for the occasional observation of posterior movement of the PSIS or posterior iliac prominence (PIP) at the extreme flexed position of the standing or seated flexion tests. As long as the sacral nutation is parallel with the forward bending spine and the sacral base tips forward by rotating on the middle transverse axis, the positive flexion test side will move the PSIS anteriorly and craniad. But at extreme flexion, with the erector spinae muscles pulling the sacrum superiorly, the base of the sacrum may move posteriorly on the normal side. The posteriorly moving sacral base takes the ilium on the restricted side posteriorly with it. Sometimes the posterior movement of the PSIS is the principal manifestation of the positive flexion test, instead of the expected superior movement.

■ Sacroiliac or iliosacral dysfunction is the usual cause of a positive Flexion/Extension Test. Occasionally the cause is neither. Respiratory restriction of the sacroiliac joint, or even cranially induced sacral oscillation may occasionally cause a positive Flexion/Extension Test. A positive flexion test may be due to sacral adaptation to a primary spinal lesion, especially dysfunction in the lumbar spine. When the spinal lesion is treated, the sacrum autocorrects and the flexion test becomes negative (normal).

Seated Flexion Test

By assessing the patient in the seated position, asymmetric iliosacral functions are minimized. The seated position increases the stability of the ilia in relation to the lower extremities by resting the ilia on the ischial tuberosities, and by buttressing them with the femurs into the acetabula. The sacrum, moving as a part of the spine between the two ilia, is still relatively free to move as compared with the two ilia. Such spine induced motion can be called sacroiliac to distinguish it from iliosacral motion (motion of one ilium in relation to the other, or in relation to the sacrum). Sacroiliac dysfunctions affect the seated flexion test more, and the standing flexion test somewhat less. Conversely, iliosacral dysfunction affects the standing flexion test more, the seated less. Lumbar dysfunction can cause a false positive Seated Flexion Test, just as it may cause a false positive Standing Flexion Test.

The Seated Flexion Test Procedure Protocol

1. The patient sits on a stable low stool without wheels. A straight chair without arms can be used, provided the seat is not contoured and does not slant, and the patient sits with the chair back to one side near a shoulder. The knees are spread shoulder width apart. The feet should be flat on the floor.

2. Sit, or kneel, directly behind the patient.

3. Instruct the patient to bend completely forward. Instruction: "*Put your feet and knees shoulder width apart, and bend forward, putting your elbows between your feet.*"

4. Place your thumbs bilaterally on the inferior slopes of the patient's gluteal tubercles (PIPs), or the inferior slopes of the Posterior Superior Iliac Spines (PSIS).

Note: A common error, when performing this test, is that the patient does not bend forward far enough. *The last few degrees of flexion are crucial to a successful test*, for this is where the slightest restriction of sacroiliac mobility will cause asymmetric motion. Therefore, the best way to perform the test is to relocate the inferior slopes of the gluteal tuberosities (PIPs), or the PSISs, with your thumbs *after the patient is fully flexed.*

5. Then instruct the patient to straighten (extend the back) "about a foot," and to stop in that position.

6. Watch your thumbs closely for any asymmetry of movement of the gluteal tuberosities or PSISs, i.e., one side moving and the other side not moving.

7. Repeat the flexion and extension movements in this small range if you are not sure of the results.

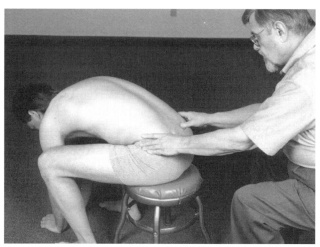

Figure 6.14. Seated Flexion Test (sacroiliac). Step 3. Patient is fully flexed, feet and knees widely apart, hands or elbows between the ankles. Doing the seated flexion test in reverse will increase the reliability of the test.

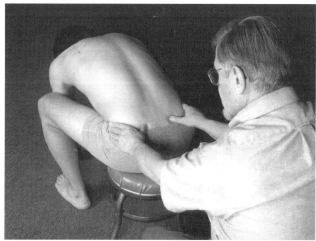

Figure 6.15. Seated Flexion Test (sacroiliac). Step 4. Find the gluteal tubercles and place the thumb pads on their inferior slopes.

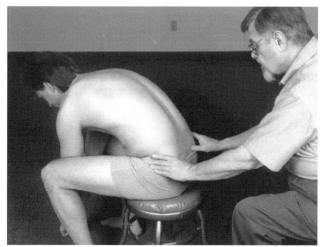

Figure 6.16. Seated Flexion Test (sacroiliac). Steps 5 and 6. Follow the gluteal tubercles as the patient begins to extend (straighten). In this part of the range of motion one is most likely to see unilateral movement of the ilium , indicating sacroiliac joint restriction on that side.

Table 6.B.

Flexion Test Results and Probable Diagnoses

PSIS/PIP Asymmetry with patient:		Probable Diagnosis
flexed standing	*flexed sitting*	
no asymmetry	no asymmetry	Normal – possible bilateral dysfunction (very rare)
no asymmetry	Left side moved – 1 to 2 mm	Sacrum Flexed Left (SFL), possibly with anteriorly rotated right innominate (AIR), or right pelvic or pubic subluxation.
no asymmetry	Left side moved – 2 to 3 mm	Sacrum Flexed Left (SFL), probably with anteriorly rotated right innominate (AIR), or right pelvic or pubic subluxation.
Left side moved 0 to 1 mm.	Right side moved – 2 to 3 mm	Sacrum Torsioned Left (STL) on the Left Oblique Axis (LOA), with probable posteriorly rotated left innominate (PIL), or left pelvic/pubic subluxation.
Right side moved 1 to 2 mm.	Right side moved – 2 to 3 mm	Sacrum Torsioned Left (STL) on the Left Oblique Axis (LOA).
Left side moved 1 to 2 mm.	Left side moved – 2 to 3 mm	Sacrum Flexed Left (SFL).
Right side moved 1 to 3 mm.	Right side moved – 1 to 3 mm	Right inferior pubic subluxation, or a combination of Sacrum Flexed Left (SFL) and anteriorly rotated right innominate (AIR).
Right side moved 1 to 3 mm.	no asymmetry	Anteriorly rotated right innominate (AIR), with probable Sacrum Flexed Left (SFL).
Left side moved 1 to 3 mm.	Right side moved – 0 to 1 mm	Posteriorly rotated left innominate (PIL), with probable Sacrum Torsioned Left (STL) on the Left Oblique Axis (LOA).
Right side moved 2 to 3 mm.	Right side moved – 1 to 2 mm	Anteriorly rotated right innominate (AIR).

Interpretation of Results

■ The bilateral PSIS (or PIP) should be pulled an equal distance *superiorly* by flexion, or *inferiorly* by extension. Anterior or posterior movements of the landmarks should be added to the linear distance of the superior-inferior movements.

■ A positive test is demonstrated when one PSIS (or PIP) is pulled (or pushed) farther after its mate has stopped moving; the side demonstrating motion, which is followed by your thumb, is the restricted (lesioned) side. It is only superficially paradoxical that the side which moves more is the restricted side. The bone moves because it is unable to allow the sacrum to move freely on it.

The seated flexion positive may be more, or less, positive compared with the standing flexion positive. To take this important variance into account, the standing and seated flexion test results can be graded as 0, 1, 2, or 3. A negative test – perfect symmetry – is graded 0. If PIP movement is 3mm ($1/8$ inch) or less on one side compared to the other, that side is grade 1 positive. Grade 2 positive would be asymmetric PIP movement $1/8$ to $3/8$ inches (3-9mm). Grade 3 would be greater than 9 mm.

Table 6.B. indicates how this information can help with interpretation of the flexion tests.

■ If a positive result is obtained, you must use other tests (tests for sacral sulci depths and sacral ILA positions, and other pelvic landmark positions) to make the definitive diagnosis; i.e., sacral torsion or flexion, or pubic or iliac subluxation, or anterior/posterior innominate rotation.

■ *Carryover factor.* As mentioned under the Standing Flexion Test, there should be some "carryover" effect from Standing Flexion to Seated Flexion testing. If the same side is positive for both standing and sitting, compare the actual distance of unilateral superior movement in order to decide whether the test is more positive standing, indicating iliosacral dysfunction, or more positive sitting, indicating sacroiliac dysfunction. If the distances are the same, there is either complete carryover, or a combination iliosacral and sacroiliac dysfunction on the same side. Evaluation of all the pelvic landmarks will resolve the question.

The Standing Flexion and Seated Flexion Tests indicate which side of the pelvis has less physiologic mobility. Usually the same side is positive in both Standing Flexion and Seated Flexion, indicating dysfunction on that side of the pelvis. Occasionally the positive side is reversed by changing from standing to sitting. In this case the positive standing side is the side of an iliosacral dysfunction and the positive seated side is the side of sacroiliac dysfunction.

■ Combinations of two or more dysfunctions are commonplace in the pelvis. Some of the dysfunctions may be latent, in the sense that evidence of them does not emerge until after another dysfunction has been treated. The evidence may emerge slowly, taking a few seconds, especially when one sacroiliac dysfunction is superimposed on another sacroiliac dysfunction.

■ Occasional complication: During forward flexion, some patients (especially obese patients) may experience sharp chest pain due to intercostal or abdominal muscle spasm. This is not serious, and clears when the patient straightens up.

The main use of the Seated Flexion Test is to grossly rule out:
1. Sacral torsion lesions (Most common sacroiliac lesion. Of these, more than 90 percent are Left-on-Left torsions in the Northern Hemisphere.)
2. Sacral flexion lesions (Of these, most will be left unilateral sacral flexion lesions in the Northern Hemisphere.)

Recall that observing paravertebral fullness for indications of vertebral segmental rotation is also a part of the Seated Flexion Test to be done and compared to observations in the standing flexed position. After assessing the PIP movement symmetry for iliosacral and sacroiliac dysfunction, the lumbars can be checked visually while they are hyperflexed both standing and sitting to note any unilateral paravertebral fullness indicative of lumbar segmental dysfunction. The seated flexed position is also an opportunity to palpate vertebral segments for more definitive diagnosis of segmental dysfunction. These diagnostic procedures have been covered in the chapters on vertebral dysfunction in Volume 2.

Biomechanical Events of the Flexion Tests

In the standing flexion test, a series of discrete events can be enumerated. These events are sequential, but they overlap to some degree.

1. Spinal flexion involves each vertebra flexing on the vertebra inferior to it, and the fifth lumbar flexing on the sacral base.

2. The sacrum nutates on the middle transverse axis. This motion begins before full spinal flexion has occurred, and may increase the pelvisacral angle up to 12 degrees.

3. The innominates flex on the femurs at the acetabular axis. This motion is almost simultaneous with sacral nutation, but slows and stops before sacral nutation is complete. The landmarks on the iliac crests, gluteal tubercles, and PSISs, move in an arc anterior and superior as the pelvis rotates on the acetabular axis. *Latissimus dorsi, quadratus lumborum*, and the *lumbodorsal fascia* are responsible for this movement of the two innominate bones. The movement is not caused by the sacrum pulling on the innominates.

4. As the sacrum nears the limit of its nutation it may reach that limit sooner on one side (the restricted side) than on the other. As the spine continues to flex and the sacrum continues to nutate, the PSIS on the restricted side will move anterior and cephalad as its innominate follows the nutating sacrum. The other PSIS does not move.

5. Occasionally the sacral nutation on the normal side converts to counternutation on the superior transverse axis. If this occurs, the PSIS on the restricted side will be carried a short distance posterior and cephalad by the counternutating sacrum.

6. When the patient begins to extend, the PSIS that moved last will move first. This unilateral movement is the criterion for a positive flexion test, regardless of the final direction of PSIS movement.

Note: The seated flexion test can be analyzed into the same sequence of events.

Effect of Pubic Subluxation on Pelvic Flexion Tests

There has been rampant confusion regarding the pelvic motion tests (e.g., standing and seated flexion tests) in relation to pubic subluxation. *Why and how does pubic subluxation affect the standing and seated flexion tests?* One point of confusion relates to the biomechanics of a positive flexion test. When the test is performed, the spine bends symmetrically forward. The sacrum simultaneously follows the spine in parallel fashion, flexing symmetrically. *The term "flexion" in this case is not defined in the craniosacral sense.* **Sacral flexion in the locomotor sense means anterior nutation of the sacral base.** In other words, the top of the sacrum tips forward when the sacrum flexes, the motion of the sacrum which accompanies forward bending of the trunk (spine). The biomechanical arthrokinematics of this motion is discussed in Chapter 2.

Some flexion versus extension confusion can be attributed to misapplying craniosacral terminology. Confusion also may arise from misapplying a rule of spinal adaptation to sacral torsion lesions. The sacral torsion rule categorically states that when the sacrum rotates, sidebends and flexes with torsion, the lumbar spine, at the lumbosacral junction, reverses what the sacrum did. *The rule does not apply to trunk forward bending, except, as explained in Chapter 2, in extreme trunk forward bending.*

The two normal sacroiliac joints permit the sacrum to nutate (literally, "nod") symmetrically in the sagittal plane through a range of 6 to 14 angular degrees independent of the ilia. Once the limit of sacral independent movement is reached, the ilia begin to follow the sacrum. If one sacroiliac joint has movement restriction, the limit is reached sooner on that side, and the ilium on that side follows the sacrum unilaterally while the sacrum continues to flex symmetrically on the normal sacroiliac side without disturbing the ilium on that side. **The side of unilateral iliac movement is the positive side of the flexion test, indicating restricted sacroiliac movement on that side.**

How does pubic subluxation cause a flexion test positive, regardless of whether the subluxation is inferior or superior?

When a pubic bone is pulled and held out of normal position by its abdominal or thigh muscle attachments, the ilium becomes slightly misaligned *on that side of the sacrum*. The physiologic flexion movements of the sacrum described above must occur on specific axes established by precisely located pivot points within the sacroiliac joints. With slight misalignment of the hip bone on the sacrum these pivots are disrupted and physiologic movement is no longer possible.

Some joint play remains, however, and the impaired sacroiliac joint is not rigidly ankylosed. Regardless of whether the hip bone is cocked back by superior pubic subluxation or cocked forward by inferior subluxation, the movement impairment due to pivot disruption has the same effect on the flexion test, making it positive on the side of abnormal pubic bone position.

The standing flexion test is based on the superior moving sacrum being able to pull an ilium with it after the sacrum has flexed with the trunk as far as it can go freely in relation to the ilium. Freedom of the sacrum to move on the ilium should be the same on both sides. When there is less mobility on one side, the sacrum can drag the ilium with it as it continues to move on the freer side. Lewit (1991) refers to this as "the overtake phenomenon," which he describes as "...on standing or sitting the (left) superior posterior iliac spine is usually the lower, but overtakes the right on stooping, becoming the more cranial of the two... the sacrum must lie asymmetrically between the ilia in such a way as to create more tension on the (left) side...; as a result, the posterior superior iliac spine (PSIS) follows the sacrum more promptly in stooping, causing the 'overtake.'" The word "promptly" may be ill-chosen to describe the standing or seated flexion test results, since the "overtake" we are interested in occurs toward the end of the "stooping" (forward bending), not at the beginning. Lewit's "overtake" is undoubtedly an entirely different phenomenon, in light of its evanescent nature – less than 20 seconds. The standing and seated flexion test results are more stable and reproducible.

Other Mobility Screening Tests
Stork Test

There are countless tests that require the patient to stand on one leg. The Trendelenburg one leg stand is classically used to detect *gluteus medius* paresis. The patient position is the same in the Gillet test, with several variations in the thumb monitoring position of various pelvisacral landmarks: sacral sulcus, median crest, PSIS (one or both sides). All variations of the Gillet test are intended to show sacroiliac joint movement, or movement restriction. The version designated below as the "Fowler Test" has a promising inter-rater reliability track record.

The Fowler Test

One "stork" test can be used to test sacroiliac mobility. An alternative to the Standing Flexion test, this one was devised by Cliff Fowler, a Vancouver physiotherapist.

1. One thumb goes on the sacral median crest, and one thumb on the iliac crest (PSIS or gluteal tuberosity).

2. Patient stands on one leg on the side not being palpated, raising the thigh to a horizontal position on the test side.

3. Normal is inferior movement of the PSIS relative to the sacrum. Restriction is indicated by superior movement, or no movement, of the iliac crest relative to the sacrum.

4. To test the other sacroiliac joint, the patient stands on the opposite foot and raises the knee on the test side.

5. A left-right comparison can be made of the amount of PSIS displacement, even if both sides move in the normal direction. The side with less displacement may have a slight restriction.

Hip Drop Test

Lumbosacral sidebending symmetry can be evaluated if the patient can do this maneuver with eyes level and without losing balance and coordination. A few patients have trouble with coordination at first, but, with patience and careful instruction, they usually can master it. When the knee bends, that ilium drops as far as the fifth lumbar sidebending motion will allow it. Since the fifth lumbar sidebends away from the dropping hip, *restricted sidebending of L5 — toward the side of the hip that drops the farthest — is detected.*

The adaptive spinal curvatures, first to one side and then to the other, should be symmetrical. If not, the left and right apices can be identified by vertebral level. This information can lead to definitive diagnosis of vertebral somatic dysfunction by narrowing down the search.

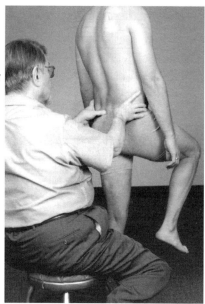

Fig. 6.17. Alternative sacroiliac mobility test. The (Fowler) Stork test. Testing sacroiliac mobility. One knee raised to right angle. With normal mobility the raised leg will push PSIS inferior on the sacrum. Palpate median crest on sacrum with one thumb and the PSIS on the raised leg side with the other.

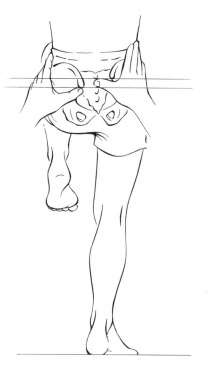

Fig. 6.18. Alternative sacroiliac mobility test. The Fowler test. One monitoring thumb goes on the iliac crest (PSIS or gluteal tubercle) on the raised leg side. The other thumb monitors the median crest of the sacrum approximately at the second sacral segment, which should be in the same horizontal plane as the PSIS.

The Hip Drop and Side Bend Tests — Comments: These are only screening tests and are insufficient as a basis for treatment. They are used simply to gain a general impression of vertebral segmental dysfunction — or the lack of it — and as an indicator that a further, more detailed examination may be required.

The "Hip Drop" Test Protocol

1. The patient stands erect, body weight is evenly distributed on both feet, feet are about 4 inches apart, and the toes are pointed straight ahead.

2. Squat, kneel, or sit behind the patient (so that your eyes are level with your hands), and palpate the highest points of the iliac crests.

3. Instruct the patient to support his entire weight on one leg while flexing the opposite knee and making a simultaneous effort to keep the upper body erect. This produces the "hip-drop" effect on the side of the flexed knee.

4. Observe the amount of hip drop, noting the amount of sidebending. Also, make special note of the location (height) and level of the apex and the depth of skin fold that occurs on that side.

5. Repeat the process for the opposite side. Make the comparison.

Interpretation of Results

■ **If the hip drop distances are equal,** the lumbosacral joint sidebends left and right symmetrically.

■ **If hip drop distances are not equal,** lumbosacral sidebending is restricted toward the side that dropped more.

■ Other spinal segmental restrictions may be suspected from variations in curve apex levels. These variations are manifestations of adaptation, which is often complex. This test is no substitute for specific segmental evaluation. Resist the temptation to overinterpret its findings.

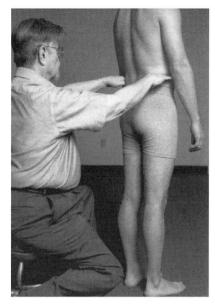

Fig. 6.19. Hip drop test. Steps 1 and 2. Place the hands on the iliac crests, eyes level with the hands, patient standing with both legs straight.

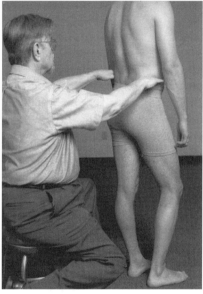

Fig. 6.20. Hip drop test. Steps 3 and 4. Patient bends one knee, assuming the "gossip" posture. Hands stay on iliac crests. Estimate distance hip drops from starting position.

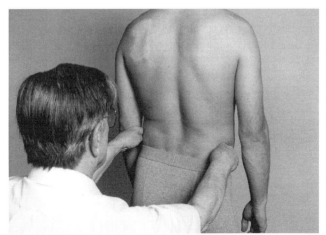

Fig. 6.21. Hip drop test. Step 4. Observing the hand for hip drop distance.

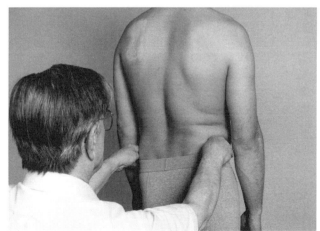

Fig. 6.22. Hip drop test. Step 5. Observing the hand for hip drop distance. Compare with step 4.

Recumbent Pelvic Mobility Tests

There are several ways to test the mobility of the pelvis with the patient recumbent. Relying on one's kinesthetic sense, the hip bones and sacrum can be pushed or pulled manually to try to create movement between the bones, and to feel it. These methods can be fairly reliable in the hands of experienced practitioners, but have poor inter-rater reliability.

Various springing tests exist: pushing on the sacrum to translate or rotate it in various directions on the ilia, or pushing on an ilium to rotate it on the sacrum. Although osteopathic physicians have used these springing tests for generations, inter-rater reliability is poorly documented. The dynamic static landmark position tests, before and after movement, presented in this text are less subjective, and, therefore more reproducible.

Functional Leg Length

Many of the manipulable disorders of the pelvis produce predictable functional leg length asymmetry. Iliosacral dysfunctions produce greater leg length asymmetry in the supine position; sacroiliac dysfunctions produce more leg length asymmetry prone. Functional leg length can be used to establish or verify a specific diagnosis of pelvic dysfunction or subluxation.

There are two types of iliosacral dysfunction – anteriorly rotated innominate and posteriorly rotated innominate. If the innominate is held in an anteriorly rotated position, then the leg on that side will be functionally longer, especially in the supine position. A posteriorly rotated innominate will shorten the leg, also especially in the supine position.

These changes in functional leg length associated with innominate rotation can be explained by the location of the innominate axis of rotation. The innominate rotates *on the sacrum* at the inferior pole of the sacroiliac joint. This innominate pivot point is posterior to the acetabulum. Thus, turning the iliac crest anteriorly on that pivot, pushes the acetabulum and leg inferiorly. Posterior rotation of the iliac crest pulls the acetabulum and leg superiorly.

In the supine position, the sacrum is resting on the examination table, and the innominates (suspended by ligamentous attachments) are free to rotate on the sacrum. Additionally, the lumbar lordosis is straightened by the forces of gravity and the anterior pressure applied to the sacral apex.

In the prone position, the pelvis rests on the ASISs and the pubic bones or abdomen. This tripod support arrangement of the two innominates limits interinnominate rotation. The lumbar lordosis is restored, and the sacrum, suspended between the ilia, is free to move in response to asymmetric lumbar loads (which are often due to tight

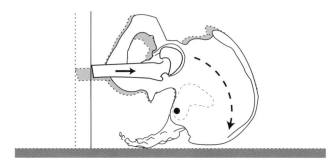

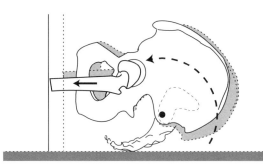

Figure 6.23. Effect of rotated innominate on leg length. The top figure illustrates the leg shortening effect of a posteriorly rotated innominate (white innominate and femur), which is superimposed on an innominate that is not rotated (grey innominate and femur). The bottom figure illustrates the leg lengthening effect of an anteriorly rotated innominate.

lumbar sidebenders). The leg is functionally shortened on the side of lumbar sidebender tightness, which tilts the whole pelvis up on that side. Thus, sacroiliac dysfunction affects functional leg length more in the prone position than in the supine.

Upslipped innominate shortens the functional leg length on that side, both prone and supine.

Dynamic Leg Length Tests

Some recumbent pelvic mobility tests depend on the ability of the examiner to change the apparent length of the legs, measured by comparing the feet or ankles with each other when the legs are straight and together. As one might anticipate, several versions and interpretations of these tests exist. In some versions, the method of changing leg lengths involves having the patient sit up from a supine position, or go supine from a sitting position. Some methods of changing leg length involve moving the leg through a circumduction pattern. Even when these methods look the same their outcomes may be different, because of variations in speed or amplitude of movement. The modifications suggested in this test should improve reliability and reproducibility.

The Dynamic Leg Length Test of Pelvic Motion Symmetry

This test is a useful alternative to the Standing and Seated Flexion tests, especially for patients who are unable to stand or sit. Although it does not distinguish between sacroiliac and iliosacral dysfunction as do the flexion tests, it can be used to confirm a diagnosis of sacroiliac *hypermobility* (or instability), which tends to restrict pelvic mobility on the side of instability in the weight-bearing condition, while demonstrating excessive mobility when tested recumbent.

The Dynamic Leg Length Test of Pelvic Motion Symmetry utilizes leg length measurement in the supine position by comparing the position of the thumbs on the medial malleoli. Because leg length is critical in this test, extreme care should be taken to insure its accuracy (Figures 6.24.A through E).

Because the sides of the table are a part of your visual field, it is important that the patient be centered and aligned on the table. Alignment of the patient's body on the table is accomplished by having the supine patient flex the knees, raise the hips off the table, and set the hips back down on the table straight. Then the examiner draws the legs out straight with the body. Before the malleoli are put close together for comparison of leg length, gently spring the legs into internal rotation to relax the hip external rotators. The malleoli are then compared by carefully pressing the side of the thumb or finger against the inferior slopes of the shelf below the bony prominence of the medial malleolus to mark identical places on each leg. Being careful to keep the legs aligned with the midsagittal plane, note any asymmetry and estimate the difference in millimeters or fractions of an inch. This is the baseline measurement.

The Dynamic Leg Length Test is based on the leg *lengthening* effect of turning the iliac crest forward by internally rotating the leg (due to the acetabulum's location being anterior to the axis of rotation in the sacroiliac joint), and the leg shortening effect of turning the ilium backward by externally rotating the leg.

To effect leg *shortening* (Figures 6.25. A through E), the ilium is rotated backward by flexing the hip and knee 90 degrees, then abducting the femur by allowing the knee of the *relaxed* leg to drop out to the side, and externally rotat-

ing the femur by lifting up on the foot. This abducted externally rotated position is held with gentle steady tension until a release is felt that allows a little extra external rotation, indicating the ilium has yielded and turned backward. It is important to be patient and wait for that release. The leg is now straightened out. Be careful to maintain the external rotation by applying steady pressure against the medial knee and lateral ankle. Avoid having to move the leg (and disturb the ilium) after it is straightened on the table, by aiming the heel to its final resting place beside the other foot. Without disturbing the ilium's new position, the malleoli are compared again. Three to six millimeters shortening is normal.

The operator then *lengthens* the leg (Figures 6.26.A through G) by flexing it again to 90 degrees and allowing the knee to drop medial, adducting the hip, then internally rotating the femur with gentle sustained tension *until the release of the ilium yielding and rotating forward is felt. (Remember ... Wait for the release!)*. Then the leg is straightened out, keeping the internal rotation tension by applying steady pressure on the lateral knee and medial ankle. Again the heel is aimed toward its final resting place and malleoli are compared once more. The total length change from shortened to lengthened is noted. It does not often exceed one centimeter. When leg length is changed more than 1.2 centimeters, it indicates sacroiliac instability.

The opposite leg is then put through the same shortening and lengthening maneuvers in order to compare the total length change of the two legs. If the totals are not equal, there is either pelvic joint restriction or hypermobility. Less than 6 millimeters of change usually indicates restriction. More than 12 mm. of change usually indicates hypermobility.

In most instances, the results of this test will agree with the results of the standing flexion or seated flexion tests. When there is paradoxical disagreement, it is usually because the standing and seated flexion tests failed to detect hypermobility, but showed restriction on the hypermobile side due to the joint wedging effect of gravity.

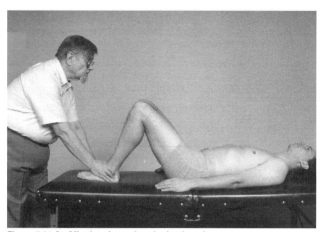

Figure 6.24.A. Aligning the patient for leg length measurements.
Feet planted firmly in the mid-line of the table, knees flexed.

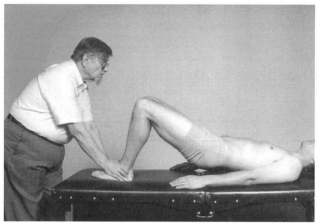

Figure 6.24.B. Aligning the patient for leg length measurements.
Raising the hips off the table to replace them in the center of the table.

Dynamic Leg Length Test Protocol

A. Patient Alignment

1. Patient is supine on the examination table with knees and hips flexed. (Figure 6.24.A.)

2. Ask the patient to *"Raise your hips off the table."* (Figure 6.24.B.)

3. Instruct the patient to let their hips back down on the examination table.

4. Operator stands at the foot of the examination table and pulls the patient's legs out straight. (Figure 6.24.C.)

5. Examiner internally rotates patient's hips by springing the toes in medially, which relaxes the external rotators. (Figure 6.24.D.)

6. Examiner measures the apparent supine leg length of the patient.(Figure 6.24.E.)

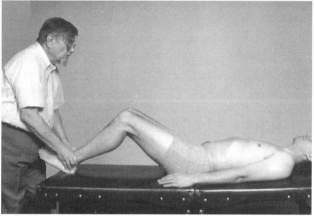

Figure 6.24.C. Aligning the patient for leg length measurements.
Passively straightening the legs in the mid-line.

Figure 6.24.D. Aligning the patient for leg length measurements.
Springing the toes in medially to internally rotate the femurs and relax the external rotators.

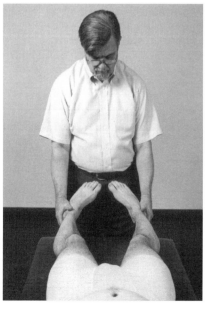

Figure 6.24.E. Measuring leg lengths – supine.
Thumbs on medial malleoli shelves to compare leg length.

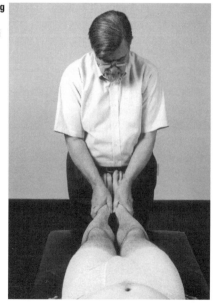

Figure 6.25.A.. The dynamic leg length test – leg shortening procedure.
Step 2. Flex hip and knee 90 degrees. Control the ankle and knee.

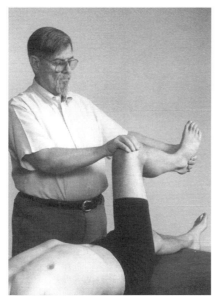

Figure 6.25.C. The dynamic leg length test – leg shortening procedure.
Step 4. Begin straightening the leg while maintaining the external rotation and abduction and aiming the foot for a resting place beside the other foot.

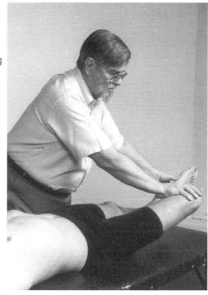

Figure 6.25.B. The dynamic leg length test – leg shortening procedure.
Step 3. Abduct the flexed hip and externally rotate the femur until the pelvic fascia yields.

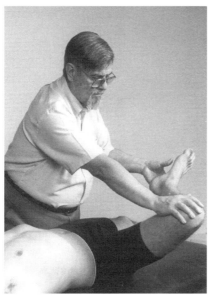

Figure 6.25.D. The dynamic leg length test – leg shortening procedure.
Step 5. Rest the leg, with that foot adjacent to the other foot.

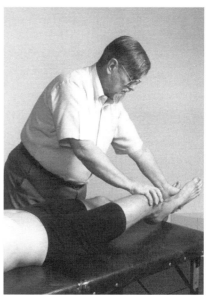

Dynamic Leg Length Test Protocol *(continued)*
B. Leg Shortening Procedure
  1. With the patient in the supine position, compare the functional leg length. (Figure 6.24.E.)
  2. One leg is passively flexed 90 degrees at the hip and knee.(Figure 6.25.A.)
  3. Abduct the flexed hip.(Figure 6.25.B.)
  4. Externally rotate the femur by raising the foot up. Wait until the fascia and innominate yield.(Figure 6.25.B.)
  5. Maintain the external rotation and slowly straighten the knee and hip, eventually resting the foot beside the other foot. (Figure 6.25.C.)(Figure 6.25.D.)
  6. Recheck leg lengths to see how much the leg was shortened. Make a quantitative decision and remember it.(Figure 6.25.E.)

Figure 6.25.E. The dynamic leg length test – leg shortening procedure.
Step 6. Recheck leg length to see how much the leg was shortened.

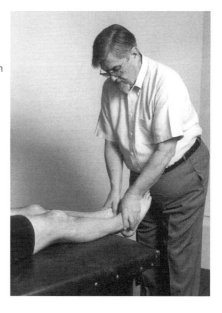

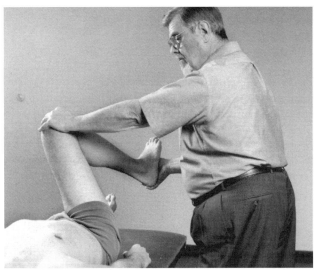

Figure 6.26.A. The dynamic leg length test – leg lengthening procedure.
Steps 1 and 2. Flex hip and knee 90 degrees. Adduct and internally rotate femur.

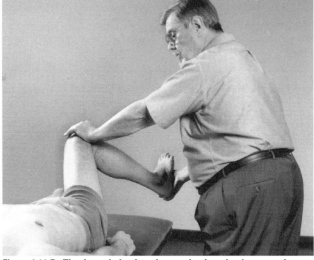

Figure 6.26.B. The dynamic leg length test – leg lengthening procedure.
Step 3. Begin to straighten leg while maintaining adduction and internal rotation tension, aiming the foot for the resting place adjacent to the other foot.

Dynamic Leg Length Test Protocol *(continued)*

C. Leg Lengthening Procedure

1. Start the leg lengthening procedure with the hip and knee flexed 90 degrees.

2. Adduct and internally rotate the femur. Wait for a release. (Figure 6.26.A. or.D.)

3. Begin to straighten leg while maintaining adduction and internal rotation tension, aiming the foot for the resting place adjacent to the other foot. (Figure 6.26.B, C, or E)

4. Lay the straight leg down on the table with the foot next to the other foot. (Figure 6.26.F.)

5. Recheck leg length to see how much the leg was lengthened. The difference between shortest and longest is the amount of length change. (Figure 6.26.G.)

D. Repeat shortening and lengthening procedures for the other leg. Compare the amount of change in leg length.

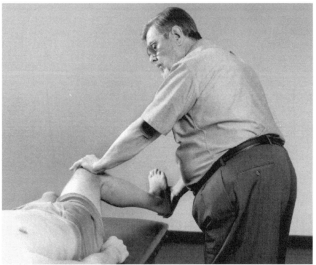

Figure 6.26.C. The dynamic leg length test – leg lengthening procedure.
Step 3. Lay the straight leg down on the table with the foot next to the other foot.

Note: Some of the illustrations on these two pages are slightly redundant. For example, Figures 6.26A and 6.26D show the same step from two different perspectives. Figures 6.26B and 6.26E are the same pose photographed from two different perspectives. These seeming duplications were included to better show the examiner's hand positions. Figure 6.26F emphasizes the importance of placing the foot so that the leg will not need to be moved for length measurement. Springing the hips into internal rotation as in Figure 6.24D should be avoided, since it can nullify the length alteration.

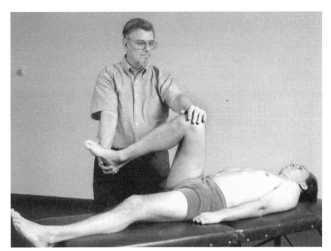

Figure 6.26.D. Steps 1 and 2.

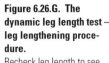
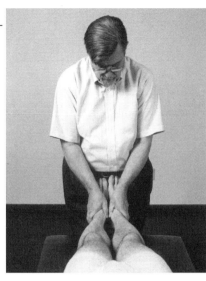

Figure 6.26.G. The dynamic leg length test – leg lengthening procedure. Recheck leg length to see how much the leg was lengthened. The difference between shortest and longest is the amount of length change.

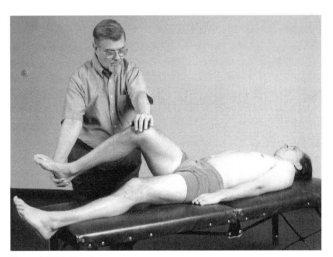

Figure 6.26.E. Step 3.

Interpretation of the Dynamic Leg Length Test

This lateralization test takes a little longer than the standing and seated flexion tests, but it can show sacroiliac *hypermobility* as well as joint motion restriction. Normal sacroiliac joints permit the test maneuvers to change functional leg length 3 to 9 millimeters. If the length changes more than a centimeter, it is evidence of sacroiliac hypermobility. The amount of length change should be the same bilaterally. If alteration of length is within the normal 3 to 9 millimeters on both sides, but one side is less than the other, that side is restricted due to sacroiliac or iliosacral dysfunction.

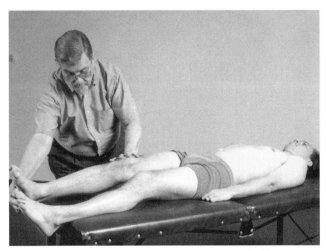

Figure 6.26.F. Step 4. Take the foot to its precise resting place beside the other foot, so that it will not have to be moved for leg length measurement.

CHAPTER 7

Subluxations and Dislocations of the Pelvis: Evaluation and Treatment

The terms **dislocation** and **luxation** are synonymous and refer to abnormal displacement of body parts or bones with associated tissue avulsion, or tearing. The term **subluxation** will be used in this text in its original orthopedic sense: a dislocation without tissue avulsion which does not spontaneously self-correct. Subluxation or dislocation of a joint not only impairs normal physiologic joint mobility, but after it is reduced (put back in place) it may be hypermobile and easier to redislocate. If this occurs in one of the pelvic joints, the other pelvic joints will be stressed in some way and may become dysfunctional. Both local symptoms, associated with the subluxated tissues, and distant symptoms, associated with postural and locomotor adaptation, are possible.

All medical students become familiar with *visceral malpositions* in the pelvis – cystocele, rectocele, uterine prolapse, and retroversions of the uterine fundus. *Bony malpositions* of the pelvis, however, have received relatively little attention from the medical professions, even though it is clear that the bones of the pelvis provide the solid framework upon which the viscera rest or hang.

As outlined in Chapter 4, there are three types of pelvic subluxation: **pubic symphyseal**, **upslipped innominate**, and **rhomboid pelvis**. The most common pelvic subluxation is misalignment of the pubic bones. When **pubic subluxation** is present, there is necessarily some *micro*-misalignment of the sacroiliac joint on the side of the abnormally positioned pubic bone. This micro-misalignment is enough to interfere with physiologic sacroiliac motion and to cause a positive flexion test, or other indication of pelvic joint motion restriction, on that side.

True sacroiliac subluxations – upslipped and rhomboid pelvis (flared) – are *macro*-misalignments of the sacroiliac joints. The most common of these is **upslipped innominate**, a shearing of the sacroiliac joint that can cause gross vertical misalignment of the sacrum and ilium. In addition, one may occasionally find a **rhomboid pelvis**, in which the anterior superior iliac spine on one side is farther lateral from the midline than the iliac spine on the opposite side, due to an arcuate displacement, in a transverse plane, of the ilium on a (rare) convex sacrum.

If screening and lateralization procedures indicate that dysfunction exists within the pelvic mechanism, the positive test result is

In this chapter:
- ■ *Pubic subluxation*
- ■ *Upslipped innominate*
- ■ *Rhomboid pelvis*
  - • *Inflared innominate*
  - • *Outflared innominate*

either due to subluxation, sacroiliac dysfunction, or iliosacral dysfunction. Assuming that non-neutral *lumbar* dysfunctions have been ruled out or eliminated, the most immediate concern is to rule out, or eliminate by treatment, dysfunctions due to subluxation. The principal reason for the primacy of this concern is the need to restore the anatomic relationships for the axes of physiologic motions. Subluxation disrupts these axes. Axis integrity is necessary, both for the correct interpretation of the bony landmarks required for accurate diagnosis, and for successful treatment of dysfunction.

Subluxations of the Pubic Symphysis
Testing for Pubic Crest Heights Asymmetry
This procedure is used to test for superior or inferior pubic subluxations (**ICD9CM 839.69**) on either the left or right side. The magnitude of misalignment may range from one to eight millimeters, but is typically 3-5 millimeters. Obviously, one millimeter would be difficult to detect visually. One might be led to suspect such an "occult" pubic subluxation if there were no other explanation found for a positive standing flexion test.

Remember that normal physiologic motion of the pubic joint occurs around the transverse axis of the symphysis pubis; i.e., the motion is rotational and in the sagittal plane. This allows for the normal iliac (innominate bone) forward or backward rotations in walking. Walking does not produce pubic subluxations.

The pubic joint is poorly reinforced with ligaments, and depends mainly on balanced tension of abdominal and thigh muscles for its alignment. The abdominal muscles (principally the *rectus abdominis*) hold each pubic bone up, preventing it from subluxating inferiorly. Thigh muscles (principally *adductors*) hold each pubic bone down, preventing superior subluxation.

The pubic bone is frequently subluxated – either inferiorly or superiorly. And **when one side is subluxated, it**

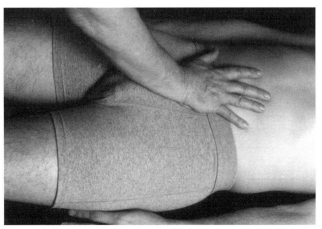

Figure 7.2. Stereognostic location of pubic brim. Start with the palm in the center of the lower abdomen, inferior to the umbilicus. Move the hand caudad until the heel of the hand or wrist bumps into the superior edge of the pubic bones.

interferes with iliosacral motion on the side of subluxation, which would cause a positive flexion test on that side. Such motion interference is thought to be due to the disruption of points within the sacroiliac joint, which normally line up on a physiologic axis for normal sacroiliac motion. With the axis disrupted, that physiologic motion cannot occur.

The Pubic Crest Heights Test
Locate the pubic crests stereognostically using the heel of your dominant hand with your palm flat on the lower abdomen, midline. Place the index finger pads on the anterior surface of the pubic bone, and with minimal pressure slide the fingers up into the abdomen to rest the finger pads on the superior point of each pubic crest. It is not necessary to push the fingers deeply into the abdomen, just enough to contact the points of the pubic crests. A little side-to-side movement of the fingertips will help you locate them precisely.

Figure 7.1. Pubic subluxation may be subluxated superiorly **(A.)**, *or* inferiorly **(B.)**, depending on which side has muscle imbalance. The size of the down and up arrows on either side of the symphysis indicate muscle balance (same size – "=" signs) or imbalance (disparate size – "+" or "-" signs). Upon initial evaluation, distinguishing between a superior pubic shear (A.) on one side versus an inferior shear (B) on the other side can be challenging, as they look the same in the body.

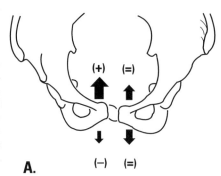

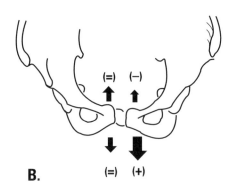

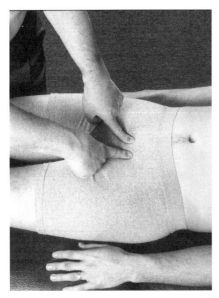

Figure 7.3. Start by palpating with the pads of the index fingers just inferior to the pubic crests on the anterior surfaces of the pubic bones.

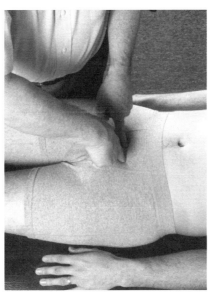

Figure 7.4. Push the soft tissues superiorly with the index fingers until they drop into the abdomen a fraction of an inch, indicating that you are on top of the pubic bone.

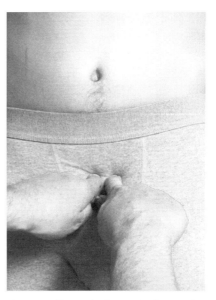

Figure 7.5. Keeping the finger pads close together, slide them side-to-side on the superior edge of the pubic bones until the prominences of the pubic crests can be identified on each side of the midline. In the above example, note the 2-3 mm. asymmetry.

The Pubic Crest Heights Test Procedure Protocol

1. The patient is supine.

2. You stand on one side with your dominant eye nearer the table.

3. The palm of your hand is placed on the patient's lower abdominal area in the midline below the umbilicus and superior to the symphysis, as shown in Figure 7.2. (This is done to save you and the patient embarrassment caused by probing about the groin with your fingertips.)

4. Once the symphysis is located, place your two index fingertips side by side at the anterior center of the mons pubis (Figure 7.3), gently sliding your fingers superiorly to push the adipose tissue out of the way so that bilateral contact can be established on the superior surfaces of the crests, and then sliding your fingers back and forth laterally to ensure comparison of identical points of each crest, as shown in Figure 7.4. The fingers should be kept parallel and about a half inch apart at the tips. At that distance apart the fingertips should be resting on the pubic crests at this time.

5. Look at your fingertips from a vertical perspective. Compare the heights (Figure 7.5.).

Interpretation of Results

■ **If the pubic crest heights are at same level**, there is no subluxation.

■ **If one pubic crest is higher**, there is a subluxation. Whether it is superior on one side or inferior on the other side can be decided by the Standing and/or Seated Flexion Test, which will indicate the abnormal side of pubic malposition by a positive test result showing restriction.

Note: Students learning these methods are advised to deliberately treat the wrong side first. Nothing will happen. You will not create a lesion. The asymmetry will persist until the correct side is treated. This approach will give you the opportunity to practice both treatment procedures. It will also serve as a reality check on the validity of your Standing or Seated Flexion Test technique. However, some combinations of dysfunctions in the pelvis may have unpredictable effects on the flexion tests. Do not take the reality check too seriously. ***Example:*** You have tested the pubic crests and learned that the right pubis is higher. With only this information, you don't know whether a right superior subluxation or a left inferior subluxation exists. If the standing flexion test indicates a right-sided lesion, the working diagnosis is a right superior subluxation. If proper treatment of the right side does not reduce the subluxation, there is probably more than one dysfunction; treat the left side and then recheck the landmarks.

■ Treatment of a pubic subluxation is done immediately following the diagnosis. If appropriate treatment does not correct the asymmetry, the flexion test misled you, and you treated the wrong side.

Recurrent pubic subluxation is usually due to neural facilitation or inhibition of the nerve supply to the *abdominal recti* and/or the medial thigh muscles, *gracilis, pectineus*, and adductors. A thorough close examination of the upper lumbar and lower thoracic spine which are the sources of innervation for the thigh muscles (obturator nerves, L_1-L_3) and abdominal muscles ($T_{10,11,12}$) is indicated. Although an actual dysfunction in these areas may not be found, adaptive scoliosis compensating for dysfunction below or above the region may be found.

Treatment Procedures for Pubic Subluxations

Treatment for Superior Pubic Subluxation

The diagnosis of superior pubic subluxation is determined by a superiorly displaced pubic crest, and a concurrent positive standing flexion test of that same side.

Protocol Task Analysis

1. The patient is supine.

2. You stand at the side of the table corresponding with the side of the lesion – towards the foot of the table, facing the patient.

3. Ask the patient to move the hips over toward your side of the table far enough that the thigh can hang off the table down toward the floor. Instruct the patient to hold the far edge of the table with one hand to resist rolling off the table.

4. The leg must hang freely, but the weight of the leg must be supported to control the amount of hip extension. This support can be provided by hooking your heel under the patient's ankle while you stand on one foot (Figure 7.6.).

5. Monitor the ASIS of the opposite side of the pelvis to determine how far the leg may be lowered. When the ASIS moves, it means the leg has dropped a little too far. Lift up on the leg with your heel.

6. Offer unyielding resistance with your hand on the patient's thigh just above the knee, and instruct the patient to flex the hip as you resist the effort. "*Raise your foot up forcibly*" (2 seconds); "*Relax*." The instruction to raise the foot up is better than asking for the knee to be lifted, for the natural tendency is for the patient to pull the ankle down against your supporting heel in order to lift the knee. The object is to co-contract the *abdominal, psoas,* and *rectus femoris* muscles strongly. It is probably this co-contraction and post-isometric relaxation which restores tension balance to the muscles of this system.

7. During post-isometric relaxation take up the slack by lowering the patient's leg with your supporting heel until the opposite side ASIS moves. Then, have the patient repeat the contraction.

8. About three repetitions are usually required for a correction.

9. Then retest.

Comments: Usually we advise repeating the treatment, if indicated, after the completion of a treatment procedure. In this case, however, the treatment procedure is so reliable that it always works, even when performed by a beginner with less than perfect technique. If the retest indicates the treatment failed, you probably treated the wrong side. The alternative explanation is that the sequence of treatment was inappropriate. This sounds reasonable, but even when spinal nerve facilitation or inhibition persists for the involved muscles' innervation, it is always possible to treat the pubic subluxation successfully, if only temporarily. Reducing the subluxation will allow for correction of other pelvic mechanics, and may possibly relieve the stresses on the upper lumbar and lower thoracic segments which generated the innervation problems which initially caused the pubic subluxation.

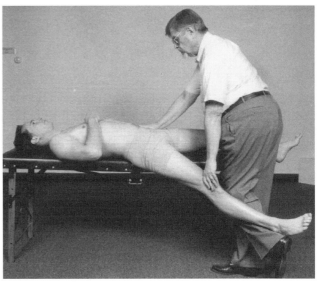

Figure 7.6. Treatment for superior pubis on the right, The suspended leg in supported on the operator's heel to prevent excess hip extension.

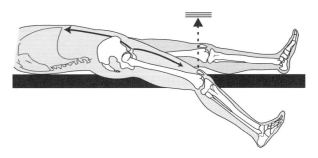

Figure 7.7. Treatment for superior pubis on the right, Simultaneous isometric co-contraction of abdominal and adductor muscles causes reflex reintegration of their motor controls. When they relax they seek their normal balanced relationship.

Treatment for Inferior Pubic Subluxation

Inferior pubic subluxation is diagnosed by an inferiorly displaced pubic crest, and a concurrent positive standing flexion test on that same side.

After the operator has introduced hip flexion on the subluxated side to the point where resistance is first encountered (thereby taking the slack out of the *gluteus maximus*), and after making a firm contact with the ischial tuberosity on the subluxated side with the wrist or back of the hand, the treatment for an inferior pubic subluxation has two principal stages: 1.) isometric contraction of the *gluteus maximus* inhibits the abdominal and adductor muscles (resulting in reflex re-integration of their motor controls), and 2.) during the relaxation phase, hip flexion is increased while the operator simultaneously pushes superiorly on the ischial tuberosity. (see Figure 7.8.)

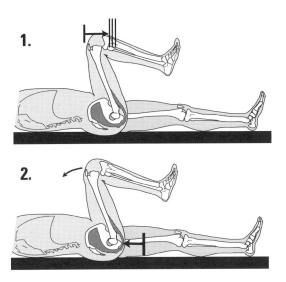

Figure 7.8. The two principal stages in the treatment for inferior pubic subluxation. During the first stage, isometric contraction of the gluteus maximus inhibits the abdominal and adductor muscles; thus reestablishing a balanced tension between the two muscle groups. In the second stage, slack is taken up through increased hip flexion while simultaneously pushing superiorly on the ischial tuberosity.

Treatment for Inferior Pubic Subluxation Procedure Protocol

1. The patient is supine.

2. You may stand on either side of the table.

3. Flex the patient's hip on the lesioned side, bringing the knee to the chest as far as is comfortable. Patients with hip joint disease may not be able to flex the hip much. It does not matter. The procedure will work anyway.

4. Straight cephalic pressure is applied to the tuberosity of the lesioned side ischium – about 5 kilograms. This pressure must be sustained throughout the procedure. Placing the knuckles of your fist down on the table as a fulcrum will allow you to easily sustain the necessary pressure using the back or the front of your wrist against the ischial tuberosity (Figure 7.9.).

5. Instruct the patient to attempt to extend the hip, while you provide unyielding resistance with your free hand on the patient's knee. "*Push your knee toward the foot of the table with four pounds (two kilograms) of force*" (2 seconds); "*Now relax.*" (Figure 7.10.) More forceful contractions are apparently not necessary. The object is to get a co-contraction of the *gluteus* and *quadratus lumborum* muscles on the same side.

6. During the post-isometric relaxation, take up the slack by increasing both the hip flexion and your cephalic pressure against the ischial tuberosity. Then, have the patient repeat the isometric contraction (Figure 7.11.).

7. Three repetitions are required for a correction.

8. Retest. See the note after the previous procedure.

Note: It is not necessary to monitor any part of the pelvis for motion during this procedure. The sense of yielding of the femur and the ischial tuberosity with hip flexion is sufficient.

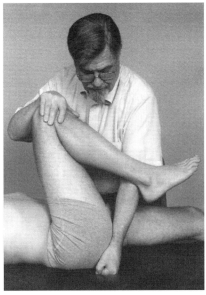

Figure 7.9. Treatment for inferior pubic subluxation on the right. Operator's fist is pressed firmly into the table below the patient's buttock. Operator's wrist contacts the ischial tuberosity firmly.

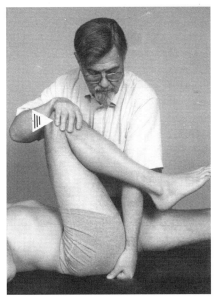

Figure 7.10. Treatment for inferior pubic subluxation. Hip extension is resisted by the operator, whose hand is on the patient's knee. Steady cephalic pressure against the ischium is maintained with the wrist.

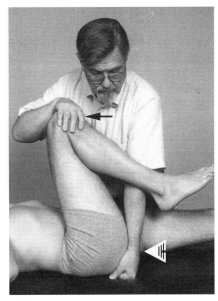

Figure 7.11. Treatment for inferior pubic subluxation. During post-isometric relaxation, the hip is passively flexed farther and pressure against the ischium is increased.

Combination Treatment for Superior *or* Inferior Pubic Subluxation

Part 1: Knees Together

1. The patient is supine.

2. You stand at either side of the table.

3. As the starting position, the patient flexes the knees and hips, keeping the knees together and allowing the feet to rest on the table, as shown in Figure 7.12.

4. You hold the knees together. Be careful how you do this. Do not put your rib cage against the patient's knee. A strong patient can break or dislocate your rib.

5. Instruct the patient to attempt to abduct the legs as you oppose the movement. "*Try to pull your knees apart*" (2 seconds); "*Now relax.*"

6. Repeat three times, and proceed to next phase – *Knees Apart*.

Part 2: Knees Apart

1. With the patient's hips and knees still flexed and the feet together, have the patient spread the knees apart as far as is comfortable.

2. Place your hand, forearm, and elbow as a brace between the patient's knees to resist hip adduction (Figure 7.13.).

3. Warn the patient that a "pop" may occur with the next step. The noise is completely benign.

4. Instruct the patient to attempt to bring the knees together as you oppose the movement. "*Try to pull your knees together*" (2 seconds); "*Now relax.*"

5. Repeat this three times.

6. Then, retest. If the treatment was not effective, use one of the more specific treatments above.

Note: This nonspecific method of treating pubic subluxation is almost as effective as the specific techniques outlined above, and it takes a little less time. It has the advantage that the patient can improvise a self-treatment for recurrent pubic subluxation, using a belt around the knees and/or a sofa cushion between the knees. A disadvantage is that, after correcting a subluxation, the side of the lesion remains unknown. When there are complex pelvic lesions, that information can be useful to explain flexion test positives and pelvic landmark findings.

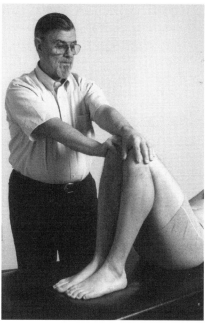

Figure 7.12. Combination treatment for superior or inferior pubic subluxation– patient's knees together.

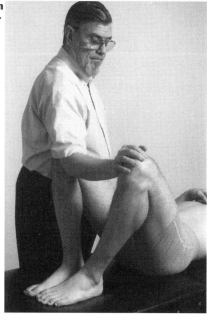

Figure 7.13. Combination treatment for superior or inferior pubic subluxation– patient's knees apart.

Upslipped Innominate Lesions

Dislocation and subluxation are almost synonymous terms, the difference being that ligaments are *torn* in a dislocation and not in a subluxation. An upslipped innominate can be either.

On the side that slips, the two ends of the sacrotuberous ligament are brought closer together, slackening the ligament. When the patient is standing, the sacrum rests too low on the ilium. The distance from the ground to the iliac crest is not altered. But when the patient lies prone, the innominate on the slipped side is superior, compared with the other innominate.

The injury was described in the osteopathic literature by Clark (1906). He attributed it, among other causes, to "...falls in the standing posture, the superimposed weight of the body driving the sacrum downward..." Fryette's term for the injury, "upslipped innominate" (1914), was objected to by Schwab (1933), who preferred to call it a "downward moved sacrum," as if it were possible, objectively or subjectively, to distinguish between the sacrum dislocated inferiorly in relation to the innominate and the innominate dislocated superiorly on the sacrum. Citing the physics of inertia, Schwab stated:

> *"In jumping, the trunk weight, together with the inertia of the sacral load, can actually cause a descent of the sacrum in relation to one or both innominates. With the patient standing erect, or examined roentgenologically erect, the two halves of the pelvis are seen to be of even height, but the sacrum is subluxated downward upon the involved side."*

That Schwab believed "downward moved sacrum" was far more common than "upslipped innominate" seems a mysterious semantic issue. He also believed that, even though "downslipped innominate" was far less common than "downward moved sacrum," it was *more* common than "upslipped innominate," in spite of the obvious auto-corrective potential of gravity.

Further semantic confusion was introduced by Greenman's (1986) description of an "inferior sacral shear:"

> *"If the relationship of the two innominates is preserved at the symphysis and with both ischial tuberosities being level against the horizontal (xz) plane, and the sacrum is found to be inferior in relation to one of the innominates, then an inferior sacral shear is present."*

It is reasonable to assume that the above description applies to examining a patient in the prone position. If so, the above criteria fit the description of a sacroiliac *dysfunction* defined in this text as "unilaterally flexed sacrum" – *not a subluxation*. Schwab did not state his criteria as explicitly as Greenman, so we cannot know, for certain, if his "downward moved sacrum" is actually a unilaterally flexed sacrum dysfunction. If it is, it would explain Schwab's statistical bias against the "rare" upslipped innominate.

The early osteopaths, in the tradition of the ancient bonesetters, tended to think of manipulating the pelvis as a process of putting bones back in place. The distinction between *dislocations* and *dysfunctions* was often blurred. Fryette (1914) conceived of four variations of upslipped innominate by failing to distinguish vertical shearing dislocations of the sacroiliac joint and anterior or posterior rotations of the innominate, which are *iliosacral* dysfunctions.

Incidence of Upslipped Innominate

Traumatic shearing dislocation of the sacroiliac joint (**ICD9CM 718.25**) can be found in about 10 percent of the general population with or without symptoms. The incidence of sacroiliac dislocation is slightly higher (10-15%) among patients with disabling low back pain. (Kidd, 1988)

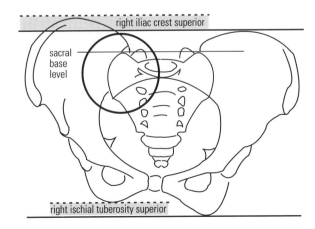

Figure 7.14. Anterior view of a right upslipped innominate – patient supine.

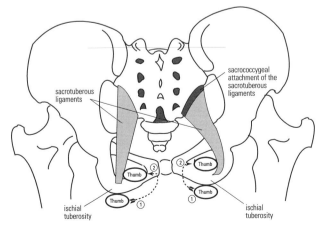

Figure 7.15. Posterior view of a right upslipped innominate – patient prone.

Table 7.A.

Age and sex distribution of patients diagnosed with upslipped innominate [N = 63/600] (Kidd, 1988)

Age	Female	Male	Number	Percent
20-30	7	4	11	17
30-40	13	6	19	30
40-50	4	8	12	19
50-60	4	2	6	10
60-70	6	3	9	14
70- +	4	2	6	10
Totals	**38**	**25**	**63**	**100**

Undoubtedly, the high incidence of this lesion can be attributed to the fact that very few of these injuries are treated appropriately. Most victims do not seek treatment at the time of the injury, typically a slip and fall (pratfall). Indeed, they are usually not aware of the severity of the damage to the sacroiliac ligaments, and are not mindful of the long-term consequences of spending the rest of their lives with their sacrum inclined to one side. The usual immediate consequence of a pratfall is more embarrassment than pain. The condition will be discovered only if it is looked for; symptoms will rarely call attention to it. It appears that many people with the condition are asymptomatic, or, at least, have symptoms not severe enough to consult a physician. Few physicians look for it; most do not know how.

Research (Kidd, 1988) indicates that the highest incidence is in the fourth decade of life, providing more than three decades of opportunity for a traumatic slip-and-fall pratfall. This suggests that some of the patients had successfully adapted to their sacral asymmetry for ten to twenty years before their adaptation decompensated.

In the author's personal clinical experience, downslipped innominate remains only a theoretical possibility. Several anecdotal cases have been reported, along with supporting – *albeit* bizarre – history. If, however, the standing flexion test was the basis for deciding the side of the lesion, the diagnosis should be considered questionable. Supine mobility tests would have made the diagnosis more believable. Still, it is troubling to explain how such a lesion could persist with standing and walking.

Diagnostic Criteria for Upslipped Innominate
The upslipped innominate injury can be detected quickly by physical examination. No technical imaging or mensuration procedures are required. X-rays may or may not show it, depending on the angle and level of the beam. Although other landmarks have been suggested, **only two physical criteria are needed for the diagnosis of upslipped innominate:**

■ Superior displacement of an ischial tuberosity in the prone position; and

■ Slackness of the sacrotuberous ligament on the same side. The normal ligament on the other side is quite taut.

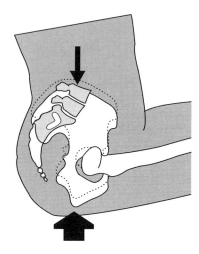

Figure 7.16. Pratfall producing an upslipped innominate. "Prat" was slang several generations ago for the lower buttocks. A pratfall is a slip-and-fall accident in which the victim lands in a sitting position, approximately. This happens frequently while walking on ice or skating.

Both must be present for an almost certain diagnosis of upslipped innominate, depending mostly on the magnitude of the asymmetry. History can be important. Intermittent migratory low back and pelvic pain is a common feature of upslipped innominate. A remembered pratfall can be significant. With more severe trauma, such as a car accident, the above findings should raise suspicion of pelvic fracture. Prone leg length and iliac crest levels measured against a horizontal (xy) plane may be added to the list of criteria, but crest levels are subject to greater measurement error than the ischial tuberosities, and leg length is influenced by variations in postural accommodation of the spine.

The distinction between luxation and subluxation of the sacroiliac joint is arbitrary. We cannot know whether ligaments have been torn [i.e., sacroiliac strain, with or without dislocation or subluxation, (ICD9CM 86.1)], or the extent of ligamentous damage without performing an autopsy. Dislocations with a tendency to frequent recurrence [unstable sacroiliac, (ICD9CM 718.35)] are probably luxations or dislocations (ICD9CM 718.85). More than 5 millimeters of displacement could be subluxation (ICD9CM 839.42). One hesitates to make the diagnosis when the displacement is less than three millimeters, and therefore possibly due to measurement error. Chronic upslipped innominate that stays corrected after treatment, i.e., is not recurrent and not a current injury, is coded (ICD9CM 718.25).

The five millimeter cutoff takes into account the standard error of measurement (i.e., the possibility of error even when the measurement technique is performed correctly). Observation of supine and prone iliac crests can be confirmatory, but there may be a larger standard error. Prone and supine leg length comparisons can also be confirmatory, but can also reflect pelvic asymmetries in other planes, as well as lumbar scoliosis. Sacrococcygeal tenderness occurs less than half the time.

If the dislocation has occurred bilaterally, the landmark findings may be symmetrical. To rule out bilateral dislocation one side must be treated experimentally, and the landmarks reexamined. This procedure should be incorporated routinely into general physical examinations. In the classroom or workshop situation students should practice the treatment procedure on seemingly "normal" classmates to rule out bilateral dislocation. The treatment procedure is nontraumatic, when performed with judicious force. There is no danger of producing a "downslipped" dislocation.

Pubic subluxation may or may not be present with upslipped innominate, either on the same side or on the contralateral side. The etiology of pubic subluxation, however, is entirely different from the traumatic etiology of upslip. Pubic subluxation is caused by abdominal-thigh muscle imbalance.

One expert in the field of manual medicine initially believed that the upslipped innominate was an undiagnosable condition after X-raying a series of patients while his thumbs were palpating the ischial tuberosities. It was then discovered that an error in technique led to the thumbs sometimes being positioned as far as two centimeters from the inferior surface of the ischium. The author, observing the technique used, noticed that the palmar stereognostic approach was not employed in locating the inferior surfaces of the ischial tuberosities, a common mistake of even highly skilled clinicians. Instead, the thumbs were simply pushed into the inferior gluteal fold.

Students should be taught to first palpate the inferior gluteal folds with the palms of the hands, which are moved in small circular motions until the stereognostic sense identifies the precise location of the inferior surface of the ischial tuberosity. The thumbs can then be placed precisely on its inferior surfaces. In placing the thumbs, care must be taken to avoid pushing the thumbs against skin tension; skin slack can be created by pulling gluteal skin down with the thumbs. The preferred method of evaluating the tension of the sacrotuberous ligaments also depends on knowing precisely where those ischial tuberosity surfaces are.

Using Mobility Tests for Lateralization and Confirmation of Upslipped Diagnosis
The use of a combination of flexion tests and the supine Dynamic Leg Length Test of Pelvic Motion Symmetry can provide supporting evidence of the diagnosis in questionable cases. The combination of standing mobility restriction and ipsilateral supine hypermobility is persuasive evidence of sacroiliac subluxation. A supine leg length changing test is a reliable method of testing nonweight-bearing sacroiliac mobility. Refer to Chapter 6, Figures 6.23.A – 6.25.G.

In the nonweight bearing supine dynamic leg length test, each side of the pelvis is subjected to controlled circumduction movements of the hip joint. These circumductions can be used to shorten the leg (with flexion, abduction, external rotation of the hip), and lengthen the leg (with flexion, adduction, and internal rotation of the hip).

The amount of leg length change on each side is compared. With the supine dynamic leg length tests, a normal pelvis will permit the leg length to change 6 to 12 millimeters. A subluxated sacroiliac joint, because it is more hypermobile under non-weight bearing conditions, will permit more than 12 millimeters. In contrast, a dysfunction due to restriction (i.e., sacroiliac or iliosacral dysfunction) will allow less than 6 millimeters' change in response to these tests. Thus, the supine dynamic leg length tests can provide supportive evidence of the presence of subluxation, by making more evident the degree of hypermobility on the side with the lesion.

Note: Before measuring supine leg length it is customary to spring the legs into internal rotation – *except when using leg length to diagnose mobility asymmetry in the pelvis.* Theoretically, the stork tests should also demonstrate hypermobility of the dislocated side, but this has not yet been tested experimentally. Of course, recumbent leg length is expected to be shortened on the side of the upslipped innominate. The change in prone leg length, before and after treatment, is an indicator of treatment success and a measure of the severity of dislocation.

Paradoxically, even though a subluxated joint is more hypermobile and tends toward instability, the standing and seated flexion tests for pelvic joint mobility almost always manifest *restricted* mobility of the subluxated side. The most likely explanation for this paradox is that supporting weight on the dislocated joint tends to jam or wedge the sacrum onto the ilium. There are exceptions, however, but they can usually be accounted for by concomitant dysfunctions on the opposite side of the pelvis (which may actually be secondary lesions compensating for the dislocation).

Sometimes the wedging effect of the weight-bearing hypermobile sacroiliac joint does not sufficiently restrict the mobility enough to affect the flexion test. In other words, hypermobility may be demonstrated both standing and supine. In this case, the flexion tests are not reliable to discriminate upslipped innominate on one side versus downslipped innominate on the other. It is best to assume that the downslipped innominate is a fictional entity, and treat the superior innominate.

Testing for Superior Subluxation or Dislocation of the Innominate (Upslipped Innominate)

Testing is a two-part procedure performed with the patient in the prone position:
A. Test for ischial tuberosity heights
B. Test for sacro-tuberous ligament tension

A. Testing for Ischial Tuberosity Heights
Procedure Protocol *(for Superior Subluxation)*

1. The patient is prone. It is important that the patient lies parallel with the table edges, which are within your visual field and helpful in making geometric judgments.

2. You stand at one side, and first place the palms of your hands over the ischial tuberosities, as shown in Figure 7.17. The hands should contact the patient at the inferior gluteal folds, and be directed anteriorly and superiorly in an effort to locate the tuberosities. Making small circular motions with the hands will help you identify the inferior surfaces of the ischial tuberosities stereognostically with the palms and heels of your hands. Novices should do one side at a time.

3. Having located the inferior surfaces of the tuberosities with the palms and heels of your hands, you should now locate the most inferior aspect of the tuberosities with your thumbs, as shown in Figure 7.18. Take care to pull some skin down from the gluteal area to create slack in the skin your thumbs are pushing into.

4. Compare the heights, observing your thumbs from directly above. You may have to step slightly toward the foot of the table in order to see your thumbs. Keep your thumbs in position for the next part of the test (sacro-tuberous ligament tension).

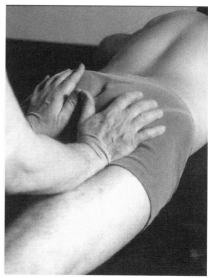

Figure 7.17. Stereognostic palpation of the ischial tuberosities for evaluating upslipped innominate – patient prone.

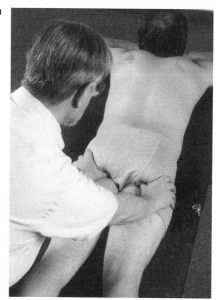

Figure 7.18. Thumbs on inferior surfaces of ischial tuberosities.

B. Testing Sacrotuberous (S-T) Ligament Tension Procedure Protocol

1. Continuing from Step 4 of Part A, you now slide the thumbs in a medial and superior direction from their inferior contacts on the tuberosities, maintaining lateral pressure with the thumb pads against the bone as in Figure 7.19. If the sacrotuberous (S-T) ligament is slack on one side, the thumb will be permitted to slide farther on that side before its progress is checked by the ligament. If one ligament is slack, the thumb on that side will slide up the ischial bone farther.

Note: The tension of the S-T ligaments can also be evaluated by gentle and intermittent pressure on the ligament halfway between the ischial tuberosity and the sacrococcygeal junction, as well as by the comparative distance that the thumb slides on each side until it is resisted by the ligament. However, the distance method is more reproducible.

2. Make the comparison between S-T ligament tension on one side with the other.

Note: The mechanism of slackening of the ligament is rendered schematically by Figure 7.15.

Interpretation of Results

■ **If the ischial tuberosities are level**, there is no luxation or subluxation, or the dislocation is symmetrically bilateral.

■ **If one ischial tuberosity is more superior**, there is a presumptive diagnosis of superior dislocation on that side, and this usually agrees with the side of the lesion as revealed by the Standing Flexion Test.

■ **Confirmation of the diagnosis is completed by assessment of S-T ligament tension**, i.e., the side of the slackened tension must correspond with the side of the more superior ischial tuberosity. A more superior ischial tuberosity with no difference in ligament tension could be the result of pelvic fracture or dysgenesis.

■ Prone leg length, taking into account any anatomic leg length difference, can be a useful diagnostic adjunct. The next task analysis describes this procedure.

■ Obviously the difficult diagnoses are the ones with very small asymmetries. It is a clinical judgment call whether to treat a 3 millimeter difference, since there could be that much measurement error in the technique. The short-term treatment, a tug on the leg combined with the patient's cough, is simple and safe, and will rule in or out bilateral dislocation. Also, the leg tug may correct and stabilize the imbalance for several days or longer. But the long-term treatment for sacroiliac instability (a Hackett belt) is quite an ordeal for the patient. The judgment call should take this into account.

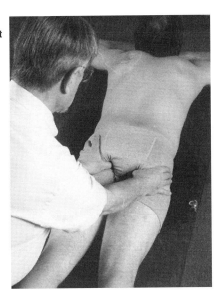

Figure 7.19. Palpating sacrotuberous ligament tensions.

Prone Leg Length Measurement

Be sure the prone patient is lying straight on the table with the feet off the end of the table. You stand at the foot of the table, and put the patient's heels together on either side of the midsagittal plane; this requires sighting up the body to be sure the legs are straight with the body and the body is straight with the table. Making sure that the ankles are flexed at the same angle, compare the positions of the plantar surfaces of the heel pads, which are more practical landmarks than the medial malleoli in the prone position.

This procedure is also used to test for functional leg shortness due to sacroiliac lesions. The mechanism of sacroiliac lesions causing a functional leg shortness requires that the lumbar spinal segments be able to adapt appropriately to the tilting of the sacral base by reversing the sacral positional asymmetry. If that adaptation requires lumbar left sidebending, the left leg will be shortened in the prone position. **The sacroiliac dysfunctions which require lumbar sidebending adaptation with consequent leg shortening are**:

1. Forward sacral torsion to the same side
2. Backward sacral torsion to the same side
3. Unilateral sacral flexion on the opposite side

Whether functional leg shortness will develop with the above lesions depends on the ability of the lumbar curvature to adapt to the tilted sacral base.

Prone Leg Length Comparison
Procedure Protocol

1. The patient is prone and lying straight, body parallel to the table edges. The feet and ankles should be off the end of the table. The face may be turned for neck comfort.

2. Put the patient's heels together in the mid-sagittal plane.

3. Be sure the ankles are flexed at the same angle.

4. Compare the heel pads, observing directly downward (Figure 7.20.).

Interpretation of Results

■ Be sure to take into account any anatomic length asymmetry before judging whether a leg is abnormally shortened.

■ Apparent shortening of a leg can be due to an upslipped innominate, a sacroiliac dysfunction, or a posteriorly rotated innominate (iliosacral dysfunction) — in which case the leg shortening will probably be greater in the supine position.

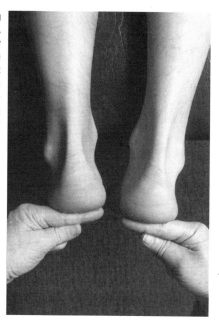

Figure 7.20. Prone leg length measurement. The left leg is apparently one centimeter short. The standing crest heights test may rule out anatomic short left leg, one centimeter. In this case, prone leg length indicates a manipulable pelvic disorder.

Treatment for Superior Innominate Dislocation *(Upslipped Innominate)*

Procedure Protocol

1. The patient lies prone with the feet and ankles off the end of the table. The face may be turned for neck comfort.

2. You stand at the foot of the table.

3. Now you will try to find the slippage plane of the sacroiliac joint. This requires abducting the leg on the side to be treated about 10 to 15 degrees. This starting position is shown in Figure 7.21.

4. The more precise the abducted position of the leg, the more effective the treatment will be. To achieve more precision, start tugging distally on the leg gently and intermittently, while you watch the patient's lumbar region. When you find the abducted angle where tugs have the least effect on the lumbar region, you are in the slippage plane of the S-I joint.

5. Now explain to the patient how and when to cough. *"I will count a rhythmic cadence to four, and I want you to cough on 'four.' Make it a single explosive — martial arts — cough, like this."* (Demonstrate.)

6. Hold the leg just above the ankle, internally rotate the leg enough to take the slack out of the hip joint capsule, and exert a slow, steady pull on the leg in the slippage plane to remove all of the slack from the hip and knees. The tensile force required is usually less than a pound; if it causes the lumbar region to move, it is too much traction, and you should back off the traction slightly and maintain it steadily.

7. Now say: *"Ready! One, two, three, cough!"*

8. Simultaneously with the cough you do a quick, sudden distraction jerk in the line of the pull on the leg. It is important that you do not back off from the localized steady traction before making the quick pull. Speed is important. Force and amplitude should be *minimal.* Ideally, the jerk should not be necessary. If the localizing steady traction is maintained precisely, the cough alone should be enough to reduce the dislocation.

9. Retest, and repeat the treatment if indicated.

10. Once symmetry is achieved and the dislocation reduced, you must find out if the reduction is stable and will support the weight of the patient. One way to do this is to have the patient stand up and walk around the treatment table, reversing directions at least once. The turns challenge the stability more than straight walking.

11. After two or three turns around the table, have the patient lie prone again for a re-check.

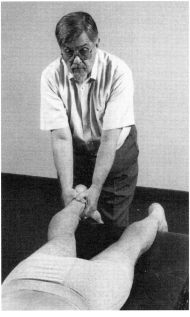

figure 7.21. Manual reduction of upslipped innominate with cough. The leg tug is both quick and low amplitude, localized by careful initial traction.

Significance of Results

■ **If the symmetry persists and the reduction is stable to the weight-bearing challenge**, further treatment will probably not be necessary, provided the patient is reasonably careful. Some activities, such as running, jumping, dancing, vacuuming, sweeping, raking, or carrying heavy loads, especially on stairs, should be restricted for about eight weeks. Low impact forms of exercise (eg., walking, Hatha Yoga, Tai Chi, etc.), are probably safe. Weekly or biweekly checkups are a good idea.

■ **If weight bearing causes recurrence of the dislocation**, the diagnosis is "unstable sacroiliac joint." The management of this problem is more complex than for a stable reduction of a subluxation. The torn ligaments must be treated just as you would treat a fractured bone, only more carefully, in the sense that reduction must be more precise. The dislocation must first be perfectly reduced, and then immobilized and stabilized (kept in the reduced position) for a period of eight weeks to allow the ligaments to heal.

■ About two-thirds of the upslipped innominate reductions stay in place once they are put in place. The recurrent ones need to be held in place by a tight elastic compressive belt long enough for the ligaments to heal, which can take 8 to 12 weeks. The belt must be worn continuously at all times unless the patient is lying down. A second belt is required to replace the wet one after a bath or shower. An elastic Hackett belt is preferred, but other elastic types can do the job as well.

■ Practitioners of prolotherapy (sclerotherapy) would probably elect to inject the sacroiliac ligaments with a sclerosing agent with the expectation that it would strengthen the joint. However, even if this is done, the joint must first be put back in place *and immobilized* for eight weeks. Outcomes comparisons have not been done to the authors' knowledge, but I suspect there would be no difference with or without injection. Healing usually occurs naturally without sclerosing the joint, provided congruent joint apposition is maintained long enough.

■ Patients with collagen disorders, such as Marfan's or Ehlers-Danlos syndrome, may take longer to heal. The most frequent reason for failure to heal in any patient is inadequate immobilization. Because ligament healing requires inflammation, aspirin or NSAIDS should be avoided, if possible. The new onset of local sacroiliac discomfort may be a sign of healing.

■ In the management of bilateral upslip it is not advisable for the surrogate to tug on the leg each time it is examined to rule out bilateral upslip recurrence; such treatment could make a hypermobile joint even more unstable by further damaging ligaments. Recurrent subluxation, if it occurs, is likely to occur on one side only. Recurrent bilateral upslip during the few hours between examinations is extremely rare. On the other hand, the surrogate should be shown how to reduce the upslip, when and if it occurs during belting, to avoid another physician's office visit. Obviously, the more often this is necessary the more jeopardy to the sacroiliac ligaments. Because of the risk of further damage to sacroiliac ligaments, repeated reduction procedures – leg tugs – should be kept to a minimum.

Sacroiliac Belt

Patient compliance is relatively poor when it comes to wearing a sacroiliac belt properly. The following program will improve compliance.

■ Explain the nature and mechanism of the lesion to the patient, using visual aids.

■ Provide the patient with an instruction pamphlet (See Appendix).

■ Make a separate appointment for belting, at which time the patient is expected to bring someone close, a relative or friend, who can be trained as your surrogate to do the diagnostic procedure detailed above, preferably twice a day, while the patient wears the belt. The training takes about ten minutes to make a confident reliable examiner out of a lay person. The landmarks to be checked at home are the ischial tuberosities, sacrotuberous ligaments, and heel pads for leg length. The patient must be prone, preferably lying across a bed.

■ The surrogate examiner is essential. If the pelvis dislocates while wearing the belt, the sooner it is discovered, the more likely the patient will learn what activity to avoid. The subluxation must be reduced, the belt tightened, appropriate measures taken to avoid another recurrence, and *the 8 week count starts over again*.

■ Two proper size belts are provided for the patient.

■ Proper skin care is important. After bathing, during the exchange of the wet belt for the dry one, the skin under the belt should be cleaned thoroughly with alcohol or soap and water. Before the dry belt is applied the skin should be dry. A lanolin- or aloe-based lotion may be applied. Additional soft padding may be needed in the areas of greatest irritation, usually near the anterior superior iliac spine.

To prevent the debilitating effects of prolonged inactivity, the immobilization, in most cases, can be achieved with an elastic sacroiliac belt. The belt must be worn very low on the pelvis, covering the area below the anterior superior iliac spine and above the greater trochanter of the femur, and should be low on the buttocks as well. Even wearing it this low, the belt tends to creep up during sitting. If it does creep up, position it lower on the buttocks. The belt must be cinched as tight as can be tolerated. In very unstable cases more than one belt at a time may be worn to increase the elastic's compression of the pelvis, required to prevent the joint from slipping out of place. Twenty to thirty minutes after the belt is applied its tightness will be noticeably lessened because of the movement of tissue fluids. It may need to be tightened.

With the belt come instructions to avoid vertical shearing forces such as jumping, dancing, jolting steps on stairs, lifting or carrying weights, and twisting movements such as sweeping or vacuuming. It often takes two weeks of life style adjustment before the patient learns what activities to avoid.

The belt must be in place at all times the patient is upright – sitting, standing, or walking. It can be loosened or removed only when the patient is lying flat. It must be worn while the patient is bathing or taking a shower. A second dry belt should be available to replace the wet belt. The belt exchange must take place while the patient is lying flat.

Unfortunately, wearing the belt is not complete insurance against recurrence of the dislocation. And if dislocation occurs during the period of healing, the time in the belt is extended, after replacement of the joint, to make the total time in place (dislocation reduced) eight weeks. The patient must be told this in advance.

The belt is moderately to extremely uncomfortable. No one wants to spend more time in the belt than is absolutely necessary. If dislocation does occur, it should be discovered as soon as possible in order to have a better chance of finding out what made it go out of place, so that one could avoid doing it again. The patient must be able to have the landmarks checked at least once a day, or preferably more often. Having this service performed at the doctor's office is inconvenient and not cost effective.

Patients must be strongly motivated to wear a sacroiliac belt. Without motivation, compliance with the therapy is highly doubtful. The reasons why it is important must be explained to the patient in detail. The clinician must be self-assured that this treatment is necessary. Ischial asymmetry that is less than 5 or 6 millimeters (one-fourth inch) may be too small to be absolutely sure of the diagnosis. Even if you are sure of the diagnosis, how sure can you be that a particular symptom or condition is caused by it? In general, it is a mistake to promise that the belt treatment will get rid of a specific symptom. Predictions are necessarily vague. No one knows how the patient's body will react to the change in sacral position, especially if the dislocation has been long-standing. Both you and the patient must believe that having a level sacral base will probably improve the quality of life in some way.

Note: In the Appendix, the reader will find a patient handout containing instructions for wearing a sacroiliac belt. The reader is welcome to copy and reproduce it for use in the practice.

Practice, Practice, Practice! In practicing the procedures related to the upslipped innominate syndrome, several related tests should be included together. At least two methods of evaluating bilateral pelvic mobility should be practiced, i.e., the Standing Flexion Test, and/or a Stork Test, and/or the maneuvers which change leg length to test pelvic mobility. If you are familiar with other tests of pelvic mobility, such as articulating the pelvis (rocking the innominates), you may wish to try those tests to see if you reach the same conclusions about the side of motion restriction. Examine ischial tuberosities, sacrotuberous ligaments, and prone leg length to check for upslipped innominate. Practice the upslipped innominate reduction procedure on a "normal" pelvis; you may discover an unsuspected (bilateral) upslipped innominate.

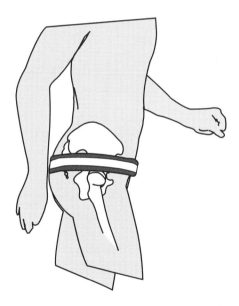

Figure 7.22. Sacroiliac belt position. The belt must necessarily be worn on the skin underneath the clothing. One type of sacroiliac belt used to stabilize a dislocated pelvis to allow the ligaments to heal is known as the Hackett belt. Healing requires 2 to 3 months of immobilization of the dislocated joint. To prevent riding up, the belt must be worn low on the pelvis, between the ASIS and the femoral trochanter. The belt is worn next to the skin under the clothing so that it does not need to be removed for excretory functions. The posterior part of the belt should be low enough across the buttock to prevent it from slipping up when the patient sits.

Rhomboid Pelvis
Testing for Inflare-Outflare Subluxations of the Innominate

Flared innominate subluxations, which Fryette (1914) referred to as "dished in" or dished out," are relatively rare. From an anatomic consideration they may be possible only with certain topologic configurations of sacroiliac joint surfaces; namely, a convex, bulged out, sacral auricular surface articulated into a concave iliac joint surface, permitting some mobility in a transverse plane. This articular morphology is uncommon. The rest of the sacroiliac joints have only infinitesimal freedom of mobility in a transverse plane. Even though they are subluxations, flare lesions are usually treated after innominate rotations, which resemble flares. Ideally, subluxations, if discovered, should be treated before any other lesions of the pelvis. Until innominate rotations are treated, medial or lateral displacement of the ASIS may not be a valid indicator of iliac flare.

As the innominate slides on the convex sacral auricular surface, moving in a transverse plane, some anterior or posterior displacement of the pubic bone on that side in relation to the other pubic bone occurs. **Outflare displaces the pubic bone anteriorly; inflare displaces it posteriorly.** This A-P shearing of the pubic symphysis is an integral part of the flare subluxation. But the displacement is quite small and nearly impossible to detect by palpation. Nevertheless, when treating an inflare, a monitoring hand may be placed on the ASIS of the opposite innominate to detect when localization positioning of the lesioned innominate has exceeded the pathologic barrier. This localizing movement is probably transmitted through the pubic symphysis rather than the sacrum.

Presumably, the same monitoring could be used in treating an outflare. The author prefers a monitoring finger in the ipsilateral sacral sulcus; it feels less awkward.

The Test for ASIS Flaring (for Iliac Flare)
Procedure Protocol
1. The patient lies supine with the umbilicus and lower abdomen exposed. Patient alignment on the table is important.
2. First, use the broadness of your palm to locate the ASIS stereognostically (Figure 7.23).
3. Then, use the thumbs to palpate the medial slopes of the ASIS, just off the inferior slopes (Figures 7.24 and 7.25).
4. Your sighting eye should be directly over the midline as you now compare the ASIS-umbilicus (or other midline landmark) distances on both sides.

Note: The umbilicus is usually a reliable midline landmark. However, scars or deformities can pull it off center. The xiphoid process may also be substituted for a midline reference point.

The Results of ASIS Flare Testing (for Iliac Flare)
■ **If the ASIS-umbilicus distances are equal,** there is no flare subluxation.

■ **If one ASIS-umbilicus distance is greater than the other,** it could mean that there is an iliac outflare of that side, or an inflare of the other side. The side may usually be determined by the standing flexion test. As in the pubic subluxations, treating the wrong side will have no effect, positive or negative.

For example, the Standing Flexion Test revealed a right-side lesion, and you have now found a greater ASIS-umbilicus distance on the right. The diagnosis is probably a right iliac outflare lesion, not a left inflare.

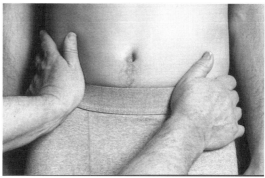
Figure 7.23. Supine stereognostic location of the ASISs.

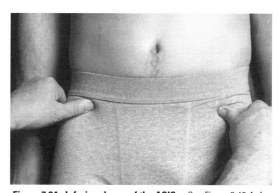
Figure 7.24. Inferior slopes of the ASISs. See Figure 8.40.A. for additional comments regarding the inferior slopes.

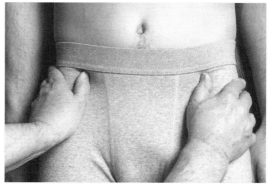
Figure 7.25. Medial slopes of the ASISs.

Treatment Procedures for Flare Lesions
Treatment for the Iliac Inflare Lesion.
Procedure Protocol

1. The patient lies supine.

2. You stand on the same side as the lesion.

3. Your one hand reaches across to support and monitor the ASIS on the opposite side. The monitoring is for the purpose of detecting movement of the opposite innominate, indicating that localization positioning for treatment has exceeded the barrier of the lesion. When you feel that motion, you must back away from it in order to be localized to the lesioned joints – sacroiliac and pubic symphysis.

4. Your other hand grasps the patient's ankle on the side to be treated. As shown in Figure 7.26, the hip of that side is flexed, then abducted and then externally rotated to a sense of barrier, as felt with the hand monitoring the opposite ASIS.

5. Figure 7.27 shows the alignment of your forearm on the patient's leg, so that your elbow rests on the medial aspect of the knee. This is important positioning to be able to resist the patient's isometric femur adduction contraction that will ensue.

6. With the positioning of the previous Step, have the patient attempt to adduct the hip as you resist the effort by offering counter-force at the knee with your elbow. This adduction effort may done with or without internal rotation of the femur. If internal rotation is added, you must resist the lateral movement of the ankle with your hand.

7. As the patient relaxes, take up the slack created by the contraction, achieving additional abduction and external rotation of the hip. Then, have the patient repeat the isometric contraction.

8. Usually, about three repetitions (steps 6 and 7) are required for a correction. Sometimes full correction does not occur until the leg is fully straightened.

9. To complete the procedure, maintain the abduction and external rotation of the hip as you straighten the leg (Figure 7.28.), and finally return the extremity to the neutral (resting) position.

10. Retest, and do additional treatment if indicated.

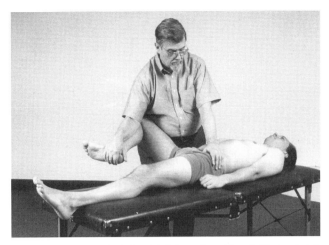

Figure 7.26. Treatment for inflared right innominate, Step 4. Monitor the left hemipelvis for localization.

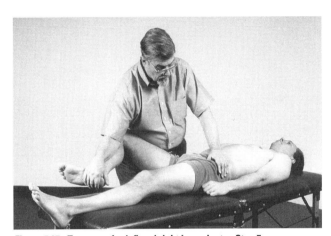

Figure 7.27. Treatment for inflared right innominate, Step 5. The abduction/external rotation tension is sustained while the leg is being straightened.

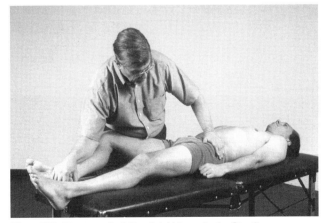

Figure 7.28. Treatment for inflared right innominate, Step 9. The patient's foot is guided to its final position, which is resting beside the other foot.

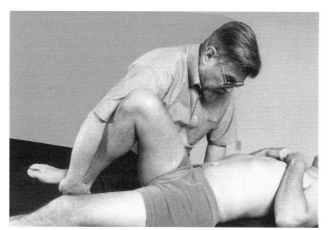

Figure 7.29. Treatment for outflared innominate on the right. The operator's monitoring hand is under the patient palpating in the sacral sulcus for localization.

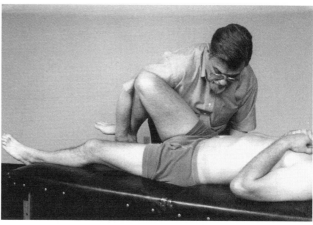

Figure 7.30. Treatment for outflared innominate on the right. The adduction/internal rotation tension is sustained while the leg is being straightened.

Treatment for the Iliac Outflare Lesion
Procedure Protocol

1. The patient lies supine.

2. You stand on the same side as the lesion.

3. Your one hand (in a forearm supinated position) reaches under patient's buttocks until your finger pads come to rest in the sacral sulcus on your side. (This will permit palpation for localization as well as applying gentle lateral traction on the PSIS, drawing it toward yourself.)

4. Your other hand grasps the patient's foot on the side to be treated by reaching across in front of the ankle to hold the medial plantar surface of the foot. (Figure 7.29)

5. As shown in Figure 7.30, the hip of that side is then flexed, adducted, and internally rotated to the sense of barrier, as perceived by the fingers in the sacral sulcus.

6. Figure 7.31 shows the alignment of your shoulder on the patient's knee. Your shoulder will resist the patient's isometric hip abduction effort.

7. While maintaining the positioning of steps 5 and 6, have the patient attempt to abduct the hip against your shoulder, while you stabilize the foot maintaining internal rotation of the femur and offering unyielding resistance with your shoulder. This abduction effort may done with or without external rotation of the femur. If external rotation is added, you must resist the medial movement of the ankle with your hand.

8. As the patient relaxes, take up the slack created by the contraction, achieving additional adduction and internal rotation of the hip, but, more importantly, sliding the outflared innominate back in place on the sacrum. Then, have the patient repeat the isometric contraction.

9. Usually, three repetitions (steps 7 and 8) are required for a correction.

10. As you complete the procedure, maintain the adduction and internal rotation of the hip as you straighten the leg, as shown in Figure 7.32.

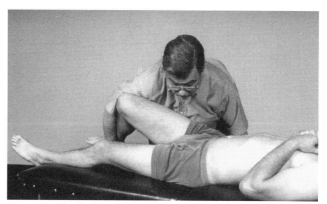

Figure 7.31. The shoulder pushes the patient's knee medially while the hand pulls the foot laterally.

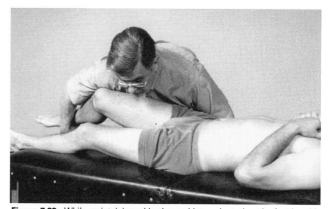

Figure 7.32. While maintaining adduction and internal rotation, the foot is guided to rest beside the other foot.

11. Retest. If indicated, repeat the treatment. Unlike treatment procedures for pubic subluxations, the flare treatments are not so forgiving – precision matters more. Thus a treatment failure does not automatically indicate that the flexion test misled you into treating the wrong (normal) side.

CHAPTER 8

Evaluation and Treatment of Pelvic Articular Dysfunction

Chapters 2 and 3 presented the normal physiologic motions of the sacrum relative to the innominates and spine, as well as the motions of the innominates relative to the sacrum and to each other. Sacroiliac or iliosacral dysfunctions occur when either the sacrum or innominates become static somewhere in the range of physiologic movement, thereby restricting the normal range or function of the joint. The purpose of this chapter is to demonstrate how to identify and treat specific dysfunctions of the pelvis which restrict the previously described normal motions. Coccygeal dysfunction will also be discussed.

In Chapter 4, sacroiliac and iliosacral dysfunctions were classified as follows:

■ **Sacroiliac Dysfunction** – *caused by spinal forces from above, altering ligamentous-articular mobility of the sacrum:*
   • Unilaterally flexed sacrum (designated left or right for the side with dysfunction – *or* may be bilateral)
   • Sacrum torsioned (designated as left or right torsioned about either the left or right oblique axis).

■ **Iliosacral Dysfunction** – *caused by abnormal movements of the lower limbs, altering osseous-articular mobility of one ilium:*
   • Anteriorly rotated innominate (designated left or right for the side of dysfunction);
   • Posteriorly rotated innominate (designated left or right for the side of dysfunction);

■ **Breathing Movement Impairments** – *caused by pelvic edema or compression of the sacroiliac joint:*
   Sacroiliac respiratory restriction (designated left or right for the side with dysfunction – *or* may be bilateral).

Valid interpretation of pelvic landmark asymmetries requires an organized sequence of examination and treatment. Landmark asymmetry can be caused by subluxation, sacroiliac dysfunction, or iliosacral dysfunction; landmarks can also be "displaced" by adaptation. Adaptations may lead to landmark positions which mimic or appear to indicate a different dysfunction than that which actually exists. To minimize the possibility of misdiagnosis or unnecessarily treating the consequences of adaptation as if they were primary lesions, a rational sequence of evaluation and treatment should be followed (see Table 8.A.). Too much or unnecessary treatment can overstress the patient, and would be an inefficient use of the clinician's time.

Sacroiliac Dysfunction

The sacrum moves adaptively in response to the forces applied to it by the movements of the spine, and to changing forces within the pelvis. The repertoire of adaptive motions for the sacrum includes nutation and counternutation, unilateral flexion, and the coupling of sidebending and rotation, i.e., torsion. **According to the Mitchell model, these variations of sacroiliac motion require multiple axes – at least two transverse axes, and two oblique axes – and the requisite bony relationships necessary for these axes to be operant.** The goal of treatment is to restore the conditions necessary for the pelvic joints to have a full range of normal articular motion.

Three types of sacroiliac dysfunction have been identified: unilaterally (or sometimes bilaterally) flexed sacrum, torsioned sacrum (which is torsioned either forward or backward about an oblique axis), and respiratory restriction of the sacrum. Both sacral torsion dysfunctions and unilateral sacral flexion dysfunctions occur frequently and are commonplace in clinical practice. The torsions outnumber the flexions in incidence – about 3:2.

Torsioned sacral dysfunction. Under normal conditions, balanced spinal sidebending usually creates torsion movement of the sacrum, as in walking. Occasionally, the sacrum may become torsioned, i.e., the sacrum becomes

Table 8.A. Treatment Sequence for Addressing Pelvic Dysfunction
Following is the recommended treatment sequence for pelvic dysfunctions; this sequence makes it possible to distinguish pelvic landmark asymmetries due to adaptation versus asymmetries due to subluxation or dysfunction:

1. **Treat non-neutral dysfunction of the lumbothoracic spine.**
   Rationale: The sacrum adapts to the forces applied to it by the movements of the spine. For example, balanced or unbalanced sidebending of the lumbars causes the sacrum to tilt sideways. If non-neutral dysfunction in the lumbars creates an adaptive lumbar curve, the effect of the curve on the sacrum could be misdiagnosed as sacroiliac dysfunction.

2. **Treat pubic or innominate subluxation.**
   Rationale: If there is subluxation or dislocation anywhere in the pelvis, then the axes about which the normal physiologic motions occur is disrupted. Therefore, subluxations must be addressed before an accurate evaluation of sacroiliac and iliosacral dysfunction can be performed. In some cases, sacroiliac and iliosacral dysfunction cannot be treated successfully until the appropriate physiologic axis has been restored.

3. **Treat sacroiliac dysfunction and breathing impairment.**
   Rationale: The three bony components of the pelvis influence each other, so that if one bone becomes dysfunctional the other two are obliged to adapt to it. The ligaments are the links which transmit the influence of one bone to the next. Sacral torsion lesions usually cause large adaptive shifts in innominate landmarks which could be misinterpreted as iliosacral dysfunction. This is why the proper sequence needs to be followed to achieve the best outcome.

4. **Treat iliosacral dysfunction; recheck sacral ILAs and sacroiliac breathing.**
   Rationale: After treating iliosacral dysfunction, it is a good idea to recheck the ILAs and sacral breathing motion to make sure that iliosacral dysfunction was not masking sacroiliac dysfunction. When one innominate rotates or displaces in relation to the other innominate, the sacrum must shift its position to equalize the sacroiliac and sacrotuberous ligament tensions. The sacrococcygeal area is strongly tethered to the ischii by the two sacrotuberous ligaments. These ligaments are quite inelastic and the bilateral tension in them tends to remain equal, except in vertical shear dislocation (upslipped innominate).

Note: In Chapter 6, we learned how to determine lateralization for dysfunctions in the pelvis. Lateralization procedures can be applied again after the more detailed examinations presented in this chapter, in order to confirm or clarify the findings of these more specific tests. These procedures may be done at any stage of the above sequence.

stuck in a torsioned position. The most common torsion dysfunction is toward the left on the left oblique axis, a *forward* variant often abbreviated Left-on-Left torsion. See Chapter 4 for a more detailed discussion of the mechanics of sacroiliac dysfunction. The high incidence of left forward torsioned sacrum on the left oblique axis suggests a ubiquitous etiology. Combining the common compensatory pattern (CCP) described by Zink (Mitchell Jr., 1984) and the phenomenon of tightness proneness of specific muscles described by Janda (1983) offers a possible etiologic explanation for Left-on-Left torsioned sacral dysfunction. Normally involved through the stance phase of the gait cycle, a disturbance in the normal cross-pattern reflex relationship between the tightness prone muscle groups, the right hip external rotators and left *latissimus dorsi/quadratus lumborum,* can account for the common torsioned sacrum lesion, without a precipitating traumatic event. In the case of a sacrum torsioned forward, a backward bending of the spine (or even a normal lordotic curve in the lumbars) in conjunction with the cross pattern reflex mentioned above establish conditions which favor the torsioned forward phenomenon. In the case of the sacrum torsioned backward (e.g., torsioned left on the right oblique axis), tightness of the left hip external rotators occurs with ipsilateral tightness of the *latissimus dorsi/quadratus lumborum,* and likely occurred when the patient was in a forward bent position.

Flexed sacral dysfunction. Some unilateral sacral flexion motion may be physiologic, but it is more likely an abnormal sacral movement in response to sidebending a dysfunctional spine. So long as sacral adaptations to spinal motion spontaneously reverse, the motions are physiologic. Typically the production of unilaterally flexed sacrum involves a traumatic force which bilaterally flexes the sacrum a lot. Following this traumatic event, only one side of the sacrum is free to extend, and the other side remains wedged.

Unilaterally flexed sacral dysfunction is much more common than bilateral, and is almost always found on the *left* side of the body, at least in the Northern Hemisphere. The diagnostic features of a left unilaterally flexed sacrum are:

- Inferior and slightly posterior displacement of the *left* ILA;
- Deepening of the *left* sacral sulcus;
- Shortening of the *right* prone leg length;
- A positive seated flexion test on the *left;* and,
- If the Sphinx test is performed, it will show only slight or no improvement of sacral asymmetry.

Already described in Chapter 3 were the paradoxical sacral motions associated with extremes of spinal flexion and extension when the sacrum *reverses* the direction of transverse axis rotation as the spinal bend approaches its limit. With extreme lordosis and a sudden increase of the weight load on the lumbosacral joint, the sacral nutation may be so extreme that it cannot spontaneously recover from the anterior nutated position. This impairment of sacroiliac function is classed, rather arbitrarily, as a sacroiliac somatic dysfunction, even though it may, in some instances, represent more of a subluxation – assuming the sacrum exceeded the physiologic range of motion in the arc of the iliac auricular surface. This dysfunction is described as **bilateral sacral flexion**. When the sacrum is flexed symmetrically, the diagnosis is more difficult than when the flexed position of the sacrum is asymmetrical. With a symmetrical bilateral sacral flexion, the diagnosis is suspected upon seeing a short distance between the PSISs with exaggerated lumbar lordosis. But it is proved by treating one side and reexamining the landmarks before treating the other side. Of course, both sides would get treated in an asymmetric bilateral sacral flexion dysfunction; the more extreme side first, leading to the discovery of the less extreme side. Bilateral sacral flexion dysfunction is very rare, probably because the two sacroiliac joint surfaces are not parallel planes. Most of the time treating one side restores symmetry to sacral position and function.

Respiratory sacral dysfunction. The breathing movements of the sacrum are also nutations. Some clinicians consider the superior transverse axis to be the respiratory axis for sacral rocking motion between the innominates. However, one radiogrammetric study demonstrated that it was not the superior transverse axis, but rather the middle transverse axis that was the operant respiratory axis (Mitchell Jr. and Pruzzo, 1979). The **middle transverse axis**, which passes through the anterior inferior aspect of the L-shaped auricular surfaces on the sides of the sacrum at the level of the S_2 segment, *is the normal pelvic respiratory axis*. With deep breathing the rocking movements of the sacrum change the pelvisacral angle an average of 1.8 angular degrees between exhalation and inhalation. Rocking of the sacrum on this axis is clearly driven by respiratory movements of the lumbar spine. Because of the location of the axis, the long and short arms of the sacroiliac articulation must permit some anterior and posterior shearing translatory play. When that joint play becomes restricted, breathing motions of the sacrum must move the entire innominate with it, greatly increasing the work of breathing. Occasionally respiratory restriction of the sacroiliac joint affects the standing and seated flexion tests. When it does, the asymmetric movement of the PIP or PSIS begins sooner than usual in the act of forward bending.

Sacroiliac Dysfunction
Evaluation for Sacroiliac Dysfunction
Sacroiliac dysfunction can be evaluated using the ILAs, sulcus depth, prone leg length, flexion tests, and the sphinx and hypersphinx tests. However, **the ILAs alone often provide enough information to discriminate between torsion and flexion dysfunction.** Torsion, being more of a *rotation* of the sacrum, displaces the ILA mostly posteriorly and only slightly inferiorly (e.g., 1.0 cm. posterior and 0.3 cm. inferior). Flexion, being more of a *sidebending* of the sacrum, displaces the ILA mostly inferiorly and less posteriorly (e.g., 0.3 cm. posterior and 1.5 cm. inferior). In those cases where the posterior/inferior comparison is ambiguous, other landmarks and tests – sulcus, leg length, flexion test – must be consulted. Remember that **the deeper sulcus and the prominent ILA are on the same side when the sacrum is unilaterally flexed, but they are on opposite sides when the sacrum is torsioned.** In sacral flexion dysfunction, the seated flexion test is positive on the side of the lesion; in torsion dysfunction the flexion test is on the side opposite the named oblique axis, e.g., left oblique axis, right positive flexion test.

The leg length indicators of sacroiliac dysfunction are caused by sidebending adaptations of the lumbar spine, the leg being shortened on the side of the shorter sidebender muscles of the spine. Leg length can be helpful in differentiating torsion from flexion dysfunctions. Left torsion on either axis shortens the left leg, whereas left flexion *appears* to lengthen the left leg (it actually shortens the right leg), assuming the lumbosacral joint functions normally. *Therefore, a left flexion should have a (neutral) left rotated fifth lumbar, and left torsion should have a right rotated fifth lumbar.* Do not forget that the fifth lumbar rotates in relation to the sacral base, not the iliac crests. It only needs to rotate enough to compensate for the sacral rotated position. Its transverse processes, therefore, may look symmetrical in relation to the iliac crests, even though it is rotated on the sacrum.

The inferior lateral angles of the sacrum are the *sine qua non* of sacroiliac diagnosis. If they are symmetrical, there is neither sacral torsion nor unilateral sacral flexion dysfunction. However, symmetry does not entirely rule out other sacroiliac dysfunctions. Symmetrical ILA positions can be found with a bilaterally flexed sacrum, or with respiratory sacroiliac restriction.

Testing for Sacroiliac Dysfunction
The Prone and Sphinx Tests for ILA Positions – Procedure Protocol

1. The patient lies prone. The face may be turned for neck comfort.

2. You stand at the side of the table so that your dominant eye is closer to the patient's feet.

3. Find the posterior surfaces of the inferior lateral angles (ILAs). You may find them by following the *median crest* of the sacrum (Figure 8.2) to its inferior bifurcation at the *sacral hiatus*, and then moving your palpating thumbs lateral past the *cornua* (Figure 8.3). Or you may use palmar stereognosis with your dominant hand to determine the most posterior portion (the fifth segment) of the sacrum and palpating just lateral to the cornua with your thumbs (Figure 8.1.). The cornua form the superior and lateral margins of the sacral hiatus, the depressed area immediately medial to the cornua. They are the bifid spinous processes of the fifth sacral segment (S_5). The ILAs are analogous to the transverse processes of S_5. (Figure 8.4.)

4. To position your dominant eye over the patient's midline, lean your body forward. To sight over your thumbnails, lower your head until your line of sight is horizontal (Figure 8.5.).

5. Compare the two ILAs, which should be level with the coronal plane. Any amount of A-P asymmetry may be significant. It is not unusual to see more than 5 millimeters ($^1/_4$ inch) of A-P asymmetry. Leave your thumbs in place on the ILAs for at least 10 seconds and observe them for slow oscillating asymmetry of similar magnitude.

6. Bring your head up and slide your thumbs down off the inferior edges of the sacrum. Sometimes you can do this by pulling the skin down over the edge of the sacrum. Be sure you do not get your thumbs on the coccyx. The edges of the sacrum are immediately inferior to the ILA posterior surfaces (Figure 8.8.).

7. With your thumbs on comparable left and right points of the inferior edge of the sacrum, thumb pads facing craniad, position your eyes directly above your thumbs, and compare the ILAs for superior-inferior asymmetry. It is not unusual to see more than 5 millimeters ($^1/_4$ inch) of inferior-superior asymmetry. Asymmetry may be as great as 20 millimeters. Again observe 10 seconds for sacral oscillation (Figure 8.9.).

8. After observing the ILA positions with the patient in the prone position, instruct the patient to *"Raise your shoulders up off the table and rest your chin in your hands."* The elbows should be directly beneath the shoulders, making the humeri as near vertical as possible (Figure 8.6.).

9. Observe the ILAs (as in Steps 1 through 7). Even if no change in ILA position has occurred, for better or for worse, it will be necessary to extend the patient's back farther. This may be accomplished with the hypersphinx position. With backward torsioned sacrum the asymmetry persists; with forward torsioned sacrum the asymmetry disappears (Figure 8.7.).

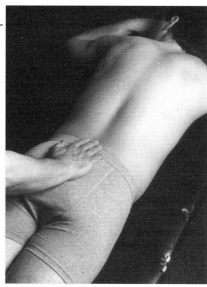

Figure 8.1. Finding the ILA with palmar stereognosis. The ILAs are at the level of the most posterior part of the sacrum. The palm detects this posterior prominence of the sacrum quickly.

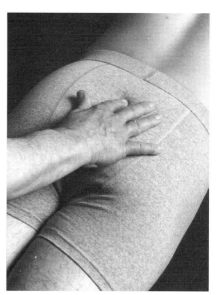

Figure 8.2. Finding the sacral hiatus by palpating the median crest of the sacrum. The median crest is the row of partly blended spinous processes. A slight side-to-side movement of the finger pad will bring this ridge to your attention. When bone is felt on either side of the finger pad, the pad is in the sacral hiatus, bounded laterally by the cornua.

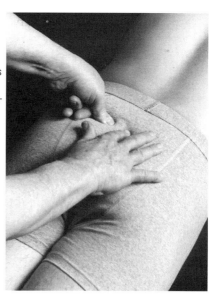

Figure 8.3. Finding the posterior surface of the ILA – just lateral to the sacral hiatus. Assume that the finger in the hiatus is at the level of S5. Even if the hiatus opens up higher on the sacrum, S4 for example, palpating the S4 alae by mistake is not a serious error. Sacral rotation will still be detected. The ILAs are lateral to the two cornua, which may be different sizes.

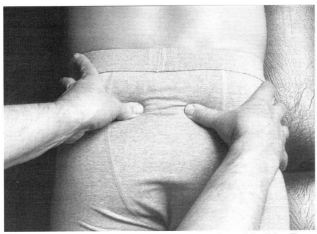

Figure 8.4. Examiner's thumbs on the posterior surface of the ILAs. The sacral cornua should be medial to the thumbs. Apply light anterior pressure to feel the hardness of the sacrum and to be sure the thumbs have not fallen off the sides of the sacrum.

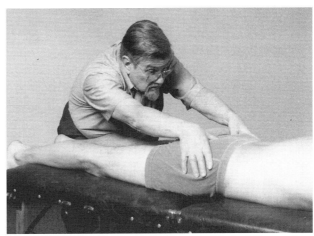

Figure 8.5. Observing the posterior surface of the ILAs for A-P symmetry with the patient in the prone position. The more horizontal the line of sight the better to detect rotated position of the sacrum.

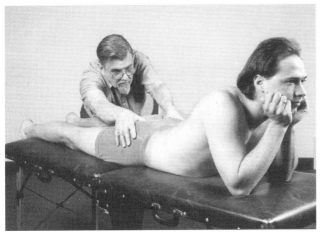

Figure 8.6. Observing the posterior surface of the ILAs for A-P symmetry with the patient in the Sphinx position. The patient's humeri should be nearly vertical for the extension effect.

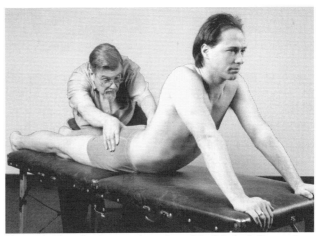

Figure 8.7. Observing the posterior surface of the ILAs for A-P symmetry with the patient in the Hypersphinx position. This position is needed to achieve maximum extension in very supple individuals.

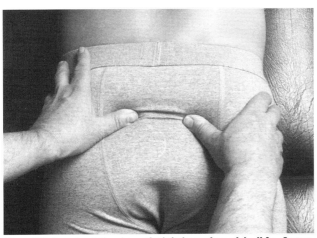

Figure 8.8. Examiner's thumbs on the inferior surface of the ILAs. Contact with the inferior surface of the ILAs should be made after examining the posterior ILA surfaces to avoid encountering the coccyx transverse processes. From the posterior surfaces, slide the thumbs inferiorly on the sacrum.

Figure 8.9. Observing the inferior surface of the ILAs for superior/inferior symmetry with the patient in the prone position. The vertical line of sight makes it easy to see sidebent position of the sacrum.

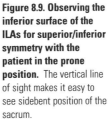
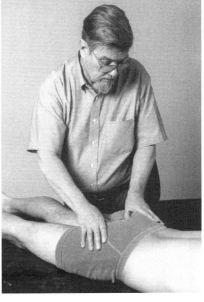

The Test for Sacral Sulci Depths
Procedure Protocol

1. Patient lies prone. The face may be turned for neck comfort.

2. Locate the gluteal tubercles by circular stereognosis (Figure 8.11.) and place the pads of your thumbs on their posterior surfaces pointed medially (Figure 8.12.).

3. Curl the tips of your thumbs medial to the iliac crests and anteriorly toward the sacrum, keeping the pads of the thumbs in contact with the iliac crests. (Figures 8.13. and 8.14.) Apply even pressure anteriorly with the tips of your thumbs. Excessive movement of the thumbs can be quite misleading.

4. The amount of thumb pad contact on the iliac crest is the *palpable* measurement of sulcus depth. Do not try to confirm it visually. Each sulcus is measured from an independent point on the iliac crest.

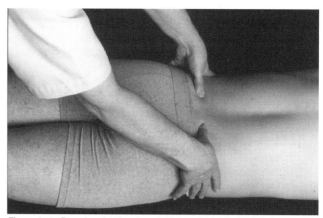

Figure 8.12. Pressing the thumb pads flat on the gluteal tubercles. Each PIP is a reference point for sulcus depth comparison, at the level of S₁.

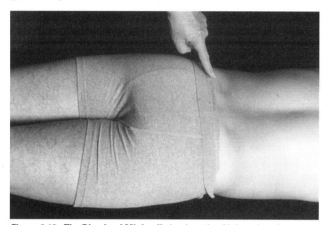

Figure 8.10. The Dimple of Michaelis is where the skin is anchored more tightly to the iliac crest at the gluteal tubercle where lumbodorsal fascia meets gluteal fascia. It is often a visible landmark.

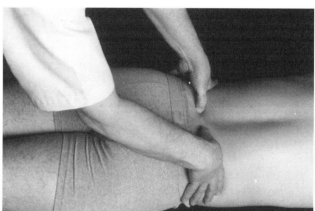

Figure 8.13. Assessing sacral sulci depth – lateral view. The thumb pads stay in contact with the iliac crests as the tips are moved medially and anteriorly.

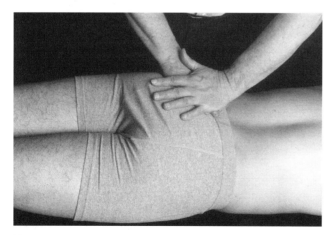

Figure 8.11. Locating the gluteal tubercle (PIP) using circular palmar stereognosis. When the dimple is not very visible, the PIP can be found by palpation with the flat of the finger pads moved passively in small circles with the other hand. The PIP should be the most prominent hard point closest to the dimple.

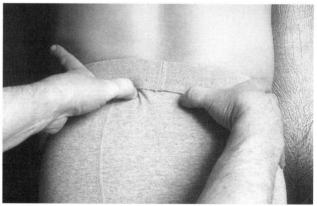

Figure 8.14. Assessing sacral sulci depth – posterior view.. Thumbs may encounter fibrolipomata in this area. They must not be mistaken for bone. Push them out of the way if they will move, or go around them. When the anterior movement of the thumbs tips is stopped by tissue, they are still more than an inch from the sacral base. We must assume equal compressibility of the soft tissues to compare sacral base position with each PIP.

Note: The frequent presence of fibrolipomata or other asymmetric soft tissue phenomena in the postsacral fascia presents a physical diagnosis challenge, which can, at times, be formidable. Fortunately, sacral base position can be deduced from other, more reliable, physical diagnosis findings by using the Mitchell model.

Because they have less overlying tissue and are more superficial landmarks, assessing relative ILA positions, on the other hand, is more visual than palpatory. The ILA positions are visual, and are compared with the cardinal coronal plane. ILA positions can be made visible simply by placing the thumbs on them where they lie superficially just under the skin overlying the most posterior part of the sacrum. Both the posterior and the inferior surfaces of the ILAs (the S₅ alae) are compared to cardinal planes of the body.

As was established in Volume 2, the most reliable way to assess range of motion is to examine the static position of a landmark before motion begins and again after motion has stopped. Before and after treatment observation of static sacral landmark positions meets the same criterion for intra- or inter-examiner reliability.

Interpretation of Results for the ILA Position and Sacral Sulci Depths Test

■ **If the ILAs are symmetrical, and remain symmetrical for 10 seconds, there is no torsion or unilateral flexion dysfunction of the sacrum.** Respiratory dysfunction or bilateral flexion dysfunction are still possibilities. Examination for respiratory dysfunction will follow treatment of iliosacral dysfunctions. Bilateral sacral flexion is treated one side at a time. The treatment of one side can rule it in or rule it out after re-examination.

■ **If the sacrum oscillates, it indicates a dysfunction in the cranial mechanism, usually in the posterior cranial fossa, or involving the temporal bone.** One full cycle of such oscillation takes about 10 seconds. Any amount of visible movement asymmetry is significant. Movements may be much larger than you would think. 5 to 10 millimeters is not uncommon, usually in the transverse plane, but sometimes in the coronal plane. Further investigation of the pelvis should be postponed until the cranial dysfunction is resolved. The absence of oscillation does not rule out cranial dysfunction.

■ **Combinations of dysfunctions may coexist.** However, one dysfunction at a time is found and diagnosed, as a rule, even when more than one coexist. All that is required for diagnosing the second, or third, dysfunction is reexamination after treatment of the first. Often it takes several seconds for the latent signs of the second dysfunction to emerge after the first dysfunction is treated.

■ **Stable, non-oscillating asymmetry of the ILAs indicates either sacral torsion or unilateral sacral flexion.** If the asymmetry is predominantly inferior, the lesion is probably unilateral sacral flexion *on* the side of the inferior ILA. If the posterior and inferior asymmetries are approximately equal in value, other tests or landmarks are needed to confirm the diagnosis.

To confirm the diagnosis of left unilaterally flexed sacrum, the right leg should be functionally shorter in the prone position; seated flexion should be positive on the left, or the sacral sulcus should be deeper on the left. If any one of these criteria is definite, the diagnosis based on ILA position is confirmed.

■ **If the asymmetry is predominantly posterior, the lesion is probably sacral torsion *toward* the side of the posterior ILA.** If the diagnosis is sacral torsion, the Sphinx Test must be performed to determine whether it is forward torsion or backward torsion. **Backward torsion** (toward the left on the right oblique axis *or* toward the right on the left oblique axis) shows maximum asymmetry in the Sphinx position. **Forward torsioned sacrum** (Left-on-Left *or* Right-on-Right) becomes symmetrical if the Sphinx position is extreme enough (hypersphinx). **A unilaterally flexed sacrum**, in most cases, changes position only slightly in the Sphinx position, but may straighten in the hypersphinx position, probably by bringing the normal side down to match the abnormal side.

To confirm the diagnosis of Left-on-Left (forward) torsioned sacrum, the left leg should be functionally shortened in the prone position; seated flexion test should be positive on the right; or the sacral sulcus should be deeper on the right; and the hypersphinx position makes the ILAs even.

To confirm the diagnosis of Left-on-Right (backward) torsioned sacral dysfunction, the left leg should be functionally shortened in the prone position; seated flexion test should be positive on the left; the sacral sulcus should be deeper on the right (because the sulcus is actually shallower on the left); and the hypersphinx position makes the ILAs worse.

■ **If the sacral sulcus of one side is deeper, and the sacral ILA of that same side is more inferior and posterior than the opposite ILA, there is unilaterally flexed sacrum on that side,** even if the inferior displacement of the ILA is equal to, or slightly less than, the posterior displacement. However, because of the ambiguities of the sulcus depth measurement, it is to be trusted less than obvious disparity in inferior *versus* posterior ILA displacement.

■ **If the deeper sulcus is on one side and the prominent ILA is on the other side, there is sacral torsion toward the prominent ILA side.** The axis must be determined with a Sphinx test. A deep sulcus on one side is indistinguishable from a shallow sulcus on the other side, just as a posterior ILA on one side looks the same as an anterior ILA on the other side.

■ **If sulcus depth is too subtle to warrant a clear decision, other tests – prone leg length or flexion tests (or other means of testing sacroiliac mobility) – are needed to confirm the diagnosis.**

The Lumbar Spring Test

This procedure was used by Mitchell, Sr. to discriminate between forward and backward sacral torsion. Forward sacral torsion slightly increases the normal lumbar lordosis. Therefore the spine does not resist anterior pressure against the back to increase lordosis in the prone position. Backward torsion slightly straightens the lumbar lordosis, causing the spine to rigidly resist anterior pressure. Even experienced clinicians had no idea what the normal rigidity of the lumbar spine was supposed to feel like. The test has been discontinued by most practitioners, and replaced with the Sphinx Test.

The Lumbar Spring Test Procedure Protocol

1. The patient is prone.
2. You stand at one side.
3. You place the heel of your hand over the patient's spinous processes of the lumbar spine.
4. You push directly downward several times, using firm but quick movements.
5. Note the reaction. Is it springy? Or unyielding?

Example: When testing the sulci depths and ILA positions, torsion to the left is discovered, i.e., sacral face is turned to the left. If that is all the information that your test has provided at that point, it could be either a Left-on-Left forward torsion or a Left-on-Right backward torsion. However, having now performed the lumbar spring test and determined that the test is negative, (i.e., the lumbar spine is springy – indicating the presence of lordosis), you may now conclude that the diagnosis is Left-on-Left forward torsion.

The Lumbar Component of Sacroiliac Dysfunction and the Sphinx Test

Any lumbar rotoscoliosis which is not in a pattern of adaptation to the sacroiliac dysfunction (lesion) should be corrected, if possible, before the sacroiliac problem is treated. This, naturally, includes all flexion or extension segmental restrictions, because they are not spontaneously reversible adaptations. Failure to treat in this sequence occasionally produces low back muscle spasm, sometimes severe.

Normal lumbar adaptation to sacroiliac lesions is a neutral (group) rotoscoliosis showing rotation (slight) in the direction of the deeper sacroiliac sulcus. The convexity of the scoliosis will be to the same side (another way of saying lateral flexion is opposite to the rotation).

Note that lumbar adaptations to sacroiliac lesions also involve moderate flexion or extension change in the lumbar lordosis. A flexed sacrum – unilateral or bilateral – increases the lumbar lordosis. Increase in lumbar lordosis is also seen with the so-called forward sacral torsions. Backward sacral torsion decreases the lumbar lordosis, rigidifying the spine in the lumbar spring test, a test originally taught by Mitchell, Sr., as a means of identifying backward torsion

lesions. However, these lumbar adaptations do not constitute flexion or extension *segmental* restrictions. All spinal adaptation occurs within the "neutral" range (i.e., not enough flexion or extension to engage a facet joint as a pivot) of spinal motion.

These increases and decreases in lumbar lordosis take place within what is considered the neutral range of lumbar positions, and therefore, are not affected by Fryette's Second Law of Physiologic Motion of the Spine, which pertains to hyperflexed and hyperextended positions of individual segments. The changes do not *directly* produce non-neutral segmental dysfunctions. The changes make portions of the spine vulnerable to trauma, which can elicit segmental impairment (dysfunction).

The sacroiliac lesion and its associated lumbar adaptation component is best considered as a unit mechanism consisting of a complex of motion restrictions. Therefore, diagnostic positional changes in forward torsioned or flexed sacrum are most marked when forward bending of the lumbars is attempted. Similarly, backward bending of the lumbars accentuates the diagnostic positional changes of the backward torsioned lesions. This suggests a better alternative – the Sphinx Test – to the lumbar spring test for differentiating forward and backward torsions. The lumbar spring test is too subjective to be reliable, and is included in this text for historical completeness only. Trunk forward bending straightens the backward torsions.

In left torsion on the right oblique axis, the left sacral base is held posterior by the lumbosacral load and the right sacral base is stabilized at the superior pole of the right oblique axis. When that load is moved farther posterior by the Sphinx position, the left sacral base is carried farther posterior, increasing the rotatory asymmetry of the ILAs.

The fifth lumbar is already forward bent on the sacrum, as well as rotated and sidebent counter to the sacrum. In both forward and backward torsioned sacral lesions, one could think of the lumbosacral joint as being screwed down tight. Under these circumstances, any positional change of L_5 will be followed by the sacrum.

The mechanism of the Sphinx test has been widely misunderstood. The basis for this misunderstanding is the dogmatic assertion that the sacrum and the fifth lumbar *always* move in opposite directions. To accommodate this view, the explanation for the worsening effect of the Sphinx position on the backward torsioned sacrum (torsioned left on the right oblique axis, for example) is said to be due to the additional forward displacement of the anterior side of the sacral base.

Although logically inconsistent, this idea has been widely taught. Such an anterior displacement of the anterior side of the sacral base in Left-on-Right torsion would require superimposing left torsion on the left oblique axis while the right oblique axis is still engaged and stabilized, clearly not possible. Simultaneous motion on both instantaneous oblique axes cannot occur in this universe.

Although such an experiment has not to date been done, it should be technically possible to determine which side of the sacral base moves more in the Sphinx test. The physical examination procedures presently in use are capable of reliably detecting changes in static position of landmarks (ILAs or sulci) between flat prone and prone extended (Sphinx) postures. For those who claim they can feel the motion of the sacral base, it should be pointed out that palpatory detection of bony motion while it is occurring is fraught with error due to variable compounding soft tissue events which may produce the illusion of bone movement. The disagreement over the mechanism of the Sphinx test is not about the static positions of the landmarks; it is about how they got there. Any explanation not consistent with the Mitchell theoretical model of oblique axes should either be regarded with caution, or developed into an alternative model with testable hypotheses.

An erroneous concept may support this illogical notion of movement of the right sacral base in spite of the right oblique axis. It is the mistaken assumption that the rotated position of the dysfunctional sacrum is maintained by *intrinsic* sacroiliac factors. It is not! The sacrum is kept rotated by lumbar forces. In the pelvis, the parts of the sacrum not a part of the instantaneous oblique axis are free to move about the oblique axis.

Treatment for Unilaterally Flexed Sacrum
Prone Treatment for Unilaterally Flexed Sacrum

To treat a unilaterally flexed sacral dysfunction, the patient lies prone on the table; you stand next to the lesion side of the pelvis facing the patient's side. Use the index finger of your cephalic hand to palpate the sacral sulcus on the side of the lesion, while the caudal hand abducts and adducts the patient's leg on the side of the lesion to find the loosest-packed position for the sacroiliac joint. When the loose-packed position is found, the leg is rested on the table at that angle (usually about 15 degrees of abduction). The palpating finger can detect when the superior or the inferior portion of the sacroiliac joint is being compacted. To assure yourself that such detection is possible, abduct and adduct the leg to more extreme positions and feel the joint lock and unlock above and below your finger. Then all that is required is to find the optimum position between those extremes. In the optimum position, alternating trac-

tion and compaction of the abducted leg causes the ilium to slip up and down beside the sacrum. The optimum position maximizes this slipping.

Instruct the patient to hold that leg internally rotated by pointing their toe in medially. This internally rotated leg position is maintained throughout the procedure. Rotating the leg gaps, or opens up, the posterior rim of the sacroiliac joint, creating an opportunity for the sacral base to move backward, a movement which spreads the posterior or superior iliac spines.

The index finger continues to palpate the sacral sulcus while the other hand applies a ventral springing pressure to the ILA on the side of the lesion with 1-2 kilograms of force, varying the angle of pressure slightly until the sulcus palpation indicates that the direction of force is the direction of greatest freedom of sacral movement.

About 10 kilograms of steady pressure is applied to the ILA at an angle which allows the freest sacral motion, and is sustained while the patient step breathes to full inhalation. The sacrum will be felt to move with breathing, as the ILA goes anteriorly and the base comes posteriorly. Hold the sacrum with steady ventral pressure on the ILA while the patient's breath is exhaled. Before the next breath is taken in, check to be sure the pressure is still in the freest plane of the sacroiliac joint, changing slightly the angle of anterior pressure. Do the breathing sequence three times, each time increasing sacral extension (counter nutation) during inhalation, and maintaining steady anterior pressure on the ILA through the exhalation phase. Recheck the ILA inferior edges with the patient prone to assess the effect of treatment.

Occasionally unilateral sacral flexion dysfunction can be resistant to treatment. Usually treatment failure can be attributed to imprecise loose-packing position, or inappropriate direction of force application. Most of the time the lesion forgives sloppy technique, and corrects anyway. When you have been as precise as you can and the lesion persists, you need another treatment strategy. An effective alternative method involves using isometric contractions of the piriformis muscle on the side of the lesion to help break the seal on the sacroiliac joint. Once the seal is broken, loose-packing positioning is easier to arrange. Seated hyperflexion with deep breathing can be an effective self-treatment for recurrent sacral flexion dysfunction, provided it is done frequently enough. These two options will be described after the first treatment protocol.

Prone Treatment of a Unilaterally Flexed Sacrum – Procedure Protocol

1. The patient lies prone. The face may be turned for neck comfort. Usually a pillow is not comfortable for the patient.

2. You stand facing the pelvis on the same side as the lesion.

3. Place a palpating finger in the sacral sulcus on the side of the lesion. This will allow you to feel iliac motion on the sacrum, and then sacral motion on the ilium. (Figure 8.15.).

4. Now, passively abduct the hip on the involved side to the loosest-packed position of the sacroiliac joint (approximately 15 degrees). The leg should be slightly lifted off the table, to avoid grinding the patella on the table. Test the looseness of the joint by slipping the ilium up and down, using the leg for control. Then internally rotate the same hip. Have the patient maintain this abducted, internally rotated position, as shown by (Figure 8.16.).

5. Place a constant pressure downward (anterior) on the inferior lateral angle on the side of the lesion, using the heel of your hand with a straight arm force. Alter the direction of the force (medial-lateral and superior-inferior) slightly from a straight vertical until you are sure you are pushing in the freest plane of the sacroiliac joint, as determined by your palpating finger in the sacroiliac sulcus. (Figures 8.17. and 8.18.)

6. Instruct the patient to take a deep breath and hold it; assure maximum inhalation by having him attempt to take in still more air. "*Take your breath in and hold it. Add some more. And still more. Now breathe out.*" This is called "step breathing."

7. After the fullest possible breath, have the patient release the breath ("*Breathe out*") while you sustain your downward (anterior) pressure on the inferior lateral angle to prevent the sacrum from flexing. (Figure 8.18.B.)

8. Repeat steps 5, 6, and 7 three times. After each repetition check to be sure your pressure is still following the freest plane of joint motion. As the sacrum slides up the auricular surface of the ilium, the bevel of the joint surfaces may change. You must follow those changes to avoid pushing bone into bone.

9. Then retest the inferior lateral angles' inferior edges for symmetry. Repeat the treatment, if indicated. Steps 4, 5, and 8 are the critical ones, in terms of precision.

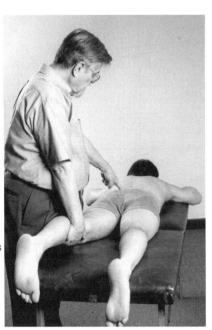

Figure 8.15. Palpating in the sacral sulcus to find the slippage plane (with the corresponding sacroiliac joint in the loose-packed position) as the leg is abducted. The finger in the sacral sulcus senses whether the joint is pinched together superiorly – too much abduction – or inferiorly – too much adduction. When the joint is loose-packed, slight longitudinal tugs and compaction on the leg will produce palpable movement at the sulcus, which is not sensed when leg position is not correct.

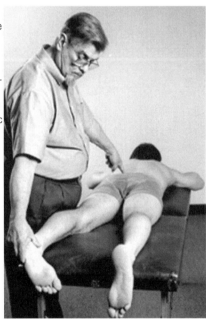

Figure 8.16. Once the appropriate abduction angle is found, the leg is rested on the table at that angle, and the patient is asked to hold the leg internally rotated during the procedure. The internal rotation serves to slightly gap the sacroiliac joint posteriorly, thereby facilitating sacral extension.

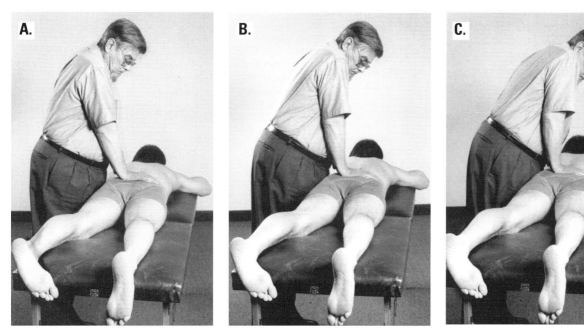

Figure 8.17. A, B, and C. Still palpating the sulcus for joint motion, anterior intermittent pressure is applied to the left ILA, varying the direction of the pressure from medial (A) to vertical (B) to lateral (C) to determine the average flexion/extension plane of the sacroiliac joint in which the sacrum moves most freely.

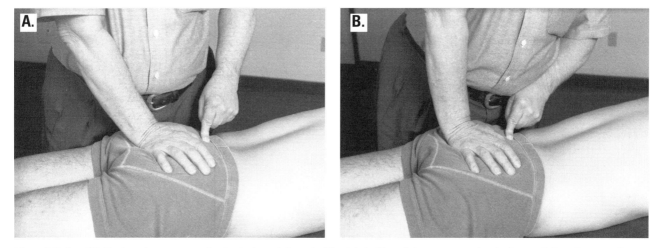

Figure 8.18. A and B. The intermittent pressure direction is also varied superior (A) to inferior (B), until the greatest sacral motion is sensed. Once the proper direction of pressure is found, steady pressure in that direction is applied while the patient step breathes. At maximum inhalation the sacral pressure may get a little extra kick before the patient exhales. Between breaths, the sacrum is not allowed to nutate. As counternutation progresses, the joint plane may change slightly. Continuous monitoring at the sacral sulcus will tell if and when this occurs.

Alternate Prone Treatment of a Resistant Unilaterally Flexed Sacrum

If correction is not accomplished with the preceding procedure, it can be modified to enhance its effectiveness. The first 5 steps are the same, but after Step 5 the sulcus palpating hand is moved to the ipsilateral ILA and pushes anteriorly at the same angle as already determined. This frees the other hand to resist external rotation of the femur.

The patient's leg on the side of the lesion, already abducted to loose-pack the sacroiliac joint, is held in an internally rotated position by bending the knee to 90 degrees and moving the foot laterad. The internal rotation gaps the sacroiliac joint posteriorly, easing the posterior motion of the sacral base. (Figure 8.19.)

After step-inhalation (Step 6), have the patient hold the breath and externally rotate the femur against your unyielding resistance: "Pull your foot against me toward the other side with five pounds of force." (Wait 2 seconds) "Now, relax and exhale." During Steps 5 and 6, while maintaining pressure on the ILA, apply intermittent anterior impulses to the ILA, and then hold the anterior pressure steady during the exhale. Three repetitions are recommended.

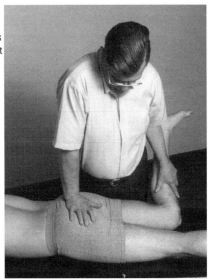

Figure 8.19. Treating resistant unilaterally flexed sacrum. Operator's right hand and elbow resist external rotation of the femur.

Self Treatment for Recurrent Unilaterally Flexed Sacrum

Flexed sacrum lesions may be recurrent in patients with chronic postural faults, including persistent lumbar lordosis. Chronic cranial or upper cervical dysfunction can also cause recurrent sacroiliac dysfunction. Maintaining physiologic pelvic mobility may be important in long term management of such postural or craniocervical problems.

A simple daily stretch can help prevent frequent recurrences of unilaterally flexed sacrum. The patient sits with the feet flat on the floor, knees shoulder width apart. After bending forward, attempting to get the elbows between the feet, the patient takes 3 deep breaths. After each breath is exhaled completely, the patient attempts to increase the flexion. (Figure 8.20.) This attempt may be helped by pulling on the chair legs with the hands.

This technique takes advantage of the paradoxical counternutation effect of trunk hyperflexion described in Chapter 2.

If repeated often enough (i.e., more than once a day), this procedure may correct the flexed sacrum before it becomes firmly wedged and locked.

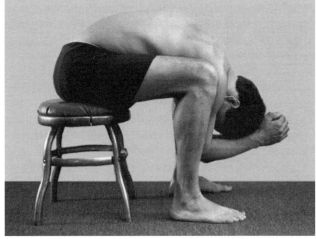

Figure 8.20. Prevention and self-treatment of recurrent flexed sacrum. The stretched out sacrospinal muscles pull the sacrum cephalad along the curved auricular surfaces at the sacroiliac joint.

Treatment for Sacral Torsion Dysfunctions
Diagnostic Criteria for Torsioned Sacrum
There are four possible torsions — forward left (the most common), forward right, backward left, and backward right. The following is a summary of the diagnostic findings of sacral torsion:

■ **All left torsions should have a fifth lumbar rotated right and sidebent left, unless L₅ is also dysfunctional.** The rotation of the fifth lumbar is relative to the sacrum, which, of course, is rotated to the left. Thus the fifth lumbar may appear nearly symmetrical when compared with the cardinal planes of the body. Conversely, all right torsions should have a fifth lumbar which behaves opposite to that which is described above.

■ **All torsions on the left axis should have a positive right seated flexion test.** The theoretical explanation to account for this is the action of the *piriformis* muscle in creating and stabilizing the oblique axis. *Piriformis* does this by pulling the sacrum down obliquely against the inferior pole of the iliac auricular surface. The fixation of this pivot point causes the flexion test to be positive on that side. Conversely, all torsions on the right axis should have a positive seated flexion test on the left.

■ **Forward torsions straighten in the Sphinx position and worsen with forward trunk bending. Backward torsions get worse in the Sphinx position** and straighten with forward trunk bending. Hyperflexion can have the reverse effect in some patients.

■ **Prone leg length is shortened on the side of the posterior ILA.**

■ A curious alteration of prone ankle resting position is often seen with forward torsion – the heel is spontaneously adducted, causing the foot to appear supinated. This phenomenon, the "cocked-heel sign," disappears as soon as the torsion is treated.

■ **The side of the posterior ILA is the side the sacrum is rotated toward.**

■ **The deeper sacral sulcus is on the opposite side from the posterior ILA.**

■ **With torsion one ILA is usually more posterior than inferior,** compared with the other side. At times the ILAs may be nearly equal, depending on the amount of spinal flexion or extension.

Note: Watch for sacral oscillation, indicating cranial dysfunction.

■ The ILA and sulcus depth findings look the same in forward torsioned as in backward torsioned sacrum to the left (as well as to the right). Without the Sphinx test it is not possible to tell whether asymmetric landmark (ILA or sulcus) displacement is forward on one side or backward on the other.

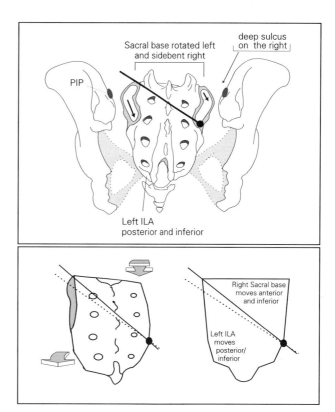

Figure 8.21. Sacrum torsioned left on the left oblique axis (Left-on-Left).

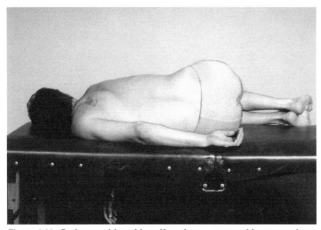

Figure 8.22. Patient positions himself on the treatment table – posterior view. The patient lies on the same side as the involved oblique axis, spine rotated so that the chest is on the treatment table, left arm resting on the table, and right hand reaching toward the floor.

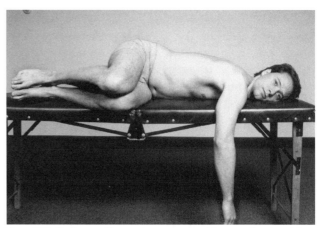

Figure 8.23. Patient position on the treatment table – anterior view. The patient's knees are forward about 6 inches past the table edge.

Treatment Techniques for Forward Torsioned Sacrum

Mitchell Sr. Procedure Protocol for Treatment of the Forward Torsioned Sacrum (Left-on-Left) Protocol Task Analysis

1. The patient lies on the side that corresponds to the involved axis, with the arm on that side behind the back (recall that the oblique axes are named left or right for the superior end of the axis). The hips and knees are flexed to 90 degrees. The knees are together and about 6 inches (15 cm.) beyond the edge of the table. The trunk is rotated so that the chest approximates the table surface. The arm closest to you hangs over the table edge; the other arm rests on the table behind the back. If there was a pillow on the table, remove it before positioning the patient. Instruct the patient: *"Please lie on your left side with your left arm behind your back, and your knees drawn up to me."* (Figures 8.22 and 8.23.)

2. Operator stands facing the patient's hip with his/her own right ankle, knee, and hip slightly flexed.

3. Lift the patient's knees up from the table and rest them together against your inguinal ligament at the top of your anterior thigh. If you bend your knee and raise the heel, the thigh provides a good supporting surface to rest the patient's knee on. You will need to lean your body weight forward. You should be able to take your hands off the patient's legs and control them with your hips. The knees must be raised far enough to bring the patient's shoulder and chest off the table. This gives the patient room to rotate the spine to derotate the lumbosacral joint. With very flexible patients, the knees must be raised higher and can be supported against your abdomen or chest. Shorter operators can support the patient's knees on the abdomen, or even the chest. (Figure 8.24.)

4. With the left hand the operator holds the patient's feet by the heels, which are together.

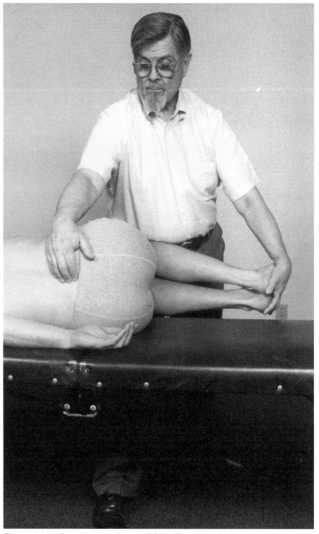

Figure 8.24. Operator starting position. The patient's knees are lifted up and rested on the operator's right anterior thigh. The lumbosacral joint is palpated to find the mid-neutral range between flexion and extension.

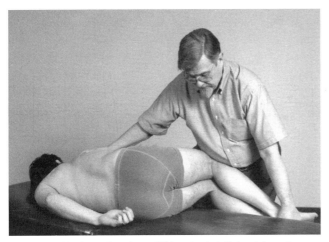

Figure 8.25. Trunk rotation phase. With each exhale (3 times) the patient reaches the right hand closer to the floor, rotating L5 to the left in neutral. The operator's hand on the shoulder is for encouragement, not forceful passive rotation. The left rotation to L5 must be maintained.

5. Operator's right hand palpates the lumbosacral interspinous ligament while slightly flexing and extending the patient's hips using a side-to-side action of his/her own pelvis. Lumbosacral pinching and gapping should be felt between the spinous processes. This insures that the lumbosacral joint is in its neutral range. Stop the positioning in mid-neutral and stabilize the legs and pelvis in that position. (Figure 8.24.)

6. Have the patient breathe in and out, and, *after* exhaling, reach for the floor with the forward hand, bringing the shoulder and chest closer to the table and derotating the lumbosacral joint. (Figure 8.25.) Repeat the breathing and reaching three times. "*Breathe in and out and hold your breath out. Reach for the floor. Breathe in and out again and reach for the floor. And once more.*" Maintain that position while the next step of the procedure is executed.

7. Operator holds the patient's right shoulder forward, maintaining trunk left rotation, and lowers the patient's feet several inches, usually below table level, or as far as hip anatomy allows. This has the effect of externally rotating the right (top) thigh and internally rotating the left. (Figure 8.25.)

8. Hold the feet at the comfortable limit of thigh rotations, and ask the patient to push the feet up against your unyielding resistance (toward the ceiling): "*Lift both feet toward the ceiling with 5 to 10 pounds (5 kilograms) of force,*" as you oppose the motion. After 2 or 3 seconds of isometric contraction, have the patient relax. Take up the slack by again lowering the feet, as in Figure 8.26. Repeat this three times.

9. Assist the patient back into a prone position and reexamine the inferior lateral angles. Repeat the entire treatment if indicated. The technique is quite effective even in the hands of inexperienced therapists, and rarely needs to be repeated. Apparent treatment failure should suggest misdiagnosis rather than poor technique.

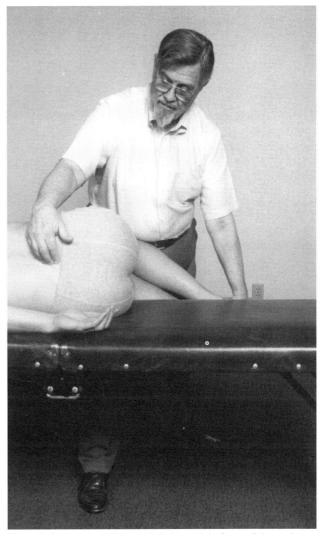

Figure 8.26. Gently lower the patient's feet toward the floor until they are hanging in a relaxed manner. (**Note:** Do not push them down!) With the patient in this position, the operator holds the feet firmly to resist the patient pushing the feet up toward the ceiling, which (in the above example) isometrically contracts the right hip internal rotator muscles and the left hip external rotator muscles; both muscles are antagonists to the right *piriformis*.

Practice this procedure on treatment tables. You may practice these examination and treatment techniques safely on any consenting partner, adult or child. The procedures are not capable of producing dysfunction. If you use a torsion treatment on a unilateral sacral flexion, the ILA asymmetry will not change. Even if your subject does not have the signs of unilateral sacral flexion, treat one side and reexamine the ILAs. You may discover an unsuspected bilateral sacral flexion!

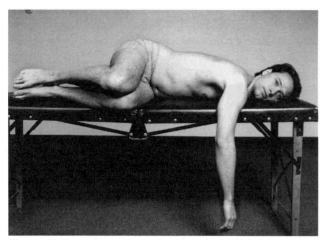

Figure 8.27. The starting position for the patient with the Mitchell, Jr. technique is the same as it was for the Mitchell, Sr. technique for treatment of Left-on-Left torsioned sacrum.

Mitchell Jr. Treatment of the Forward Torsioned Sacrum — Operator Seated Method

Treating a forward torsioned sacral dysfunction with the therapist seated is especially useful for treating the larger, older, or obese patient because it provides better support for the patient's legs. The method is the same as Mitchell, Sr.'s method except that you sit on the edge of the table. Figure 8.27 shows the patient's starting position.

For the treatment of forward sacral torsion, the patient lies on the table in the lateral Sims' position *on the side of the named oblique axis,* hips and knees flexed to 90 degrees, chest down, hands off the table. You sit on the table near the patient's buttocks facing the same direction as the patient and support the patient's thighs on your thigh. Your foot should be on a stool or chair to slightly elevate the patient's knees. Hold the patient's feet together by the heels and allow the feet to lower to a relaxed position. Ask the patient if he or she is comfortable and not lying on any tender points. If necessary, adjust the patient's position for comfort. Slightly flex and extend the patient's hip while palpating the lumbosacral interspinous space for the gapping and pinching of the neutral range of motion. Be sure the lumbosacral joint is in neutral. Next, have the patient inhale and exhale three deep breaths, reaching the forward hand progressively toward the floor *after* (not during) each exhalation. Next, ask the patient to push the feet up toward the ceiling against your unyielding hand with 5 to 10 kilograms of force for 2-3 seconds and then to relax. After complete relaxation, allow the feet to descend to the beginning of resistance. Do this leg action three times, and then assist the patient to the flat prone position on the table. Recheck the ILAs.

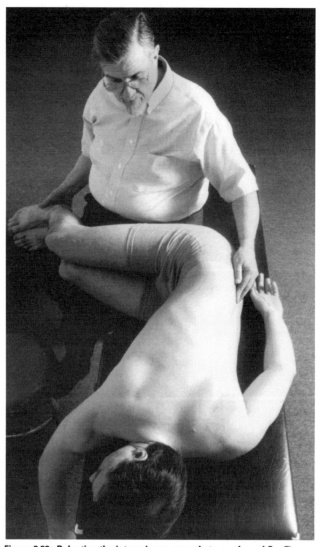

Figure 8.28. Palpating the interspinous space between L$_5$ and S$_1$. The foot of the operator's supporting knee is propped up on the rung of a stool.

Mitchell Jr. Treatment Procedure Protocol for Sacrum Torsioned Forward

1. The patient's starting position is the same as in the first alternate method, lying on the side of the involved axis. (Figure 8.27.)

2. You sit on the edge of the table facing the same way as the patient.

3. Lift the patient's knees up from the table and rest the knees, legs and feet in your lap. Your foot closer to the patient must be on a low stool or the rung of a chair (Figure 8.29.). This will enable you to raise your leg under the patient's thigh by flexing your ankle. Raising the patient's knees can result in additional room for the patient's shoulders and chest, thereby allowing for greater rotation of the spine (in order to derotate the lumbosacral joint) as the patient reaches his hand toward the floor. With very flexible patients the knees must be raised higher, and a higher stool may be needed. You must spread your knees so that the patient's feet hang free of support.(Figure 8.30.)

4. Palpating the lumbosacral junction for neutral positioning is shown in Figure 8.28.

5. Your other hand stabilizes the legs in your lap, grasps both heels together (Figures 8.28 and 8.29), and passively flexes the hips (together), until you feel gapping movement at the lumbosacral junction, indicating that the joint is in neutral. You may need to inch your buttocks toward or away from the patient to accomplish this. Be sure the lumbosacral joint is not at its flexion barrier.

6. The breathing and reaching the hand toward the floor is the same as Step 6 in the previous procedure. The patient's forward hand should continue to stretch toward the floor. (Figure 8.30.)

7. Next, using the hand that is holding the heels, lower the feet as far as gravity will take them. It should not be necessary to straighten the knees in order to lower the feet. You may need to move your knees farther apart to provide space for the patient's feet.

8. Hold the feet down with your hand and instruct the patient to "*Lift both feet toward the ceiling with 5 to 10 pounds (5 kilograms) of force*," as you oppose the motion. After 2 or 3 seconds of isometric contraction, have the patient relax. Take up the slack by again lowering the feet, as in (Figure 8.31.). Repeat this three times.

9. Assist the patient back into a prone position and reexamine the inferior lateral angles. Repeat the entire treatment if indicated. The technique is quite effective even in the hands of inexperienced clinicians, and rarely needs to be repeated. Apparent treatment failure should suggest misdiagnosis rather than poor technique.

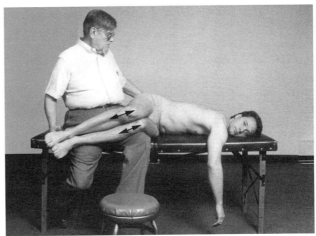

Figure 8.29. Testing for the pinching-gapping effect at the L_5–S_1 interspinous space caused by flexion and extension of the hips (see arrows) produced by side-to-side movement of the operator's supporting leg. The pinching and gapping indicates that the lumbosacral joint is still in its neutral range for trunk rotation, the next step.

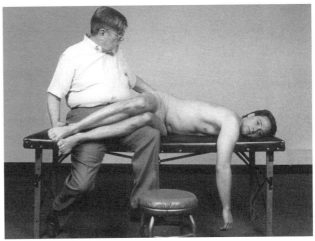

Figure 8.30. Elevating the knees with the supporting leg to create available rotation space for the patient's trunk rotation effort: *"Inhale... Exhale ...Reach your right hand toward the floor."*

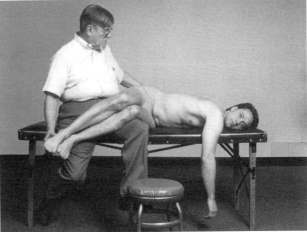

Figure 8.31. Lower the patient's feet gently and hold them down firmly to resist the isometric upward pushes of the hip rotators.

Self Treatment of Forward Torsioned Sacrum

The following procedure is a self-treatment technique for forward sacral torsion. The seated version presented here is very similar to the recumbent versions, except the patient's position is rotated 90 degrees. To better understand the mechanics of this technique, try to visualize the treatment table turned on end against the patient's side (the side of the involved sacral axis). The technique may be done with or without the assistance of a therapist. Each of these options will be represented by **a. with the therapist,** *or* **b. without the therapist.**

Self Treatment Task Analysis

1. The patient sits on a firm chair or low stool with the feet on the floor, ankles and knees together.

2.a. You stand in front of the patient astride the patient's knees. Ask the patient to "*slump*" (eliminate the lumbar lordosis).

2.b. The patient allows the back to sag, eliminating the lumbar lordosis.

3. The patient puts both hands to the side of the lap corresponding to the side of the oblique axis.

4.a. Say to the patient, "*Breathe in and out and reach your forward hand toward the floor.*" Use your hand to hold the shoulder back, preventing trunk flexion.

4.b. The patient breathes in and out and reaches the forward hand toward the floor, holding his or her own shoulder back by putting the hand on that side behind the chair seat to prevent full trunk flexion.

5. The breathing and reaching is repeated three times. The forward hand is left stretching toward the floor.

6.a. Clamp your knees together on the patient's knees, and use your knee to push the patient's knees away from the reaching hand. The patient's feet should remain in place firmly flat on the floor. Move the knees sideways until you meet resisting tension. Stop there.

6.b. The patient uses the reaching arm to push the knees sideways until a twisting tension can be felt at the lumbosacral joint and stops there.

7.a. Tell the patient, "*Push your knees back against my knee with 10 pounds (5 kilograms) of force.*" (Wait 2 seconds.) "*Stop pushing and relax.*" Resist the patient's push with your knee. The patient's feet should remain in place as a fulcrum on the floor.

7.b. The patient uses the reaching arm to resist the 2-second push of the thighs, then stops.

8. Slack is taken up and steps 6 and 7 are repeated three times.

9. Unfortunately, the patient cannot examine his or her own ILAs, but the therapist should recheck them.

Note: Patients can use this technique as a daily home treatment, if recurrent forward torsion dysfunction is found on sequential office visits, at least until the underlying postural or habitual etiology is found and corrected. This procedure may also be done as an operator guided technique. See the **a.** options in the task analysis.

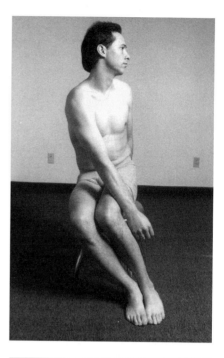

Figure 8.32. A. Self-treatment for Left-on-Left torsioned sacrum – frontal view.

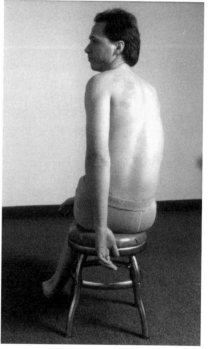

Figure 8.32. B. Self-treatment for Left-on-Left torsioned sacrum – posterior view.

Treatment Techniques for Backward Torsioned Sacrum

The treatment for backward sacral torsion is not nearly as strenuous for the therapist as the forward torsion treatments. The patient does most of the work. This technique can turn you into a savior in the eyes of the patient, who often presents this lesion as a very painful and crippling disorder. Typically, the patient limps into the office with the trunk bent forward and to the side, often with a hand on the lower back. This habitus, which simulates psoas spasm, is pathognomonic.

The Sphinx position, customarily used to confirm this diagnosis, may be too painful for the patient. An improvised modification of the Sphinx test involves leaving the patient standing while resting the hands on the treatment table. The examiner stands behind the patient to monitor the ILAs while the patient raises or lowers the shoulders with the supporting hands. This small range of trunk bending may be enough to demonstrate improving or worsening asymmetry of the ILAs, sufficient to discriminate forward from backward torsion.

Even though severely and painfully disabled, the patient will be able to lie on his side, and will tolerate the localizing positions of the treatment procedure. This procedure involves isometric contractions of hip abductors and lumbar sidebender muscles on the same side. It is stipulated that *piriformis* functions as a hip abductor in the treatment position. Thus the reflexly shortened muscles, *piriformis*, *latissimus dorsi* and *quadratus lumborum*, contract isometrically, then relax and permit lengthening. In left torsion on the right oblique axis these shortened muscles are on the left (uppermost) side, and their tension is believed to maintain the backward torsion dysfunction.

The patient lies *on the side of the oblique axis,* **with the pelvis as close as possible to the anterior edge of the table.** Operator should stand close enough to the table to prevent the patient rolling off the table. The patient's legs are arranged with the top foot resting on the table in front of the bottom leg, and the bottom leg extended at the hip far enough to initiate pinching action (motion) at the lumbosacral interspinous space. The therapist then stabilizes the pelvis in its lateral recumbent position. The patient's top arm is behind the back reaching toward the back edge of the table. The patient's face is turned over the top shoulder. The therapist then asks the patient to inhale and exhale deeply, increasing the trunk twist after each exhalation. Next, the top foot is brought forward off the table by passively straightening the knee, taking care not to alter the flexion angle of the hip. The therapist asks the patient for three successive 5-to-10-kilogram (11 to 22 pounds) pushes to raise the top foot toward the ceiling against the unyielding therapist's hand. During the relaxation after each push the leg is allowed to lower to the beginning of tension. The patient is assisted back to the prone Sphinx position for recheck of the ILAs.

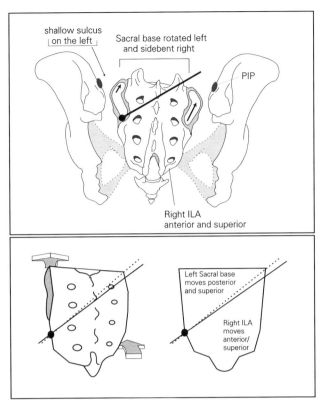

Figure 8.33.A. Osteokinematics and bony positions of a Left-on-Right backward torsioned sacrum.

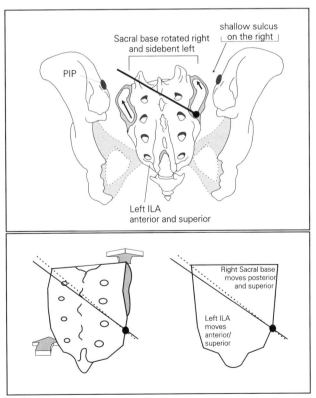

Figure 8.33.B. Osteokinematics and bony positions of a Right-on-Left backward torsioned sacrum.

Treatment for Backward Torsioned Sacrum
Procedure Protocol

1. The patient lies lateral recumbent on the side which corresponds to the involved oblique axis. This means that a patient having a "Left-on-Right" (left torsion of the right oblique axis) lesion, as shown in Figure 8.34., would lie on the right side. Pillow support for the head and neck is inappropriate, since it interferes with rotating the head and shoulders.

2. You stand at the side, facing the patient, to ensure that the patient does not roll off the treatment table.

3. The starting position is shown by Figure 8.34.. **The patient lies with the pelvis as close to the edge of the table as possible.** The top foot rests on the table in front of the bottom foot. The knees may be *slightly* flexed.

4. With one hand palpate the interspinous space at the lumbosacral junction as shown in Figure 8.35.

5. With your other hand move the bottom leg posteriorly, hyperextending that hip until movement is felt at the lumbosacral junction. (Figure 8.35.) The leg will remain in this extended position throughout the rest of the procedure. You may remove your hand from the leg.

6. Palpation at the lumbosacral junction with your finger is still needed. You may leave your finger there, or substitute a finger on the other hand.

7. Stabilize the pelvis with your forearm to prevent it from rolling as the trunk is twisted. This is shown in Figure 8.36.

8. Instruct the patient to *"Breathe in and out, and after exhaling, to let the top shoulder turn back, rotating the trunk."* Repeat the breathing and twisting three times, or until the patient can grasp the back edge of the table and hold on to it. Be careful not to relinquish any pelvic alignment for the sake of greater truncal rotation. Older patients may not be able to rotate the trunk far enough to reach the table edge. Hanging the arm back with the shoulder abducted will maintain fifth lumbar derotation, which is the purpose of trunk rotation. More supple patients may be able to reach the table edge before they are fully rotated. In this case, moving the hand along the table edge toward the foot will maintain increasing amounts of rotation (Figure 8.37).

9. Maintaining trunk rotation, and pelvic alignment, bring the patient's top foot off the table by straightening the knee *without flexing the hip.* (Until now this foot has rested on the table in front of its mate.) Maintaining pelvic alignment, place your hand (which has been palpating the lumbo-sacral junction) on the foot, leg, or knee to resist abduction of the top leg (Figure 8.38.).

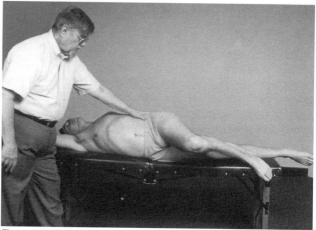

Figure 8.34. Patient's starting position for treatment of Left-on-Right torsioned sacrum. It is important for the patient to lie with the pelvis very close to the front edge of the treatment table, in order for the upper hip to be adducted in the final steps of the procedure without losing lumbosacral extension.

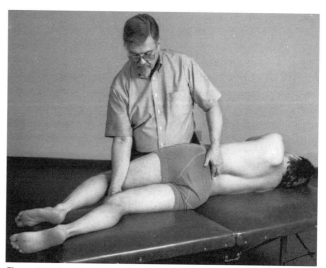

Figure 8.35. Introduce extension at the lumbosacral junction by sliding the patient's bottom leg backward. The operator stands close to the table to prevent the patient from rolling off. Palpate the lumbosacral joint as you extend it to the end of its neutral range.

10. Instruct the patient to *"Raise the knee toward the ceiling"* with 5 to 10 pounds (2 to 5 kilograms) as you oppose the motion. After 2 or 3 seconds of isometric contraction, have the patient relax. Take up the slack by lowering the foot toward the floor, as in Figure 8.39. The leg should not be forced down. It is often necessary to request additional relaxation: *"Really relax!"* Repeat the isometric contraction (resist), relax (take up the slack) three times.

11. Assist the patient back into the Sphinx position for reexamination of the ILAs.

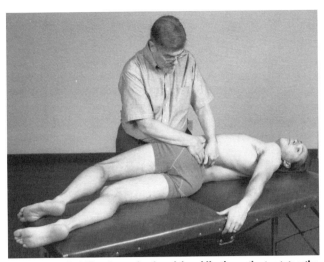

Figure 8.36. Stabilize the patient's pelvis while the patient rotates the trunk to the left. The legs are arranged with the top foot resting on the table in front of the bottom foot.

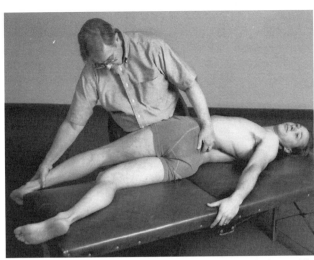

Figure 8.38. Moving the top foot off the table by extending the knee without flexing the hip. This precaution is to preserve the extended neutral position of the lumbosacral joint.

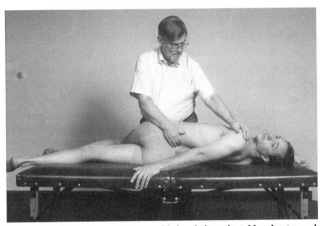

Figure 8.37. Having the patient move his hand along the table edge toward the foot will increase trunk rotation.

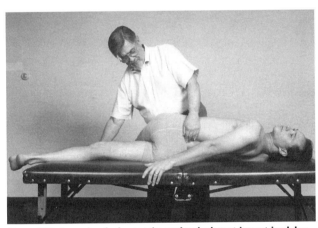

Figure 8.39. Lowering the leg to take up the slack post-isometric abduction.

Rotated Innominate Dysfunctions

There are only two iliosacral dysfunctions: anterior innominate and posterior innominate. The diagnosis of innominate rotation dysfunction is based on asymmetric positions of the anterior superior iliac spines (ASISs). Superior-inferior comparisons are made of the two ASISs in a coronal plane. With the patient supine, locate the anterior superior iliac spines with palmar stereognosis, place the thumb tips on the inferior slopes of ASISs, and assess inferior-superior symmetry. Check supine leg length. Consider the flexion test results to determine the side of the lesion.

ASIS anterior-posterior and superior-inferior position evaluation should be evaluated *after* the sacroiliac dysfunctions, especially the torsion lesions, have been ruled out or treated and resolved. In the presence of sacroiliac dysfunction, the innominates naturally assume an adapted position relative to each other. There is no reason for these adapted positions to be maintained after the sacroiliac dysfunction is no longer present. As an example of the difference between ASIS asymmetry due to adaptation and that due to iliosacral dysfunction, forward sacral torsion dysfunction causes superior-inferior malalignment of the ASISs on the order of 2 or 3 centimeters. In contrast, an anteriorly rotated innominate (an iliosacral dysfunction) typically displaces an ASIS a centimeter or less.

Note: ASIS misalignment is naturally associated with PSIS misalignment. When the ASIS goes caudad, the PSIS of the same innominate goes cephalad. Both ASIS and PSIS may be cephalic with upslipped innominate.

Recall from Chapter 2 that **movement of the ilium on the sacrum requires only one axis (actually, a pivot point)**. Motion of the ilium on this pivot point (iliosacral motion) requires adaptive motion in other parts of the pelvis to equalize tensions in the ligaments – i.e., around a transverse axis through the pubic symphysis, and through the sacrum on the contralateral oblique axis (see Torsions).

The innominates rotate in relation to each other on the transverse pubic axis to adapt to sacral torsion. This adaptive rotation of the innominates normally displaces the ASISs more than rotated lesions of the innominate.

The features of innominate rotation are:
- The more inferior ASIS is also more anterior.
- The supine leg length will be shortened on the posteriorly rotated innominate side, or lengthened on the anterior side.
- There should be no concomitant pelvic subluxation or sacroiliac dysfunction.
- The standing and seated flexion tests should indicate iliosacral restriction on the side of the dysfunction. Posterior innominate on the left (PIL) looks the same as anterior innominate on the right (AIR), except that the flexion tests are positive for iliosacral restriction on the left instead of the right. AIR is more common than PIL.

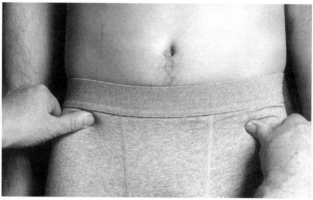

Figure 8.40.A. Observing the thumb pads where they contact the inferior slopes of the ASISs. Belt lines should not be used to determine superior/inferior symmetry. Keep the sides of the table in your visual field, taking care that the patient is aligned on the table.

Figure 8.40.B. Observing the index finger pads on the anterior points of the ASISs for A-P symmetry. Anterior rotated innominate displaces the ASIS inferiorly *and* anteriorly.

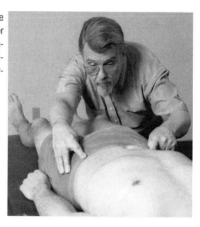

Evaluating for Rotated Innominate

Evaluation for Anterior or Posterior Rotated Innominate Procedure Protocol

1. The patient lies supine. Examiner stands with dominant side next to the patient.
2. Examiner places palms on each side of the anterior pelvis and slides the skin around in small circles to locate the bony prominences of the ASISs.
3. Examiner's thumbs contact the inferior slopes of the ASISs firmly (Figure 8.40.A.).
4. Observing the thumbs from above at arm's length, examiner determines if they are in the same or different transverse planes. Estimate the approximate asymmetry in centimeters or fractions of an inch.
5. Place the pads of the index fingers on the anterior points of the ASISs.
6. Observe the fingers with a horizontal gaze. Determine if they are in the same coronal plane (Figure 8.40.B.).

Interpretation of Results

If one ASIS is both inferior and anterior, either that innominate is rotated anteriorly or the other innominate is rotated posteriorly. The standing flexion test should be positive on the lesioned side. If the asymmetry is more than 1.5 cm., recheck for sacral torsion dysfunction.

Treatment Techniques for Anterior Rotated Innominate

Three techniques for treating anterior innominate will be presented: lateral recumbent, prone, and standing. Certainly more methods could be devised. However, it should be pointed out that supine techniques have presented localization and axis control problems, and indirect techniques (Lippincott, 1948) have been primarily successful in those dysfunctions showing very small and subtle positional asymmetry. The following methods were selected for their potential for success. The first method – **the lateral recumbent technique – is, by far, the most successful.** Even then, only partial success may be achieved when treating very chronic rotation dysfunctions. Several treatments may be required for complete correction. In this regard, the anterior innominate lesion may resemble some somatic dysfunctions of the appendicular skeleton. In the treatment of spinal segmental dysfunctions a reasonable expectation is one hundred percent correction with one treatment.

The force of isometric contractions in these procedures is fairly large, five to twenty pounds (2 to 10 kilograms). None of the muscles employed activate the sacroiliac joint directly. However, when the joint is localized to its pathologic barrier, the action of the muscles serves to gap the joint in some direction, freeing it for rotatory motion. Failures or partial failures of treatment can be attributed to:

1. extreme chronicity;
2. imprecise localization; or
3. inadequate contraction force.

In the event of treatment failure, especially in cases that resist skillful high velocity low amplitude thrust technique, it is prudent to schedule repeat treatments at another time, rather than to attempt to immediately repeat the treatment. Between treatments the patient can gently stretch the iliosacral ligaments using the "Hard Way Shoe Tie" automanipulation. If the treatment is excessively strenuous or too forceful (over 200 foot/pounds of angular torque), sacroiliac hypermobility may result. When treating patients with inborn errors of collagen metabolism – e.g., Ehlers-Danlos syndrome or Marfan's syndrome – the angular torque should probably be kept under 40 foot/pounds (5 kilograms of pressure against your resistance). Foot/pounds of angular torque are calculated by multiplying the pressure at the knee by the distance from the knee to the sacroiliac joint.

Lateral Recumbent Technique for AIR

The patient lies on the left side. A pillow may be provided for neck comfort. The therapist guides the patient's right knee with the right hand while palpating in the sacroiliac sulcus for iliosacral motion. After the hip is fully flexed by placing the patient's foot on the therapist's hip, which is used to push against the foot to cause hip flexion, the innominate commences to rotate posteriorly. The knee is guided to find the plane of freest rotation in the sacroiliac joint, usually in the direction of slight abduction. The innominate is moved to the end of the rotation range to the barrier, and held there. The patient pushes the knee three times up and then three times down against the therapist's hand; each two- or three-second forceful (2 to 5 Kg) push is followed by a short period of relaxation during which the iliosacral rotation is carried to the new barrier by farther flexing the hip in the freest plane of the sacroiliac joint.

The forces generated by these muscle actions apply tensions at approximately right angles to the sacroiliac joint. Nevertheless, when the ilium is repositioned for localization, it is rotated on the inferior transverse axis by additional flexion of the hip. Remember that the sacroiliac joint is passive, and the muscle contractions indirectly apply forces to the ligaments of the joint in order to loosen it for mobilization.

Because AIR is frequently a chronic resistant lesion, a third step is usually necessary. This step requires a contraction of the hip extensor muscles (three times). In order to be able to resist the action of these powerful muscles, the therapist needs maximum mechanical advantage. This is the reason the third step is always done last, after the adduction and abduction steps. To further increase the therapist's mechanical advantage, the hand which has been used to guide the knee is moved to the patient's rib cage by placing the arm between the knee and the ribs. From this position the therapist can usually resist a very forceful extension push, in case he forgets to tell the patient how much force to use (about 10 Kg.). Again relocalization to the barrier is done during each relaxation phase. Rechecking the ASISs is done with the patient supine.

Lateral Recumbent Treatment for Anterior Innominate Right (AIR) Procedure Protocol

1. The patient lies on the noninvolved side, lesioned innominate up. A pillow may be provided for neck comfort.

2. You stand at the side of table, in front of the patient, facing the patient.

3. Your one hand holds and guides the knee on the side to be treated. The patient's bare or stockinged foot is against your hip or thigh. The starting position is shown by Figure 8.41. The leg on the involved side is positioned by flexing the hip and knee of that side to about 90 degrees.

4. Your other hand palpates the sacral sulcus for iliosacral motion.

Note: By this placement of your hands (Steps 4 and 5), it is possible to guide the leg through the plane of the freest iliac rotation, and stop the movement before the ilium moves the sacrum.

5. Maintaining the localized position described above, with your hand supporting the medial aspect of the knee, have the patient attempt to *adduct* the femur against your unyielding resistance and then relax. "*Try to pull your knee down toward the floor using about 10 pounds of force.*" (Wait 2-3 seconds.) "*Now relax.*" (Figure 8.42.)

6. Take up the slack created by this isometric contraction, achieving additional hip flexion, as shown in Figure 8.42. However, you must continue to monitor the sacrum. As in Step 4, you want that point just before the sacrum begins to move. Be sure you are turning the ilium in the plane of freest movement by varying the abducted position of the thigh. Usually, the farther back the ilium rotates the more abduction is required. Then have the patient repeat the isometric contraction (adduction) three times, taking up the hip flexion slack during each post-isometric relaxation.

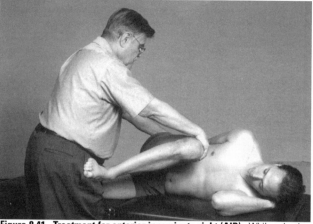

Figure 8.41. Treatment for anterior innominate right (AIR). While palpating the sacral sulcus for joint motion, the right knee is guided into hip flexion following the freest sacroiliac slippage plane. The patient's foot stays on the operator's hip.

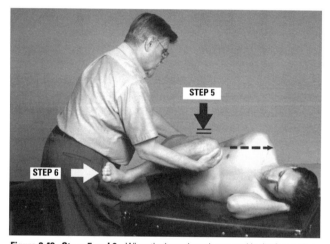

Figure 8.42. Steps 5 and 6.. When the innominate has turned in the freest plane as far as it can without the sacrum following, the hand on the knee resists isometrically a moderate force contraction of the hip adductors. The fingers are on the medial side of the knee (Step 5) to resist the downward push of the knee. After relaxation, the operator takes up slack in innominate rotation by pushing his hip against the patient's foot (Step 6) and guiding the knee superior and laterally to follow the rotation plane of the sacroiliac joint.

7. You resist the upward push of the knee with your hand on the lateral aspect of the knee, as shown in Figure 8.43., and instruct the patient to *abduct* the hip. "*Push your knee toward the ceiling.*" Have the patient relax after a 2- or 3-second contraction, then take up the slack by flexing the hip and rotating the ilium around its transverse axis, achieving a new localized position. Repeat the maneuver a series of three times. This step is like Steps 5 and 6, except that *abduction* is substituted for adduction.

8. At this point, the patient's hip flexion should be sufficiently increased to permit you to place your arm between the knee and the patient's ribs, as shown in Figures 8.44 and 8.45. This makes it easier for you to resist the extension effort. Ask the patient to extend that hip as you resist the effort. "*Push your foot against me.*" If you feel really secure, you can encourage the patient to push harder. "*Try to push me across the room with your foot.*" With your hand holding the patient's rib cage you are in a position to resist a surprising amount of force. In this technique, the more forceful the better, since the object of the contractions is to gap the sacroiliac joint, increasing its freedom of movement.

9. As usual, three repetitions of isometric contraction, post-isometric relaxation, and relocalization may be needed for a correction. However, the palpating finger in the sacral sulcus may detect a significantly large amount of movement during one of the post-isometric relocalization maneuvers. Whenever this occurs, at whatever stage of the procedure, further treatment of the rotated innominate is usually unnecessary.

10. Recheck the supine ASIS symmetry. If the asymmetry persists, and you felt no significant release of motion, you probably should repeat the procedure, and assume that localization was not precise enough the first time. If you felt a release, but some asymmetry persists, it is probably best to teach the patient the standing procedure to be done daily at home between visits to your office. Very chronic innominate rotation dysfunctions sometimes correct in stages. In this regard, this dysfunction is somewhat unique. Nearly all other somatic dysfunctions can be expected to correct completely with Muscle Energy Technique in one treatment procedure.

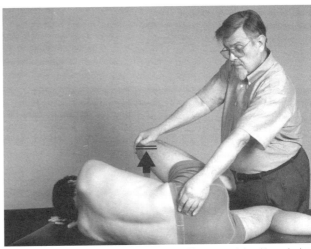

Figure 8.43. Resisting isometric abduction. The operator's hand is on the lateral side of the knee. The left hand monitors the sacral sulcus. Step 7.

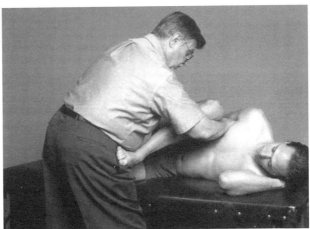

Figure 8.44. Step 8. It is always best to save this step for the last, after the operator's mechanical advantage has increased by preliminary hip flexion.

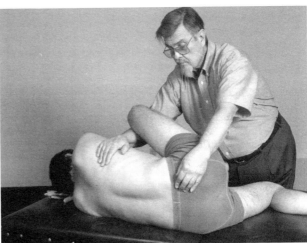

Figure 8.45. Taking up the slack after the extension effort is done with pressure of the hip against the foot.

The Prone Treatment for Anterior Innominate (AIR)

Mitchell, Sr.'s technique for treating anterior innominate was performed with the patient prone. The technique has fewer steps, but is not quite as effective as the lateral recumbent technique.

Procedure Protocol

1. The patient is prone, lying close to the edge on your side of the table, and should be able to hang the leg down off the table. Only half of the pelvis (the normal half) rests on the table.

2. You stand on the side to be treated, slightly behind the buttocks level of the patient.

3. The starting position is shown in Figure 8.46.A. The knee of the hanging leg is flexed to approximately 90 degrees, so that the foot can be placed on your nearer knee. You can secure the patient's foot there by clamping the foot between your knees.

4. Your hand grasps the flexed knee, further securing the foot on your knee by pulling it back against your knee, and guiding the patient's knee with your hand in the freest plane of innominate rotation, usually slightly abducted.

5. Your other hand palpates the sacral sulcus to detect iliosacral rotation motion, as you guide the leg through the plane of freest posterior iliac rotation, pushing against the foot with your knee by bending your knees. Stop the movement before the ilium moves the sacrum.

6. Maintaining the position described above, have the patient attempt to extend that hip as you resist the effort. *"Push your foot back against me with about twenty pounds of force."* (Wait 3 seconds.) *"Now relax."*

7. During the post-isometric relaxation, take up the slack created by the contraction, achieving additional hip flexion, but continuing to monitor the sacrum, stopping the posterior rotation of the innominate before the sacrum moves with it. Then, have the patient repeat Steps 5 and 6 a series of three times.

8. Retest with the patient in the supine position for measurement of ASIS symmetry. Additional treatment, if indicated, should be done at another time.

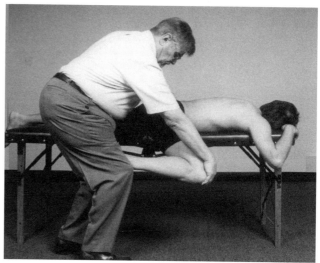

Figure 8.46.A. Prone treatment for AIR. While the foot is against the left knee, the right knee contacts the foot laterally to stabilize its position. Slight increases in the patient's hip flexion is achieved by slightly bending the resisting knee during post-isometric relaxation. Palpating the sacral sulcus facilitates guiding the innominate in its freest plane. A sustained compressive force from the patient's knee into the acetabulum stabilizes the inferior transverse axis for innominate rotation.

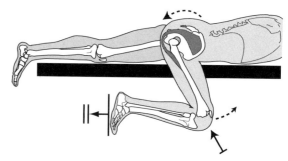

Figure 8.46.B. Prone treatment for AIR. Although this procedure closely resembles the treatment for inferior pubic subluxation, with the patient turned from supine to prone, certain key elements of the procedure are much easier to implement prone than supine. Stabilizing the inferior transverse axis, upon which the innominate must turn, is accomplished by proximal pressure through the flexed femur into the acetabulum, which pulls the innominate down on the sacrum. Hip extension effort is easier to resist and control with the knees. Most important, the sacral sulcus is accessible to palpation for localization.

Self Treatment for Anterior Innominate Right Standing Technique

The "Hard Way Shoe Tie" is an alternative self-treatment technique for the treatment of recurrent AIR. The patient stands with the right foot in the seat of a chair, and then reaches both hands toward the left foot. Staying in this maximum flexed position, the patient takes three deep breaths, and, following each exhalation, stretches the hands closer to the left foot. This may be done as a daily exercise, one to six times daily.

Self Treatment Procedure Protocol for Anterior Innominate on the Right (AIR)

1. Put your right foot on a chair or low stool.
2. Try to "tie your left shoe laces" with your left knee straight.
3. If you cannot reach your foot, breathe in and out and try again.
4. If you still cannot reach your foot, breathe in and out and try again.
5. If you still cannot reach your foot, stop and try again later.
6. If you can reach your foot, you probably do not need the treatment.

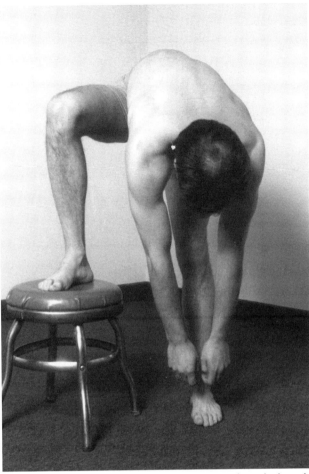

Figure 8.47. The Hard Way Shoe Tie for self treatment of anterior innominate right lesion.

Treatment of Posteriorly Rotated Innominate
Treatment for Posterior Innominate Left (PIL)

The patient lies prone on a low table, near you. You stand at the patient's right side. Bring your left hand from the lateral side of the left knee underneath the knee just below the patella. By keeping your left elbow straight, leverage is increased and muscle effort conserved, thereby allowing you to lift the leg with your weight instead of your arm muscles. When you lift the patient's left leg off the table by the proximal tibia, the patient must keep the leg relaxed so that the weight of the foot keeps the knee extended. If the knee is not kept extended, you must hold the leg farther up toward the axis of rotation, losing some of your leverage.

Rest your right hand on the lateral-superior aspect of the crest of the left ilium – as far as possible from the inferior transverse axis. This serves both to assist rotating it anteri-

orly, and to monitor the freest plane of rotation during relocalization to the barrier. The freest plane of motion is controlled by the angle of abduction of the leg being lifted. Lift the leg off the table. This is done most easily by standing as close as possible to the patient's head and leaning your trunk toward the head end of the table. Feel the anterior rotation of the left innominate and adduct or abduct the leg to find the plane which maximizes it. While keeping the left ilium at its anterior rotation barrier, i.e., before the sacrum and the rest of the pelvis moves, you resist while the patient, on request, pulls the left leg toward the table with 5 to 10 kilograms of force. After complete relaxation, the left ilium is relocalized to the new barrier by pushing the crest forward and raising the leg farther.

Prone Treatment for Posterior Innominate
Procedure Protocol

1. The patient is prone, preferably on a very low table. It helps if the patient lies close to the edge of the table as near as possible to you.

2. You stand at the side of the table *opposite to the lesion.*

3. Your hand grasps the anterior aspect of the knee on the side to be treated. Avoid reaching under the knee from the medial aspect. Reach over to the far side, turn your palm toward you, and come underneath the knee just distal to the patella. Keep your elbow straight.

4. Your other hand is on the lumbar flank, with the thenar eminence contacting the posterior iliac crest on its most superior lateral aspect (Figure 8.48).

5. Lift the leg, extending the hip, by keeping your elbow straight and leaning your body toward the head of the table. If the knee bends, ask the patient to relax the leg and let the weight of the foot keep the knee straight. Find the angle of abduction which maximizes the sense of anterior rotation of the iliac crest felt by your hand on the crest. Go to the limit of anterior rotation in this plane, stopping before the sacrum is dragged along by the ilium. This sense of barrier is monitored indirectly as the sense of changing hysteresis is felt through the iliac crest.

6. Maintaining the extended position described above, have the patient attempt to flex that hip, as you resist the effort. Then, have the patient relax. *"Pull your leg toward the table with about ten pounds of force."* (Wait two seconds.) *"Now relax."*

7. During post-isometric relaxation take up the slack created by this isometric contraction, achieving additional anterior rotation of the innominate in the freest plane of the joint.

8. Usually, three repetitions are required for a correction. When a release occurs, you may feel it, but it is often too subtle to feel. Always recheck the ASIS symmetry in the supine position, and do additional treatment if indicated. The same considerations apply here as applied to the treatment of AIR, but chronicity is less of a problem.

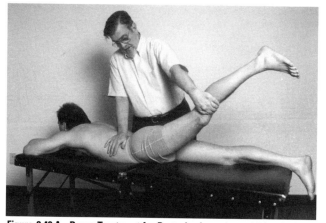

Figure 8.48.A. Prone Treatment for Posterior Innominate. Lifting the leg is much easier if you hold it below the knee (longer lever) and use your body weight instead of your muscles. The long lever principle also applies to the hand on the iliac crest. Remember the rotation axis is at the inferior pole of the sacroiliac joint. The right hand stabilizes it.

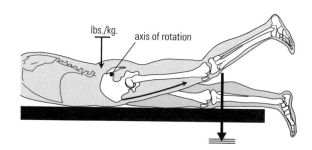

Figure 8.48.B. Mechanics of prone treatment for posterior innominate. Visualizing the inferior transverse axis helps in keeping it stable. The patient's *rectus femoris* isotonic contraction assists the operator's anterior pressure on the iliac crest to turn the innominate anteriorly.

DESIGN YOUR OWN TECHNIQUE

By now the reader should have a firm enough grasp of the basic principles of Muscle Energy Technique to deal effectively with clinical problems in many contexts. For example, many therapists are not tall enough to perform the preceding procedure comfortably. If you are too short, or your table is too high, you may need to do this procedure with the patient lying on the side. How would you modify the technique to observe the principles implicit in the preceding description? To wit: **(1)** What is the easiest way to support and control the leg while extending the hip with slight abduction? **(2)** Where will you place your hand to monitor the freest plane of iliosacral rotation and to get maximum leverage on the crest to turn it forward to the barrier? **(3)** What body position will give you the most mechanical advantage? **(4)** What pertinent muscle contractions will you ask the patient to perform – taking into account your ability to resist leg movement and the conservation of your own effort? Are there alternatives to isometric hip flexion? Remember how the muscle groups were used to treat AIR. If you thought this out for yourself, you probably arrived at a technique similar to the second alternative procedure described next.

Lateral Recumbent Treatment for Posterior Innominate
Procedure Protocol

1. The patient lies on the noninvolved side. A pillow should be provided for head and neck comfort.

2. You stand at the side of the table, behind the patient.

3. The starting position is shown by Figure 8.49. The top leg is extended and slightly abducted at the hip, so that it clears the other lower extremity. This is best accomplished by supporting the flexed knee with your hand and arm and stepping back.

4. Your hand on the iliac crest (superior to the PSIS for maximum leverage) feels for the freest plane of anterior rotation of the innominate on the sacrum. Your arm should be nearly horizontal, or even pushing slightly up on the iliac crest.

5. Your supporting hand, using an underhand grip, since it must both support and provide resistance, varies the abduction of the femur to find the plane of maximum anterior rotation, which is stopped at the barrier, before the sacrum moves with the ilium.

6. Maintaining the position described above, have the patient attempt to flex the hip as you resist the effort. Have the patient relax. "*Pull your knee forward.*" (Wait two seconds.) "*Relax.*" A sensible alternative is to ask the patient to abduct the leg. The weight of the leg can be sufficient counterforce for this effort, sparing the therapist. "*Lift your knee toward the ceiling.*" Resisting adduction would be more strenuous, but is a rational option.

7. Relocalize to the new anterior rotation barrier by extending the hip in the freest plane of the sacroiliac joint. Have the patient repeat Steps 4, 5, and 6 for a series of three.

8. Usually, three repetitions are required for a correction. When a release occurs, you may feel it, but it is often too subtle to feel. Always recheck the ASIS symmetry in the supine position, and do additional treatment if indicated.

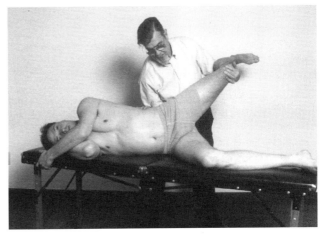

Figure 8.49. Lateral Recumbent Treatment for Posterior Innominate. Avoid pressing medially on the iliac crest by keeping your elbow low. The hand on the iliac crest is as far superior as possible, to achieve maximum leverage for rotation on the inferior transverse axis.

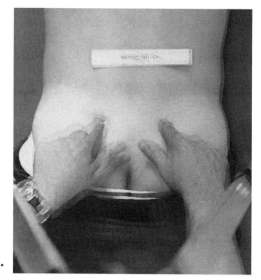

A.

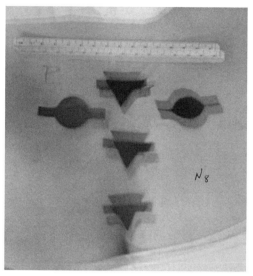

B.

Figure 8.50. A. and B. Two methods of observing sacroiliac respiratory movement. The above pictures are deliberate double exposures to simultaneously show inhaled and exhaled positions of the landmarks. In (A) the index fingers are on the two posterior superior iliac spines to follow them while the patient takes a full breath. Respiratory restriction on one side makes the PSIS on that side move more than the one of the other side, as indicated by the double exposure photographic technique. With deep inhalation, the caudal linear movement of the hand should be about 3 millimeters greater than the caudal movement of the PSIS. In (B), double exposure photography and markers on the skin over the gluteal tubercle and over the median crest of the sacrum were used to demonstrate and compare the inhaled and exhaled positions of the sacrum relative to the ilium. Notice that on the right the marker for the sacrum and the gluteal tubercle moved in parallel fashion and the corresponding markers on the left did not move, indicating normal respiratory movement on the left and restricted movement on the right. In practice, clinicians would use their hands and fingers, in place of the markers, to evaluate these relative respiratory movements.

Sacroiliac Respiratory Dysfunction

Pursuant to the numerous references in this text to respiratory movement of the sacroiliac joints, we will now present a clinical method for examining and evaluating that movement. Its most obvious clinical relevance is in terms of its impact on the efficiency of respiratory-circulatory mechanisms of the entire body. Consider the additional work of breathing imposed by loss of respiratory mobility of a sacroiliac joint. Each breath would then move the mass of one-half of the pelvis back and forth; and this happens 23,000 times a day!

Respiratory movement in the sacroiliac joints can be examined by direct visual inspection. The flexion tests, dynamic leg length tests, or stork tests are of little use in evaluating pelvic respiratory movement, because they are rarely affected by respiratory impairment. One could miss any impairment during a craniosacral examination by simply not looking for it. In most instances the skin overlying the gluteal tubercle, at the dimple, is tightly adhered to the tubercle and moves with the iliac crest. Similarly, the skin overlying the median crest of the sacrum moves with the sacrum. Skin marker ink marks, or adhesive stickers, put on the skin over these landmarks will allow you to observe the relative movements of the sacrum and ilia which occur with a deep breath. Of course, if you don't have stickers or a skin marker, you can use your thumbs. Inhaling deeply displaces the markers inferiorly, but **the marker on the sacrum should move 3 millimeters farther inferiorly than the markers on the dimples.** If there is respiratory restriction on one side, that dimple will move more inferiorly than the one on the normal side with deep inhalation.

Figure 8.51. Drawings showing axis of rotation for sacroiliac respiratory motion. Respiratory axis of sacrum (level S$_2$) for exhalation/inhalation. Regarding the diagram (which views pelvis from the left side), the following points are noted: **1.** The sacral apex moves anteriorly during inhalation, posteriorly during exhalation; **2.** Sacral motion (viewed from left side) is a clockwise motion during inhalation with its axis near S2; **3.** Ilial motion (viewed from left) is also a clockwise motion during inhalation with its axis through the PSIS. **4.** Research data indicate that normal sacral excursion averages about 3 mm. greater than the ilia in respiration.

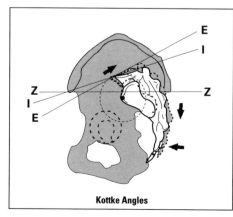

Kottke Angles

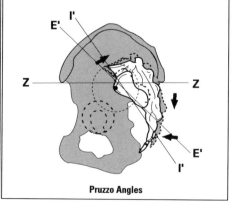

Pruzzo Angles

Testing Sacroiliac Respiratory Motion
Procedure Protocol

1. Patient lies prone.
2. You stand at the side of the table, leaning slightly forward to put your dominant eye vertically directly above the sacrum.
3. Place your thumbs or index fingers on the inferior slopes of the gluteal tubercles at the dimples (the Bilateral Dimple test – Figure 8.50.A).
4. Instruct the patient to take a deep breath. *"Take a deep breath. Let it out."*
5. Allow the tubercles to move your thumbs in the same way that you allowed your fingers to be moved by ribs to test rib respiration.
6. Watch the movement of your thumbs for asymmetry. If there is asymmetry, the side that moved more inferiorly with inhalation is the side of sacroiliac respiratory restriction.
7. If the movements are symmetrical, respiratory sacroiliac movement may be normal, or there could be bilateral restriction.
8. To test one side for restriction, place one thumb on the inferior slope of a gluteal tubercle and the other thumb on the median crest of the sacrum, and have the patient take a deep breath. If the sacrum moves less than 3 millimeters more inferiorly than the tubercle, respiratory motion is restricted on that side. This test may also be used to confirm the bilateral dimple test (Figure 8.52) .

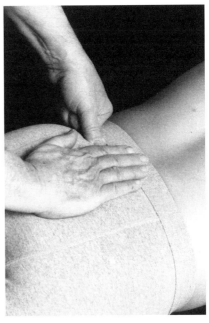

Figure 8.52. Sacroiliac respiratory restriction may be bilateral and symmetrical. Both iliac crests and the sacrum will, in this case, move parallel with each other. Motion restriction can be detected by observing the same breathing movement of the hand on the sacrum and the thumb or finger on the iliac crest landmark.

Treating Restricted
Sacroiliac Respiratory Motion

J. Gordon Zink, the conceptual pioneer of respiratory-circulatory technique, treated the sacroiliac joint with the patient lying on the side. With one hand on the sacrum he circumducted the hip, and the innominate with it, starting from a flexed, internally rotated, adducted position, passing through abduction, and ending with an adducted, extended, externally rotated position. The monitoring hand on the sacrum made for precise execution that almost always produced an articular "pop" from the sacroiliac joint.

The Muscle Energy adaptation of Zink's technique derives from Thomas Schooley's inventive suggestion (personal communication). The sacrum is monitored with the patient lying supine, as in craniosacral technique. The circumduction is done in stages, pausing at each restriction, and releasing it with isometric MET. The procedure has elements of the Dynamic Leg Length Tests and the treatments for inflared and outflared innominates, with the addition of the monitoring hand under the sacrum. (Figures 8.53. through 8.55.)

Treatment of Restricted Sacroiliac
Respiratory Motion
Procedure Protocol

1. Patient lies supine with the knees bent, feet on the table.

2. While the patient raises the hips off the table, you reach between the legs and put your hand on the posterior surface of the sacrum.

3. The patient then rests the pelvis on your hand, and straightens the legs.

4. Your free hand now passively moves the leg on the side of the restriction. Starting with internally rotated adduction, the hip is flexed until the ilium begins to move the sacrum. Back away from that barrier slightly, and ask the patient to abduct the knee against your resisting hand (or shoulder). "*Push your knee out to the side, laterally.*" (Wait 2 seconds) "*Relax.*" (Figures 8.53., 8.56., and 8.57.)

5. During post-isometric relaxation, take up slack by increasing adduction to round out the circular path of circumduction. This has the effect of gapping the sacroiliac joint posteriorly. Steps 4 and 5 may be repeated as often as necessary.

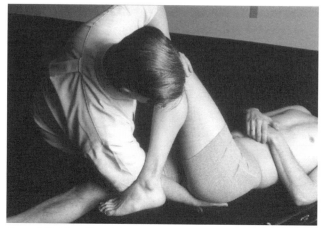

Figure 8.53. The adducted/internally rotated phase of innominate circumduction.

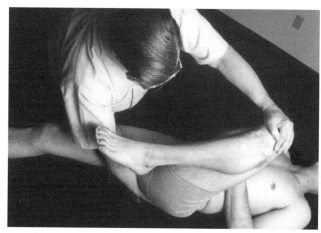

Figure 8.54. Full hip flexion, between the adducted and abducted phases

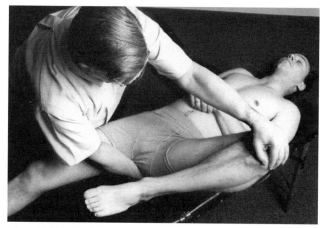

Figure 8.55. Abduction/external rotation going toward hip extension.

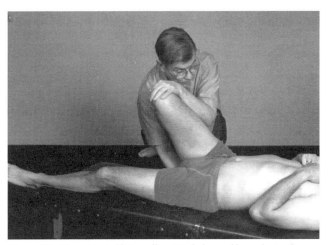

Figure 8.56. The adducted/internally rotated phase of innominate circumduction encounters restriction.

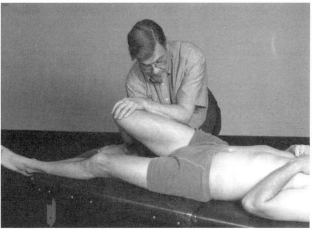

Figure 8.57. Increasing adduction during the post-isometric relaxation phase.

6. Continue on around the circumduction path, gradually reducing adduction and internal rotation as you approach hyperflexion, and beginning external rotation and abduction after you pass hyperflexion. If you encounter an interruption in the "roundness" of the circumduction path, pause at that location and have the patient do 2 or 3 isometric contractions and releases. If the interruption is near the hyperflexed position, have the patient use extension efforts (Figure 8.54.). If the interruption occurs during the externally rotated abducted phase, have the patient adduct against your resisting hand (Figure 8.55.). This would have the effect of gapping the sacroiliac joint anteriorly. As you straighten the leg toward extension, muscle actions tend to gap the sacroiliac joint superiorly; with hyperflexion, the inferior part of the sacroiliac joint gaps. Sometimes you may even get a "pop," especially going through the abducted phase.

7. Have the patient lie prone for reexamination. If you practice this procedure on a presumed normal subject, you may unexpectedly discover bilateral sacroiliac respiratory restriction.

Coccygeal Dysfunctions

Asymmetry of the coccyx is sometimes associated with coccydynia (painful coccyx), but it is usually a painless condition. Persistent coccydynia is relatively rare, and may be caused by inflammation in or around the coccyx. The cause of the inflammation may be local, as, for example, a pilonidal cyst, but is usually generated by more distant pathology. Lumbosacral dysfunction is a common etiology. The *ganglion impar,* located on the anterior surface of the coccyx, is a point of confluence of the two sympathetic ganglionated chains. Aphysiologic conditions such as inflammation or congestion in the vicinity of the *ganglion impar* can cause functional disturbances in the pelvic organs, and can be the source of causalgic pain syndromes.

Positional asymmetry of the coccyx is sometimes experienced as a generally mild discomfort. Even though it may be asymptomatic, it implies a disturbance in respiratory-circulatory mechanics in the pelvis which can have long-term pathologic consequences for the pelvic viscera. When discovered, it should be treated.

The coccyx is composed of three to five small mobile segments, vestigial vertebrae. It provides attachment for a significant portion of the pelvic diaphragm muscles – *coccygeus* and *levator ani.* These are the muscles which move the coccyx. However, since tail wagging is not an important human social function, as it is in dogs, their contribution to human wellbeing is more basic. The **levator ani** lifts the anus at the end of defecation, and assists in the control of defecation.

But its name belies its most important function – massaging the plexus of veins in the ischiorectal fossa, a major factor in accelerating the flow of venous blood from the pelvis. Arising from lines of attachment above the obturator foramina and from the sacrotuberous ligaments, the levator ani muscles form the medial walls of the ischiorectal fossae. The lateral walls extend anteriorly to the pubic bones and posteriorly to the sacrotuberous ligaments. The internal obturator muscles are a part of the lateral walls. Within the ischiorectal fossae are the pudendal nerves, arteries, and large plexuses of veins which function like a heart ventricle when the levators ani squeeze them up against the lateral walls. This "systole" of the ischiorectal fossae is a passive action of the levators caused by inhalation. "Diastole" occurs with exhalation, as the veins in the fossae fill up again.

If the coccyx is found to be rotated, it indicates that the tension in the pelvic diaphragm muscles is out of balance, and the basketlike shape of the levator ani muscles is distorted. Usually that distortion is directly related to altered configuration of an ischiorectal fossa on one side. The ischiorectal fossa may be deformed one of two ways: (1) venous plexus engorgement or (2) obturation or partial obliteration. Obturation may occur with sustained inhalation, as in anxiety states, and may persist due to surface adhesion of the levator ani to the obturator fascia. The dictionary defines obturation as stopping up, obstructing, or closing.

Logically, it seems that engorgement would tend to rotate the coccyx toward the side of engorgement, whereas obturation would tend to rotate the coccyx away from the involved ischiorectal fossa. If this is the case, engorgement occurs more frequently than obturation. **Empirically, treating the ischiorectal fossa on the side of coccygeal rotation straightens the coccyx most of the time.** And when it does not, treating the contralateral fossa does straighten it.

A manual treatment technique for the ischiorectal fossa was used by Mitchell, Sr., who called it "the pants-on treatment for hemorrhoids." The treatment consists of patiently and insistently wedging the fingertips into the ischiorectal fossa from a point just medial to the tuberosity of the ischium until movement of the levator ani can be felt with quiet breathing. The procedure can take a minute or more, and can make your fingers very sore. However, the time can be shortened considerably by applying Muscle Energy principles.

Having the patient cough causes abrupt contractions of the levator ani, which speeds up the decongestion of the engorged venous plexus or helps break the surface tension seal on the obturator fascia.

Often the wedging treatment can be avoided altogether by having the patient do a short series of Kegel's exercise contractions, about thirty repetitions. Kegel's exercises, for readers who have not studied gynecology, are rhythmic contractions and relaxations of the pelvic diaphragm muscles. Explaining to a patient how to do the exercise is made more difficult by the fact that it cannot be demonstrated and must be described in words. It seems that everyone understands the expression, *"Pull your anus in and let it go."* About one contraction per second is an appropriate rate.

Evaluation for Coccygeal Dysfunction
Examining the Coccyx for Rotation
Procedure Protocol

1. Patient lies prone.

2. You stand at the side of table looking straight down at the pelvis.

3. Identify the inferior lateral angles of the sacrum (S_5 segment) by stereognosis.

4. Keep your thumb pads facing into the pelvis and your thumb tips one centimeter (half-inch) apart on each side of the midline just inferior to the S_5 segment. Press your thumbs antero-superiorly into the gluteal muscle mass until your feel the hardness of the coccygeal transverse processes.

5. Observe your thumbs for symmetry, just as you would observe any other vertebra for rotation. Rotation of the coccyx is described in relation to the sacrum.

6. Feel and observe each segment of the coccyx until you come to its tip. Usually rotation begins with the first coccygeal segment, but there can be "intracoccygeal" rotation – second segment rotated on the first segment, for example.

7. Also observe the coccyx for anteflexion or lateral deviation. Either of these positional faults may be due to pelvic diaphragm tension. Any coccygeal positional fault may be labeled and treated as coccygeal dysfunction. Positional faults which persist after treatment may be due to old fracture or ankylosis.

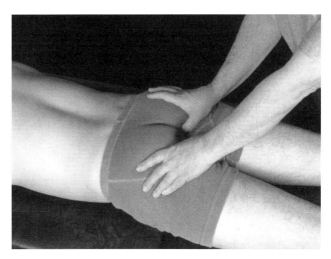

Figure 8.58. Palpating the coccyx. The coccyx may consist of as many as five vertebrae. Palpate their transverse processes for rotated position, sidebent position, or excessive flexed or extended position. Finding (by palpating) the coccyx rotated to one side is an indication that one side of the pelvic diaphragm does not work as well as the other side. The impaired side may be paralyzed, inhibited, or adhered to the obturator fascia by surface tension. Twenty or thirty repetitions of Kegel's exercise will usually straighten the coccyx. More important than the restoration of coccyx alignment is the restoration of the venous/lymphatic pumping action of the pelvic diaphragm's respiratory motions which prevents passive congestion of the pelvic organs and supportive tissues.

Treatment for Coccygeal Dysfunction
Ischiorectal Fossa Technique Procedure Protocol for Treatment of Coccygeal Dysfunction

1. The patient lies on the side with a pillow supporting the head and neck for comfort. The hips and knees are flexed to right angles. The side to be treated may be up or down, but treating it in the down position is often more uncomfortable for the patient.

2. With palmar stereognosis identify the inferior surface of the ischial tuberosity.

3. Slide your fingertips superiorly along the medial surface of the ischium, aiming the line of pressure toward the sacral base. It helps to keep two or three of your fingers straight and pressed tightly together for rigidity. It also helps if your elbow, forearm, wrist and hand are in a straight line. Your fingernails should be as short as possible.

4. After your fingertip meets soft tissue resistance, keep it there, and ask the patient to cough once. After the cough, increase the pressure a little to move farther up into the ischiorectal fossa. Repeat the cough as needed.

5. Keep going up into the ischiorectal fossa until your fingers (usually the backs of your fingers) can detect breathing motion of the *levator ani* muscle with quiet breathing. Do not instruct the patient to breathe in order for you to see if you can feel it. Quiet, resting respiration should be palpable. If it is not, go higher into the fossa. Be patient! It takes time.

6. As you go up into the fossa, explore anteriorly and posteriorly for obturation. Remember that the potential space of the ischiorectal fossa extends from the pubic ramus back to the sacrotuberous ligament.

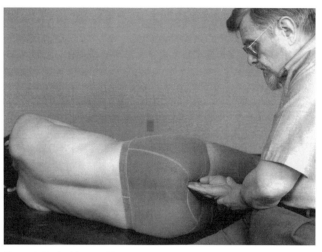

Figure 8.59. Ischiorectal fossa technique. Keep your fingers straight and pressed against each other for structural reinforcement of your hand. Stay close to the ischial bone. Fred Mitchell, Sr. referred to this procedure as "the pants-on treatment for hemorrhoids." While not a "cure" for hemorrhoids (varicose rectal veins), it does reduce the pressure in these veins, and tends to prevent internal hemorrhoids from becoming external hemorrhoids.

Kegels Exercise

The "pants-on-treatment" is usually moderately uncomfortable. It can often be avoided by having the patient do thirty repetitions of Kegels exercise. These exercises were named for the gynecologist who invented the bivalve vaginal speculum. As an exercise to decongest the pelvis, it would be almost as beneficial for men as for women. It is an exercise which is difficult to demonstrate, but it can be described in words. It is repetitious one-second contractions of the levator ani. You simply pull your anus in and then let it go. This is almost an involuntary movement following a bowel movement. More than the *levator ani* is involved. The *coccygeus* and *transversus perineii* muscles also participate.

As a part of a daily exercise regimen, it can prevent degenerative diseases of the pelvis, including hemorrhoids, visceral prolapses such as cystocele or rectocele, rectal prolapse, prostatic hypertrophy, and dysmenorrhea.

Thirty repetitions of Kegel's exercise will usually straighten a rotated coccyx. When Kegel's exercise fails to correct coccyx position, the ischiorectal fossa technique ("Pants-on treatment for hemorrhoids") should be employed.

It is rarely necessary to manipulate the coccyx with an index finger in the rectum. When this becomes necessary, it is best, and more comfortable for the patient, to use indirect ligamentous release technique (Sutherland) instead of direct articulatory technique.

In general, coccydynia is a symptom of lumbosacral adaptive stress, not coccygeal dysfunction.

Table 8.B. Pelvic Diagnosis Table

Characteristics of Pelvic Somatic Dysfunction

The following chart provides one-sided examples of the principal lesions of the pelvis (top horizontal row) in the MET model, and the diagnostic landmark findings (left-side column) associated with them. Contralateral findings can be extrapolated by reversing the results.

The landmark positions and/or specific test results affected by a given diagnosis	DIAGNOSIS							
	Anatomic short leg on left	Pubic Crest inferior on right	Upslipped Innominate on right	Sacrum Torsioned Left-on-Left	Sacrum Torsioned Left-on-Right	Sacrum Flexed on Left	Anterior Innominate on Right	Iliac Flare Lesion on Right
Standing Iliac Crest Heights – side with inferior displacement	Left side	Variable	Not Applicable	Variable – favors left	Variable	Variable – favors right	Variable	Not Applicable
Pubic Crest Heights – side with inferior displacement	Not Applicable	Right side	Not Applicable	Not Applicable	Not Applicable	Not Applicable	Not Applicable	Not Applicable
Prone Ischial Tuberosity – side with superior displacement	Not Applicable	Not Applicable	Right side	Not Applicable	Not Applicable	Not Applicable	Not Applicable	Not Applicable
Sacrotuberous Ligament Tension – side with laxity	Not Applicable	Not Applicable	Right side	Not Applicable	Not Applicable	Not Applicable	Not Applicable	Not Applicable
Standing Flexion Test – PSIS demonstrating a positive	Not Applicable	Right side ++	Right side ++	Right side +	Left side +	Left side +	Right side ++	Right side ++
Seated Flexion Test – PSIS demonstrating a positive	Not Applicable	Right side +	Right side ++	Right side ++	Left side ++	Left side ++	Right side +	Right side +
Posterior ILA displacement	Not Applicable	Not Applicable	Not Applicable	Left side ++	Left side ++	Left side +	Not Applicable	Not Applicable
Inferior ILA displacement	Not Applicable	Not Applicable	Not Applicable	Left side +	Left side +	Left side ++	Not Applicable	Not Applicable
Posterior ILA displacement in Sphinx position	Not Applicable	Not Applicable	Not Applicable	Symmetrical	More Posterior	Not Applicable	Not Applicable	Not Applicable
Deeper Sacral Sulcus	Not Applicable	Not Applicable	Not Applicable	Right side	Right side	Left side	Not Applicable	Not Applicable
Fifth Lumbar Rotated to the ...	Not Applicable	Not Applicable	Not Applicable	Right side	Right side	Left side	Not Applicable	Not Applicable
Short leg with patient prone	Left side	Variable	Right side	Left side ++	Left side ++	Right side ++	Left side +	Left side
Short leg with patient supine	Left side	Variable	Right side	Left side +	Left side +	Right side +	Left side ++	Not Applicable
PSIS position with patient prone – inferior side	Not Applicable	Variable	Variable	Left side ++	Left side ++	Not Applicable	Left side +	Not Applicable
ASIS position with patient supine – inferior side	Not Applicable	Right side	Variable – favors left	Right side ++	Right side ++	Not Applicable	Right side +	Not Applicable

Appendix A

YOUR DISLOCATED PELVIS
or
LIFE WITH A SACROILIAC BELT

You have been found to have a sacroiliac subluxation, which is a minor dislocation of your pelvis. This common dislocation is described as "an upslipped innominate," a vertical shear of the sacroiliac joint with damage to the ligaments of the joint and inferior displacement of the sacrum on the ilium. It is detected by observing malalignment of your ischial tuberosities while you are lying prone (chest down), and by palpating slackness of the sacro-tuberous ligament on the side of the superior tuberosity.

The treatment for your pelvic joint dislocation requires that you wear a sacroiliac belt at all times when you are not lying flat in bed. This means, of course, that you will bathe or shower in the belt and have a second dry belt to put on after the bath. It also means the belt must be in place and tight before you get out of bed. Many patients who get up in the middle of the night have simply slid the belt up around the waist where it is loose. Then, when they have to get up they only have to push the belt down in place. The belt is only an aid to help hold the pelvic bones in place while the ligaments of the joint heal. Healing takes two to three months if, and only if, the bones are held precisely in place without interruption. The belt should be worn low on the pelvis, between the anterior superior iliac spine and the trochanter of the femur, and should come down low on the buttocks so that it does not ride up when you are sitting.

The dislocated sacroiliac joint is not a direct source of pain; the pain is generated by the postural adaptation to the altered position of the sacrum.

Living with a sacroiliac belt is no picnic. The dislocation may occur again and again, in spite of wearing the belt. If it does, the cause must be determined and avoided in order to insure that the reduction remains stable for a minimum of two months. Common causes are 1. Belt too loose, 2. incorrect lifting, 3. jolts from sitting down or going down stairs incorrectly, or 4. trunk-twisting movements such as running a vacuum cleaner, sweeping or raking. Patients need a lot of encouragement and support while undergoing this therapy. It is common for dislocations to occur during the first two weeks of wearing the belt. Patients become discouraged when they realize that the two months starts over again with each dislocation event. It often takes about two weeks to learn how to live with the belt so that it can do the job. Once healed, the joint is usually as strong as an uninjured sacroiliac joint.

Therefore, it will be important that someone in your family is trained to make the measurements to determine if your pelvis is in place or not. The examination technique requires that the patient lie prone (face down) with the body in straight alignment. The examiner locates the ischial tuberosities (the pelvic bones you sit on) using the *palms* of both hands. Then each thumb is placed on the most caudal (toward the feet) surface of each ischial tuberosity and the thumbs are observed from above the prone patient to compare their positions – superior or inferior – in relation to each other. The tension of the sacrotuberous ligaments is compared by sliding the thumbs off the tuberosities in a medial, superior, and slightly posterior direction following the ischial bone. The ligament with less tension will permit the thumb to slide farther around the bone on that side. Superior displacement of the ischial tuberosity (more than a quarter inch) combined with slackness of the sacrotuberous ligament on the same side makes the diagnosis of an upslipped innominate. This determination should be made more than once a day, so that you will know if your pelvis goes out of place and why it went out of place, if it did. You can then take precautions to avoid dislocating the pelvis while you are wearing the sacroiliac belt.

Skin care is important. After bathing, during the exchange of the wet belt for the dry one, the skin under the belt should be cleaned thoroughly with alcohol or soap and water. Before the dry belt is applied the skin should be dry. A lanolin- or aloe-based lotion may be applied. Additional soft padding may be needed in the areas of greatest irritation, usually near the anterior superior iliac spine.

The compensatory dysfunctions in other regions of the body may be treated during the belting period, provided the treatment procedure does not risk dislocating the joint again. Inflammation encourages ligament mending, so if your lower back and buttocks get sore, it could be a good sign. Avoid taking aspirin or NSAIDS for pain. A balanced diet usually provides the necessities for healing: protein, zinc, manganese, vitamins A and C. A good supplement might help. Consult your physician.

Good luck!

Appendix B: Of Clinical Interest

Autonomic Effects

In discussing physiologic variations of human bodies, A. Hollis Wolf once observed that clinical outcomes can be profoundly influenced by the genetically inherited physiologic predispositions mediated by the autonomic nervous system. Patients with a tendency to predominantly sympathetic nervous system reactions to stress exhibit a physical habitus in which the trunk of the body outgrows the limbs and neck. Such patients react to stress with hypertension, and have an increased susceptibility to heart attacks, for examples. Patients whose parasympathetic nervous system dominates their reactions to stress are more prone to chronic illness, allergies, and more often die of cerebral vascular accidents. Wolf cautioned that vigorous manipulative treatment of the thoraco-lumbar region of the body could make a sympathetic dominant patient feel worse and a parasympathetic dominant patient feel better. In contrast, vigorous treatment of the sacrum or cranium could make the parasympathetic dominant patient feel worse, and the sympathetic dominant patient feel better. The parasympathetic dominant patient's physical habitus is one in which the pelvis and lower limbs and the cranium have outgrown the rest of the body, resulting in a person with a large head, large eyes, large pelvis and legs in proportion to the abdomen, thoracic area, and upper limbs.

The peripheral distributions of the parasympathetic nervous system arise from the cranium and the pelvis; the sympathetic nervous outflow arises from the thoracic and lumbar spine. Mechanical and circulatory processes in the pelvis influence the functions of the parasympathetic nervous system.

The Pelvis in Obstetrics

Pelvic distortions due to subluxations and/or somatic dysfunctions can have negative effects on the course of labor and delivery. Obviously fetal lie and presentation may be influenced. Sacroiliac dysfunctions significantly deform the birth canal, negatively influencing the three stages of labor. Considering the ligamentous relaxation which is known to occur during pregnancy, it may seem strange that pelvic dysfunctions may persist in pregnancy. But this author has seen sacral torsions and unilateral flexion lesions of the sacroiliac joints in women in active labor. Interestingly, some babies are born with sacroiliac dysfunction.

Precipitous labor and deliveries with malpresentations can cause sacroiliac dysfunction. Sutherland (Wales, 1998) found what he called "depressed sacrum" in women suffering from post-partum psychosis, and claimed that correction of the sacroiliac fault using craniosacral techniques cured the psychosis. Obstetrical delivery often marks the onset of chronic low back disorders.

A history of an unstable sacroiliac joint from an upslipped innominate, even though successfully treated, may be a problem in labor and delivery. Vaginal delivery can disrupt partially healed sacroiliac ligaments, exacerbating the instability. In spite of the occasional influence of the hormone relaxin in women, pelvic subluxation appear to show no sexual preference.

Preventable Disorders of the Reproductive System

Dysfunctions and subluxations of the pelvis have mechanical, circulatory and reflex influences on the reproductive systems, male and female (Woodall, 1926). Many obstetricians and gynecologists are very conscientious about teaching their patients Kegel's exercises – rhythmically contracting and relaxing the pelvic diaphragm muscles: levator ani, coccygeus, urogenital diaphragm – which raise and lower the anus. About 7 to 10 repetitions 3 or 4 times a day are recommended. The muscles massage the large venous plexus in the ischiorectal fossa, relieving venous and lymphatic congestion in the pelvis. The exercise has the potential to relieve, or prevent, dysmenorrhea, dyspareunia, uterine malpositions and fibroids.

Prostatic hypertrophy and prostatitis are also related to pelvic congestion. Males may also benefit from Kegel's exercises! Infertility problems may be helped by manipulative treatment of the pelvis and lower back, in addition to Kegel's exercises.

Bibliography and Recommended Reading

Adams T, Heisey RS, Smith MC, Briner BJ. Parietal bone mobility in the anesthetized cat. *J Am Osteopath Assoc,* 1992; 92(5):599-622. Reports a device used to measure intercranial bone articular motion.

Alexander, FM. *The Alexander Technique: The Original Writings of F. M. Alexander.* Larson Publications. 1997

Anson BJ, Ed., *Morris's Human Anatomy,* Twelfth Edition, New York, Blakiston Division, McGraw-Hill Book Company, 1966:

Basmajian JV: *Muscles Alive.* Fourth Edition. Baltimore, Williams & Wilkins, 1978. A classic in muscle electrophysiology.

Arbuckle, B. *Collected Writings of Beryl Arbuckle, DO.* Indianapolis. American Academy of Osteopathy. 1986.

Barral, JP and Mercier, P. *Visceral Manipulation.* Seattle, Eastland Press, Inc., 1988.

Barral, JP and Mercier, P. *The Thorax.* Seattle, Eastland Press, Inc., 1988.

Basmajian JV and Nyberg R (Eds.): *Rational Manual Therapies.* Baltimore, Williams and Wilkins, 1993.

Beal, MC. The sacroiliac problem: review of anatomy, mechanics and diagnosis. *J Am Osteopath Assoc* 81:667–679, 1985.

Beal MC (Ed.): *The Principles of Palpatory Diagnosis and Manipulative Technique.* Indianapolis, IN, American Academy of Osteopathy, 1992. Important work in physical diagnosis.

Bogduk N, & Twomey LT. *Clinical Anatomy of the Lumbar Spine.* 2nd Ed., Melbourne, Churchill Livingstone, 1991 The scientific bases of manual therapy.

Bourdillon JF: *Spinal Manipulation.* 3rd Edition. London, William Heinemann Medical Books, Ltd., 1982. An MD explains and describes osteopathic manipulative treatment.

Bowles CH: Functional orientation for technic (Report on a functional approach to specific osteopathic manipulative problems developed in the New England Academy of Applied Osteopathy during 1952-1954). Part I 55:177; Part II 56:107; Part III 57:53.

Bowles, CH: Functional technique: A modern perspective. *J Am Osteopath Assoc,* 80:326-331. Jan.81.

Burke RE and Edgerton VR: Motor unit properties and selection in movement. In Wilmore JH (Ed): *Exercise and Sport Science Reviews.* New York, Academic Press, 1975.

Burke RE, Levine DN, Zajac FE III, Tsairis P, and Engel WK: Mammalian motor units: physiological-histochemical correlation in three types in cat gastrocnemius. *Science* 174:709-712, 1971.

Burns, Louisa: *Pathogenesis of Visceral Disease Following Vertebral Lesions.* Kirksville. Journal Printing Co. 1948.

Butler DS: *Mobilization of the Nervous System,* Melbourne, Churchill Livingstone, 1991.

Cailliet R: *Low Back Pain Syndrome,* (2nd edn.) Philadelphia, FA Davis, 1968.

Cathie AG: Testing for regional motion. *DO,* June 1969.

Cathie AG: Papers Selected from the Writings and Lectures of Angus G. Cathie, DO, M.Sc. (Anatomy), FAAO. Indianapolis IN, *American Academy of Osteopathy Yearbook,* 1974.

Chapman F, Chapman AH, and Owens C: *Chapman's Reflexes.* Salisbury, NC, Rowan Printing Company, 1932. (See Owens, Charles, 1937.)

Clark, ME. *Applied Anatomy.* Journal Printing Company. Kirksville, Missouri, USA. 1906

Colachis SC, Worde RE, Bochtal CO and Strohm BR Movement of the sacroiliac joint in the adult male: a preliminary report. *Archives of Physical Medicine and Rehabilitation,* 44, 490. 1963

Cramer A, *Iliosakralmechanik.* Asklepios 6, 261. 1965

Cyriax J: *Textbook of Orthopaedic Medicine,* Vol. 1. London, Cassell, 1977.

DeGowin EL, DeGowin RL: *Bedside Diagnostic Examination.* Fourth Edition. New York, Macmillan Publishing Co., Inc., 1981.

DiGiovanna EL, Schiowitz S (Eds.): *An Osteopathic Approach to Diagnosis and Treatment.* Philadelphia, J.B. Lippincott Company, 1991. Second Edition, Philadelphia, Lippincott-Raven, 1997.

DonTigny RL: Mechanics and treatment of the sacroiliac joint. In: Vleeming A, Mooney V, Dorman T, Snijders CJ and Stoeckart R (eds): *Movement, Stability and Low Back Pain.* Edinburgh, Churchill Livingstone. ch38, p461. 1997.

Dorman TA. Storage and release of elastic energy in the pelvis: dysfunction, diagnosis, and treatment. *J. Orthop. Med.* 14:2, 1992.

Downing CH: *Principles and Practice of Osteopathy.* Kansas City, MO, Williams Publishing Company, 1923.

Dunnington WP: A musculoskeletal stress pattern: observations from over 50 years' clinical experience. *J Am Osteopath Assoc,* 42:437-440, 1964.:

Dvorak J, Dvorak V: *Manual Medicine: Diagnostics.* Georg Thieme Verlag, Stuttgart • New York; Thieme-Stratton, Inc. New York. 1984 2nd Edition, 1990.

Edgerton VR, Gerchman L, and Carrow R: Histochemical changes in rat skeletal muscle after exercise. *Exp Neurol* 24:110-123, 1968.

Emminger E: Die Anatomie und Pathologie des blockierten Wirbelgelenks. *Therapie über das Nervensystem,* vol.7, Chirotherapie-Manuelle Therapie, Ed. Gross,D. Stuttgart: Hippokrates, 1967.

England R: The first rib: Some clinical and practical considerations. *Academy of Applied Osteopathy Yearbook,* 1964, 112-124.

England R: The second rib: Some clinical and practical considerations. *Academy of Applied Osteopathy Yearbook,* 1967, 89-117.

Farfan HF: *Mechanical Disorders of The Low Back.* Philadelphia, Lea & Febiger, 1973.

Farfan HF: Muscular mechanism of the lumbar spine and the position of power and efficiency. *Orthopedic clinics of North America,* 6, 1975:135-144.

Ferguson AB: The clinical and roentgenographic interpretation of lumbosacral anomalies. *Radiology* 22:548-588. 1934.

Fisk JW: *The Practical Guide to Management of the Painful Neck and Back; Diagnosis, Manipulation, Exercises, Prevention.* Springfield, IL, Charles C. Thomas, 1977.

Flynn TW (Ed.): *The Thoracic Spine and Rib Cage, Musculoskeletal Evaluation and Treatment.* Newton, MA, Butterworth-Heinemann, 1996.

Fortin JD, Pier J, Falco F: Sacroiliac joint injection: pain referral mapping and arthrographic findings. In: Vleeming A, Mooney V, Dorman T, Snijders CJ and Stoeckart R (eds): *Movement, Stability and Low Back Pain.* Edinburgh, Churchill Livingstone. ch22, p271. 1997.

Frigerio NA, Stowe RR, Howe JW: Movements of the sacroiliac joint. *Clinical Orthopedics and Related Research,* 100:370–377, 1974

Fryette HH: *Principles of Osteopathic Technic.* Carmel, CA: Academy of Applied Osteopathy, 1954. 2nd printing 1966 (Now American Academy of Osteopathy, Indianapolis, IN)

Fryette HH. Physiologic movements of the spine. *Academy of Applied Osteopathy Year Book.* 1950. p. 91.

Fryette HH: Four innominate lesions – their cause, diagnosis and treatment. (drawings by C.H, Morris, D.O., Chicago). *J Am Osteop Assoc* 14:105-114, 1914. Reprinted in *Academy of Applied Osteopathy Yearbook,* 1966.

Frymann VM, King HH (Ed.): *Collected Papers of Viola Frymann.* Indianapolis, IN, Academy of Applied Osteopathy, 1997.

Fulford RC. *Dr. Fulford's Touch of Life.* New York. Pocket Books. 1996.

Gaymans F: Die Bedeutung der Atemtypen für Mobilization der Wirbelsäule. *Manuelle Medizin,* 18, 96.

Gilliar WG: Neurophysiologic aspects of the thoracic spine and ribs. In Flynn TW (Ed.): *The Thoracic Spine and Rib Cage, Musculoskeletal Evaluation and Treatment.* Newton, MA, Butterworth-Heinemann, 1996.

Goodridge JP: Muscle energy technique: definition, explanation, methods of procedure. *J Am Osteop Assoc* 81(4): 249–254, 1981.

Gowitzke BA and Milner M: *Understanding the Scientific Basis of Human Movement.* 2nd Edn. Baltimore, Williams & Wilkins, 1980.

Gracovetsky S: Linking the spinal engine with the legs: a theory of human gait. In: Vleeming A, Moomey V, Dorman T, Snijders CJ and Stoeckart R (eds): *Movement, Stability and Low Back Pain.* Edinburgh, Churchill Livingstone. ch20, p243. 1997.

Gracovetsky S: *The Spinal Engine.* Vienna, Springer-Verlag 1988.

Grant, JCB: *A Method of Anatomy,* Baltimore, Williams and Wilkins, 1952.

Grant JH: Osteopathic roentgenology. *Academy of Applied Osteopathy Yearbook,* 1961, 87 – 89.

Grant R (Ed.): *Physical Therapy of the Cervical and Thoracic Spine.* 2nd Edition. New York, Churchill Livingstone, 1994.

Greenman, PE. Innominate shear dysfunction in the sacroiliac syndrome. *Manual Medicine* (1986) 2:114-121

Greenman, PE. Structural diagnosis in chronic low back pain. *Manual Medicine* (1988) 4:114-117

Greenman, PE.: *Principles of Manual Medicine.* Baltimore. Williams & Wilkins, 1989. 2nd Edition, 1995.

Grieve GP: *Modern Manual Therapy of the Vertebral Column.* Edinburgh, Churchill Livingstone, 1986.

Guy AE: Vertebral mechanics - Part II. Indianapolis IN, *Academy of Applied Osteopathy Yearbook,* 1949, 98-104.

Hackett GS: *Ligament and Tendon Relaxation Treated by Prolotherapy,* 3rd edn. Springfield, IL, Charles C. Thomas, 1958.

Halladay, HV: Applied Anatomy of the Spine. Second Edition. In *Yrbk Acad Appl Osteop,* 1957.

Hallgren RC, Greenman PE, Rechtien JJ: Atrophy of suboccipital muscles in patients with chronic pain: A pilot study. *JAOA,* vol. 94, no 12: 1032-38, 1994.

Hickey DS, Hukens DW: Relation between the structure of the annulus fibrosus and the function and failure of the intervertebral disc. *Spine,* 5:106, 1980.

Hollinshead,WH: *Textbook of Anatomy,* Hagerstown, MD 21740, Harper & Row, 1974.

Hoover HV: Basic physiological movements of the spine. *Academy of Applied Osteopathy Yearbook of Selected Osteopathic Papers,* Indianapolis, IN., American Academy of Osteopathy, 1969. p125.

Hoppenfeld, S: *Physical Examination of the Spine and Extremities.* New York, Appleton-Century-Crofts, 1977.

Inman VT, Ralston HJ, Todd F: *Human Walking.* Baltimore, Williams & Wilkins, 1981.

Janda V: Muscle weakness and inhibition (pseudoparesis) in back pain syndromes. In: Grieve GP (ed) *Modern Manual Therapy of the Vertebral Column.* Edinburgh, Churchill Livingstone, ch19, p197, 1986.

Janda V: Muscles, central nervous motor regulation, and back problems. In Korr IM (Ed): *Neurobiologic Mechanisms in Manipulative Therapy.* New York and London, Plenum Press, 1978.

Janda V: On the concept of postural muscles and posture in man. *The Australian Journal of Physiotherapy* 29:83-84, 1983.

Janda, V. (Two videotapes): *Sensory Motor Stimulation* & *Muscle Length Assessment,* made in Australia and available from OPTP, Minneapolis, MN. 1996

Janda V: Evaluation of muscular imbalance. In Liebenson C (Ed.), *Rehabilitation of the Spine: A Practitioners Manual.* Baltimore, MD, Williams & Wilkins, 1996.

Janda, V.: Rational therapeutic approach to chronic back pain syndromes. In *Procedings of the Symposium: Chronic Back Pain, Rehabilitation and Self-help.* Turku, Finland. 69-74. Dec. 12-13, 1985.

Jirout J: The normal mobility of the lumbo-sacral spine. *Acta Radiol.* 47:345, 1957.

Jirout, J. The dynamic dependence of the lower corvical vertebrae on the atlanto-occipital joints, *Neuroradiology,* 6: 249. 1974.

Jirout, J. Radiographic signs of the function of the intrinsic muscles of the spine. In *Back Pain, an International Review,* p.391. Eds. Paterson, JK and Burn, L. Dordrecht, Boston, London: Raven Press.1990

Johnson, Stanley, MD – personal communication, 1966. Demonstrated *in vivo* inherent cranial motion using strain guages and a modified EKG machine.

Johnston WL: Segmental behavior during motion. I. A palpatory study of somatic relations. II. Somatic dysfunction, the clinical distortion. *J Am Osteop Assoc* 72:352-361,1972. III. Extending behavioral boundaries. *J Am Osteop Assoc* 72:462-475, 1973.

Johnston WL, Friedman HD: *Functional Methods: A Manual for Palpatory Skill Development in Osteopathic Examination and Manipulation of Motor Function.* Indianapolis, IN, American Academy of Osteopathy, 1994.

Jones LH: *Strain and Counterstrain.* Indianapolis, IN. American Academy of Osteopathy, 1981.

Jones LH, Kusunose R, Goering E: *Jones Strain-Counterstrain.* Boise, ID, Jones Strain-Counterstrain, Inc.,1995.

Judovich B, Bates W: *Pain Syndromes – Diagnosis and Treatment.* 4th Edition. Philadelphia, F.A. Davis Co., 1954.

Kapandji IA: *The Physiology of the Joints* (3 Volumes). Edinburgh, London and New York, Churchill Livingstone, 1979.

Keller HA: A clinical study of the mobility of the human spine, its extent and its clinical importance. *Arch.Surg.,* 8:627, 1924.

Kendall FP, McCreary EK, and Provance PG: *Muscles Testing and Function,* 4th Edition. Baltimore, Williams and Wilkins, 1993.

Kidd, RF. Pain localization with the innominate upslip dysfunction. *Manual Medicine* 3:103-105 1988.

Kimberly PE: Michigan State University College of Osteopathic Medicine Muscle Energy Tutorials.

Kimberly PE: *Outline of Osteopathic Manipulative Procedures.* Kirksville, MO, KCOM Press, 1980.

Knott M, Voss DE: *Proprioceptive Neuromuscular Facilitation: Patterns and Techniques,* 2nd edn. New York, Harper and Row, 1968.

Korr D: Principles of osteopathic manipulation. A rationale. Part I. *Osteop Ann* 12:10-26,Jul 84.

Korr IM: The sympathetic nervous system as mediator between the somatic and supportive processes. In *The Physiological Basis of Osteopathic Medicine.* New York. The Postgraduate Institute of Osteopathic Medicine and Surgery, 1970.

Korr IM: NINCDS Monograph No.15, *The Research Status of Spinal Manipulative Therapy,* Edited by M. Goldstein. Bethesda, MD, 1976.

Korr IM: The spinal cord as the organizer of disease processes. Part 2, The peripheral autonomic nervous system. *J Am Osteop Assoc* 79:82-90, 1979.

Korr IM: Osteopathic medicine: The profession's role in society. *J Am Osteop Assoc* Vol 90, No 9: 824-837, Sep 1990.

Kottke FJ, Clayson SJ, Newman IM, Debevec DF, Anger RW, and Skowlund HV: Evaluation of mobility of hip and lumbar vertebrae of normal young women. *Arch Phys Med* 43:1-8, Jan 1962.

Kottke FJ, et al.: Changes in the pelvisacral angle with flexion and extension of the trunk. *Phy Med and Rehab. Dept. Newsletter,* U of Minnesota, 1941.

Kuchera ML, Kuchera WA: *Osteopathic Considerations in Systemic Dysfunction.* Columbus, OH, Greyden Press, 2nd. Edition, Revised, 1994.

Kuchera WA, Kuchera ML: *Osteopathic Principles inPractice.* Columbus, OH, Greyden Press, Original Works Books, 2nd. Edition, Revised, 1994.

Kuchera ML, Jungman M: Inclusion of a levitor orthotic device in management of refractive low back pain patients. *J Am Osteop Assoc* 10:673, 1986.

Larson NJ: Sacroiliac and postural changes from anatomic short extremity. *Academy of Applied Osteopathy Yearbook,* 1966, 132-133.

Lavignolle B, Vital JM, Senegas J, Destandau J, Toson B, Bouyx P, Morlier P, Delorme G, Calabet A: An approach to the functional anatomy of the sacroiliac joints *in vivo. Anatomica Clinica* 5:169-176, 1983.

Lee D: *Manual Therapy for the Thorax: A Biomechanical Approach.* Delta, British Columbia, Canada, DOPC, 1994.

Lee D: *The Pelvic Girdle: An approach to the examination and treatment of the lumbo-pelvic-hip rigion,* 2nd. Ed. Edinburgh. Churchill Livingstone, 1999.

Lewit K: *Manipulative Therapy in Rehabilitation of the Locomotor System.* London, Butterworths, 1985.

Lewit K: *Manipulative Therapy in Rehabilitation of the Locomotor System.* 2nd. Edition. London, Butterworths, Heinemann, Ltd. 1991.

Lewit K: *Manipulative Therapy in Rehabilitation of the Locomotor System.* 3rd. Edition. Oxford, Butterworths, Heinemann, Ltd. 1999.

Liebenson C (Ed.): *Rehabilitation of the Spine: A Practioners Manual.* Baltimore, MD, Williams & Wilkins, 1996.

Lippincott, HA: The osteopathic techniques of Wm. G. Sutherland, D.O. *Yrbk Acad Appl Osteop* 49:1-45, 1949

Lippincott, HA: Corrective technique for the sacrum. *Yrbk Acad Appl Osteop* 58:57ff, 1958

Lippincott, HA: The depressed sacrum. *Yrbk Acad Appl Osteop* 65 (Vol.2):206ff, 1965

Lockhart RD: *Anatomy of the Human Body.* Philadelphia, Lippincott, 1959.

Lovett RW: The mechanism of the normal spine and its relation to scoliosis. *Med. Surg. J.,* 153:349, 1905.

Lovett RW: *Lateral Curvature of the Spine and Round Shoulders.* Philadelphia, Blakiston's, 1912.

MacBain RN: The somatic components of disease. *JAOA* 56: 159-165, Nov 1956.

MacConaill MA: The movements of bones and joints. 2. Function of the musculature. *J. Bone & Jt Surg* 31-B:100-104, 1949.

MacConaill MA and Basmajian JV: *Muscles and Movements: A Basis for Human Kinesiology.* Baltimore, Williams & Wilkins, 1969.

Macrae IF, Wright V: Measurement of back movement. *Ann. Rheum. Dis.,* 28:584, 1969.

Magoun HI: A method of sacroiliac correction. *Yrbk Acad Appl Osteop* 54. 1934.

Magoun HI: *Osteopathy in the Cranial Field.* 3rd Ed. Kirksville, The Journal Printing Company, 1976.

Maigne R: *Douleus d'Origine Vertébrale et Traitments par Manipulations.* Paris, Expansion Scientifique, 1968.

Maitland GD: *Vertebral Manipulation.* Fifth edition, London, Butterworth & Co. (Publishers) Ltd,1986.

Marcus A: *Musculoskeletal Disorders: Healing Methods from Chinese Medicine, Orthopaedic medicine, and Osteopathy.* Berkeley, North Atlantic Books, 1998.

Mennell JMcM: *Joint Pain.* Boston, Little Brown, 1964.

Mitchell FL Sr: The balanced pelvis and its relationship to reflexes. *Academy of Applied Osteopathy Yearbook,* 1948: 146-151.

Mitchell FL Sr: Structural pelvic function. *Academy of Applied Osteopathy Yearbook,* 1958: 71-90. (Reprinted with revised illustrations in *Academy of Applied Osteopathy Yearbook,* 1965, vol 2: 178-199.)

Mitchell FL Jr., Pruzzo N: Roentgenographic measurement of sacroiliac respiratory movement. AOA Research Conference, Chicago, March 1970.

Mitchell, FL and Pruzzo, NA: Investigation of Voluntary and Primary Respiratory Mechanisms, *J. Am.Osteo.Assoc.* 70:1109-1113, June, 1971. Demonstrated a movement response in the sacroiliac joints to the demands of voluntary respiratory inhalation and exhalation.

Mitchell, FL Jr, Moran PS & Pruzzo NA: *An Evaluation and Treatment Manual of Osteopathic Manipulative Procedures.* Kansas City, MO. Institute for Continuing Education in Osteopathic Principles, 1973. (out-of-print)

Mitchell FL Jr.: The training and measurement of sensory literacy in relation to osteopathic structural and palpatory diagnosis. *JAOA* Vol 75, No 10, June 1976, 874-884.

Mitchell FL Jr, Roppel RM, St Pierre N: Accuracy and perceptual decisional delay in motion perception, abstracted. *JAOA* 1978; 78:149-150.

Mitchell, FL, Jr. Voluntary and involuntary respiration and the craniosacral mechanism, In *Collected Osteopathic Papers,* Tilley, M, Ed., Insight Publishing Co., New York, 1979.

Mitchell FL Jr: Towards a definition of somatic dysfunction. *Osteop Ann* 7:12-25, 1979. Reprinted in *J Soc Osteopaths,* Maidstone, Kent, U.K. Summer 1980.

Mitchell, FL Jr (ed) Moran PS & Pruzzo NA: *An Evaluation and Treatment Manual of Osteopathic Muscle Energy Procedures.* Valley Park, Missouri. Institute for Continuing Education in Osteopathic Principles, 1979. (out-of-print)

Mitchell FL Jr: Voluntary and involuntary respiration and the craniosacral mechanism. *Collected Osteopathic Papers,* M. Tilley, ed., New York, Insight Publishing Co., Inc., 1979.

Mitchell FL Jr: The respiratory-circulatory model: Concepts and applications. In *Concepts and Mechanisms of Neuromuscular Functions.* Greenman PE (Ed.). Berlin. Springer-Verlag. 1984.

Mitchell FL Jr: Concepts of muscle energy. In *Proc of the 5th International Conference Inter. Fed of Orthopedic Manipulative Therapists (I.F.O.M.T.),* 1985, 1 – 6.

Mitchell FL Jr: Elements of muscle energy technique. In Basmajian JV, Nyberg R (Eds): *Rational Manual Therapies.* Baltimore, MD. Williams & Wilkins, 1993, 285 – 321.

Mitchell, FL Jr., Mitchell PKG: *The Muscle Energy Manual, Volume One: Concepts and Mechanisms, the Musculoskeletal Screen, Cervical Region Evaluation and Treatment.* East Lansing, MI, MET Press, 1995.

Mitchell, FL Jr., Mitchell PKG: *The Muscle Energy Manual, Volume Two: Evaluation and Treatment of the Thoracic Spine, Lumbar Spine, & Rib Cage.* East Lansing, MI, MET Press, 1998.

Mitchell, FL Jr., Mitchell PKG: *The Muscle Energy Manual, Volume Three: Evaluation and Treatment of the Pelvis and Sacrum.* East Lansing, MI, MET Press, 1999.

Morris, JM, Lucas, DB and Bressler, B. Role of the trunk in stability of the spine. *Journal of Bone and Joint Surgery,* 43A, 327. 1961.

Nachemson AL: Lumbar spine instability: a critical update and symposium summary. *Spine,* 10:290–291, 1985.

Nachemson AL: Physiotherapy for low back pain. A critical look. *Scand. J. Rehabil. Med.,* 1:85, 1969.

Nachemson AL: A critical look at the treatment for low back pain. The research staus of spinal manipulative therapy. Bethesda, MD, DHEW Publication NO. (HIH) 76-998:21B, 1975.

Neumann HD: *Introduction to Manual Medicine.* Berlin, Heidelberg, Springer-Verlag, 1989. 4th Edition, 1994.

Neumann HD: *Manuelle Medizin: Eine Einfuehrung in Theorie, Diagnostik und Therapie.* 5th edn. Berlin, Heidelberg, Springer-Verlag, 1999.

Northup,TL, D.O., Sacroiliac lesions primary and secondary, *Academy of Applied Osteopathy Yearbook,* 1943-44, pp. 54-55.

Owens, Charles: *An Endocrine Interpretation of Chapman's Reflexes.* 1937. (Reprint available from Indianapolis, IN, American Academy of Osteopathy.)

Patia AE, Ed. *Advances in Psychology, Volume 78: Adaptability of Human Gait.* Amsterdam. Elsevier Science Publishers. 1991.

Patterson MM: The reflex connection: History of a middleman. *Osteop Ann* 4:358-367, 1976.

Pearcy MJ: Stereo radiography of lumbar spine motion. *Acta Orthop. Scand.,* 56:212 [Suppl.], 1985.

Pearcy MJ, Tibrewal, SB: Axial roation and lateral bending in the normal lumbar spine measured by three-dimensional radiography. *Spine,* 9(6): 582, 1984.

Penning L: Normal movements of the cervical spine. *Am. J. Roentgenol.* 130:317, 1979.

Penning L, Wilmink JT: Rotation of the cervical spine. *Spine,* 12(8):732, 1987.

Pettman E: The "functional" shoulder girdle. In *Proc of the 5th International Conference Inter. Fed of Orthopedic Manipulative Therapists (I.F.O.M.T.),* 1985, 81 – 94. (Published by Inter. Fed. of Orthopedic Manipulative Therapists, #2 Landing Rd., Whakatane, New Zealand.)

Porterfield JA, DeRosa C: *Mechanical Low Back Pain – Perspectives in Functional Anatomy.* Philadelphia, W. B. Saunders Co., 1991.

Porterfield JA, DeRosa C: *Mechanical Neck Pain – Perspectives in Functional Anatomy.* Philadelphia, W. B. Saunders Co., 1995.

Pottenger, Francis. *Symptoms of Visceral Disease.* Philadelphia. Saunders. 1941.

Pruzzo, NA. Use of the the anode heel effect in lumbosacral radiographs. (Master's thesis)[cited in 1971 *J Am Osteop Assoc*]

Retzlaff EW, Mitchell FL Jr. (eds.): *The Cranium and Its Sutures.* New York, Springer-Verlag, 1987.

Reynolds, H.M.: Three dimensional Kinematics in the pelvic girdle, *J. Am.Osteo.Assoc.* 80:277-280, December, 1980. Demonstrated in a fresh unembalmed cadaver movement of the sacrum on the ilium in response to flexion and abduction of the femur at the hip. The movement is predominantly flexion and extension, or as Kapandji (1974) described nutation and counternutation at the sacroiliac joint.

Roppel RM, St Pierre N, Mitchell FL Jr: Measurement of accuracy in bimanual perception of motion, abstracted. *J Am Osteop Assoc* ;77:475. 1978.

Rose J and Gamble JG. *Human Walking,* 2nd Ed. Baltimore, Williams & Wilkins, 1994.

Roy R, Ho KW, Taylor J, Heusner W, and Van Huss, W: Observations on muscle fiber splitting produced by weight lifting exercise. Abstract. American Osteopathic Association Research Convention, 1977.

Ruddy TJ: Osteopathic rhythmic resistive duction therapy. In *Academy of Applied Osteopathy Yearbook.* 1961, 58–68.

Ruddy TJ: Osteopathic rapid rhythmic resistive technique. In *Academy of Applied Osteopathy Yearbook.* 1962, 23–31.

Ruddy TJ: Osteopathic manipulation in eye, ear, nose, and throat. In *Academy of Applied Osteopathy Yearbook.* 1962, 133–140.

Saliba VL, Johnson GS, Wardlaw CF: Proprioceptive Neuromuscular Facilitation. In Basmajian JV, Nyberg R (eds.): *Rational Manual Therapies.* Baltimore, Williams and Wilkins, 1993.

Schildt, K., Untersuchungen zum Entwicklungsstand der Motorik bei Kindergartenkindern. In *Functional Pathology of the Motor System. Rehabilitacia,* Suppl. 10-11, p.166. Eds. Lewit, K. and Gutmann, G. Bratislava: Obzor. 1975.

Schneider W, Dvorák J, Dvorák V, Tritschler T. *Manual Medicine: Therapy.* Stuttgart, New York, Georg Thieme Verlag, 1988.

Schooley, TF: The osteopathic lesion. *Academy of Applied Osteopathy Yearbook,* 1970.

Schooley, TF: *Osteopathic Principles and Practice.* Indianapolis, IN. American Academy of Osteopathy, 1987.

Schwab, WA. Principles of Manipulative Treatment – The Low Back Problem (Part X). *J Am Osteop Assoc,* Feb. 1933.

Selye, Hans. *Stress in Health and Disease.* Butterworths, Boston, 1970.

Sherrington CS: On reciprocal innervation of antagonist muscles. *Proc. R. Soc.* Lond. [Biol] 79B:337, 1907.

Skládal et al, The postural function of the diaphragm, *Çeskoslovenskà Fysiologie,* 19, 279, 1970.

Smidt GL: Interinnominate range of motion. In: Vleeming A, Mooney V, Dorman T, Snijders CJ and Stoeckart R (eds): *Movement, Stability and Low Back Pain.* Edinburgh, Churchill Livingstone. ch13, p187. 1997.

Solonen, JA: The sacroiliac joint in the light of anatomical, roentgenological and clinical studies. *Acta Orthopaedica Scandinavica,* Suppl. 27. 1957

Spackman Robert: *Two Man Isometric Exercise For the Whole Man.* Dubuque, Iowa, W.C. Brown, 1964.

Steindler A: *Kinesiology of the Human Body.* Springfield, IL, Charles C. Thomas, 1955.

Still AT. *Philosophy of Osteopathy.* Kirksville, Missouri. Published by the author. 1899.

Still AT: *Autobiography.* Kirksville, MO, 1908 (Reprint available from Indianapolis, IN, American Academy of Osteopathy).

Still AT: *Osteopathy: Research and Practice.* Seattle, Eastland Press, 1992. (Originally published by the author, Kirksville, MO, 1910)

Stoddard A: *Manual of Osteopathic Technique.* Second Edition. London, Hutchinson, 1966.

Stoddard A: *Manual of Osteopathic Practice.* London, Hutchinson, 1969.

Strachan WF, Beckwith CG, Larson NJ, Grant JH: A study of the mechanics of the sacroiliac joint. *J Am Osteop Assoc* 37:576-578, 1938.

Sturesson, B, Selvic, G, and Uden, A. Movements of the Sacroiliac joints. A roentgen stereophotogrammetric analysis. *Spine* 14(2), 162-165. 1989

Sutherland WG: *The Cranial Bowl.* Published by the author, 1939. Reprinted by the Cranial Academy, Indianapolis IN, 1948.

Travell JG and Simon DJ: *Myofascial Pain and Dysfunction: The Trigger Point Manual.* Baltimore, Williams & Wilkins, 1983.

Travell JG and Simon DJ: *Myofascial Pain and Dysfunction: The Trigger Point Manual. Volume Two: The Lower Extremities.* Baltimore, Williams & Wilkins, 1992.

Truhlar RE: *A.T. Still in the Living.* Chagrin Falls, OH, Published by the author, 1950.

Twomey LT, Taylor JR: *Physical Therapy of the Low Back.* Melbourne, Churchill Livingstone, 1994.

Van Buskirk RL: Nociceptive reflexes and the somatic dysfunction: a model. *J Am Osteop Assoc* 90, no 9, 792-809, Sept 1990.

van Wingerden JP, Vleeming A, Snijders CJ, Stoeckart R: A functional - anatomical approach to the spine-pelvis mechanism: Interaction between the biceps femoris muscle and the sacrotuberous ligament. *Eur Spine J.* Vol 2: 140-144, 1993.

Vleeming A, Pool-Goudzwaard AL, Stoeckart R, van Wingerden JP, Snijders CJ: The posterior layer of the thoracolumbar fascia. *Spine* Vol 20, No. 7: 753-758, 1995.

Vleeming A, Mooney V, Dorman T, Snijders C, Stoeckart R (Eds.): *Movement, Stability, and Low Back Pain: The Essential Role of the Pelvis.* New York, Churchill Livingstone, 1997.

Wales AL. *Contributions of Thought: The Collected Writings of William Garner Sutherland, D.O.,* 2nd Ed. Portland, Oregon, Rudra Press, 1998

Ward R (Ed.): *Foundations of Osteopathic Medicine.* Baltimore, MD, Williams & Wilkins, 1997.

Warwick & Williams, Eds. *Gray's Anatomy,* 35th British Edition, Philadelphia, W.B.Saunders, 1973.

Weed LL: *Medical Records, Medical Education, and Patient Care: The Problem-Oriented Record as a Basic Tool.* Cleveland, OH, The Press of Case Western Univ., 1969.

Weisl, H, *The relation of movement to structure in the sacro-iliac joint,* Ph.D. Thesis, University of Manchester. 1953. An analysis of structural anatomy to verify whether it supported the contention that pelvic mobility exists.

Weisl, H. The articular surfaces of the sacroiliac joint and their relationship to the movements of the sacrum, *Acta Anat.* 20 and 22, 1-14, 1954. The topography of the auricular surfaces has hills and valleys which approximate their opposites in the other bone but are not congruous. Cross sections at three levels will show convexities changing from medial to lateral.

Weisl, H. The movements of the sacroiliac joint, *Acta Anat.* 23:80-91, 1955.

White AA: Analysis of the mechanics of the thoracic spine in man. An experimental study on autopsy specimens [Thesis]. *Acta Orthop. Scand.,* 127 [Suppl.], 1969.

White AA: Kinematics of the normal spine as related to scoliosis. *J. Biomech.* 4:405, 1971.

White AA, Panjabi MM: *Clinical Biomechanics of the Spine.* 2nd Edition. Philadelphia, JB Lippincott Co., 1990.

Willard FH: The muscular, ligamentous and neural structure of the low back and its relation to back pain. In Vleeming A, et al., (Eds.): *Movement, Stability and Low Back Pain: The Essential Role of the Pelvis.* Churchill Livingstone, Edinburgh, 1997.

Willard FH: Neuroendocrine-immune network, nociceptive stress, and the general adaptive response. In: Everett T, Dennis M, Ricketts E (eds): *Physiotherapy in Mental Health: a Practical Approach.* Oxford, Butterworth Heinemann, 1995. pp102-126.

Woodall, Percy Hogan, MD, DO, *Intrapelvic technique: or, manipulative surgery of the pelvic organs.* Kansas City, Mo., Williams Pub. Co., 1926

Wyke BD: The neurology of low back pain. In Jayson MIV (ed): *The Lumbar Spine and Back Pain.* London, Pitman Medical, 1980.

Yates HA, Glover JC: *Counterstrain: A Handbook of Osteopathic Technique.* Tulsa, OK, Y Knot Publishers, 1995.

Zink JG: Osteopathic holistic approach to homeostasis. 1969 Academy Lecture, Indianapolis, IN, *Academy of Applied Osteopathy Yearbook*, 1970, 1-10.

Zink JG: Respiration and circulatory care: The conceptual model. *Osteopath Ann* 1977: 5: 108-112.